AF530783

Research Issues in Human Behavior and Sexually Transmitted Diseases in the AIDS Era

Research Issues in Human Behavior and Sexually Transmitted Diseases in the AIDS Era

Editors:

Judith N. Wasserheit
Sexually Transmitted Diseases Branch
National Institute of Allergy and Infectious Diseases
Bethesda, Maryland

Sevgi O. Aral
Behavioral Studies Section
Division of STD/HIV Prevention
Centers for Disease Control
Atlanta, Georgia

King K. Holmes
University of Washington Center for AIDS and STDs
Seattle, Washington

Associate Editor:

Penelope J. Hitchcock
Sexually Transmitted Diseases Branch
National Institute of Allergy and Infectious Diseases
Bethesda, Maryland

American Society for Microbiology
Washington, D.C.

1325 Massachusetts Avenue, N.W.
Washington, DC 20005

Research issues in human behavior and sexually transmitted diseases in the AIDS era / editors, Judith N. Wasserheit, Sevgi O. Aral, King K. Holmes; associate editor, Penelope J. Hitchcock.
p. cm.
Includes index.
ISBN 1-55581-036-5
1. Sexually transmitted diseases—Prevention. 2. AIDS (Disease)—Prevention. I. Wasserheit, Judith N. II. Aral, Sevgi O. III. Holmes, King K.
[DNLM: 1. HIV Infections—prevention & control. 2. Risk Factors. 3. Sex Behavior. 4. Sexually Transmitted Diseases—epidemiology. 5. Sexually Transmitted Diseases—prevention & control. WC 144 R432]
RA644.V4R47 1991
616.95'105—dc20
DNLM/DLC

Printed in the United States of America

Contents

Contributors

Hortensia Amaro – Social and Behavioral Sciences Department, Boston University School of Public Health, Boston, Massachusetts 02118

Roy M. Anderson – Parasite Epidemiology Research Group, Imperial College, London University, London SW7 2BB, England

Sevgi O. Aral – Behavioral and Prevention Research Branch, Division of STD/HIV Prevention, Centers for Disease Control, Atlanta, Georgia 30333

Robert C. Brunham – Department of Medical Microbiology, University of Manitoba, Winnipeg, Manitoba, Canada R3E 0W3

Manuel Carballo – Programme on Substance Abuse, Research and Development Unit, World Health Organization, CH-1211 Geneva 27, Switzerland

Donna Cheung – Department of Anthropology, Brown University, Providence, Rhode Island 02912

Roel A. Coutinho – Municipal Health Service, 1000 HE Amsterdam, The Netherlands

Anke A. Ehrhardt – HIV Center for Clinical and Behavioral Studies, New York State Psychiatric Institute, and Department of Psychiatry, College of Physicians and Surgeons, Columbia University, New York, New York 10032

Martin Fishbein – Department of Psychology, University of Illinois, Champaign, Illinois 61820

Robert E. Fullilove – College of Physicians and Surgeons, Columbia University, New York, New York 10032

Isolde Gornemann – Social and Behavioral Sciences Department, Boston University School of Public Health, Boston, Massachusetts 02118

Sylvan B. Green – Clinical and Diagnostic Trials Section, National Cancer Institute, Bethesda, Maryland 20892

Penelope J. Hitchcock – Sexually Transmitted Diseases Branch, National Institute of Allergy and Infectious Diseases, Bethesda, Maryland 20892

King K. Holmes – Center for AIDS and STD, Seattle, Washington 98122

Edward W. Hook III – Johns Hopkins University School of Medicine and Clinical STD Services, Baltimore City Health Department, Baltimore, Maryland 21205

Robert Hornik – The Annenberg School for Communication, University of Pennsylvania, Philadelphia, Pennsylvania 19104-6220

James Jaccard – Department of Psychology, State University of New York at Albany, Albany, New York 12222

Robert B. Jones – Departments of Medicine, Microbiology, and Immunology, Indiana University School of Medicine, Indianapolis, Indiana 46233

Franklyn N. Judson – World Health Organization, Geneva, Switzerland, and University of Colorado Health Sciences Center, Denver, Colorado 80204-4507

Marie Laga – WHO Collaborating Centre on AIDS, Department of Microbiology, Institute of Tropical Medicine, 2000 Antwerp, Belgium

Susan E. Middlestadt – The Academy for Educational Development, Washington, D.C. 20037

Lucile F. Newman – Department of Community Health, Brown University, Providence, Rhode Island 02912

Maria E. M. Paalman – Dutch Foundation for STD Control, 3511 GE Utrecht, The Netherlands

Nancy S. Padian – Department of Epidemiology and Biostatistics, University of California, San Francisco, San Francisco General Hospital, San Francisco, California 94110

Peter Piot – WHO Collaborating Centre on AIDS, Department of Microbiology, Institute of Tropical Medicine, 2000 Antwerp, Belgium

Allan R. Ronald – Section of Infectious Diseases, St. Boniface General Hospital, Winnipeg, Manitoba, Canada R2H 2A6

Stephen C. Shiboski – Department of Epidemiology and Biostatistics, University of California, San Francisco, San Francisco General Hospital, San Francisco, California 94110

William A. Smith – The Academy for Educational Development, Washington, D.C. 20037

P. F. Sparling – Department of Medicine, University of North Carolina School of Medicine, Chapel Hill, North Carolina 27599-7005

Oussama Tawil – Programme on Substance Abuse, Research and Development Unit, World Health Organization, CH-1211 Geneva 27, Switzerland

J. A. R. Van Den Hoek – Municipal Health Service, 1000 HE Amsterdam, The Netherlands

A. Eugene Washington – Center for Reproductive Health Policy Research, School of Medicine, University of California, San Francisco, California 94143-0936

Judith N. Wasserheit – Sexually Transmitted Diseases Branch, Division of Allergy and Infectious Diseases, National Institute of Allergy and Infectious Diseases, Bethesda, Maryland 20892

Tracey Wilson – Department of Psychology, State University of New York at Albany, Albany, New York 12222

Sally Zierler – Department of Community Health, Brown University, Providence, Rhode Island 02912

Preface

The incidence and natural history of human disease are determined by the unique interactions among biological characteristics of the host, biochemical and physical properties of the causative agent or pathogen, and a broad range of human behaviors. For no diseases is an appreciation of this constellation of factors more critical than for sexually transmitted diseases (STDs), including human immunodeficiency virus (HIV) infection. STD transmission is tied to one of the most fundamental of all human behaviors, sexual intercourse. And STD-associated stigma often limits prevention and control efforts by adversely affecting the behavior of patients, health care providers, and policymakers alike. Furthermore, many of these infections continue to challenge our ability to develop safe vaccines and curative antimicrobial agents.

This monograph explores a new model for research which attempts to integrate biomedical and behavioral approaches for STD prevention and control. The impetus for the volume came from two interdisciplinary conferences convened in November 1989 and April 1990 by the National Institute of Allergy and Infectious Diseases (NIAID) to define a behavioral research agenda related to STDs (Appendix I, "Report of the NIAID Study Group on Integrated Behavioral Research for Prevention and Control of Sexually Transmitted Diseases"). Although the clinical, epidemiological, behavioral, and laboratory-based scientists who participated in the meetings found that bridging the languages and paradigms of these disparate fields was not easy, there was uniform excitement about the research insights and opportunities that resulted from successful interdisciplinary communication.

The monograph was written to assist other biomedical and behavioral scientists in both industrialized and developing countries in addressing STD research issues through interdisciplinary approaches and collaborations. Each chapter was authored or edited through the collaborative efforts of biomedical and behavioral researchers. The first section, "Biology, Clinical Manifestations, and Epidemiology of Sexually Transmitted Diseases including HIV Infection: Implications for Interventions and Behavioral Research," contains three chapters that provide behavioral scientists with potentially useful background information on biomedical aspects of these diseases. Similarly, "Approaches to Changing Human Behaviors: Implications for Design of Interventions for Control of Sexually Transmitted Diseases including HIV Infection" contains three chapters that introduce biomedical investigators to the theoretical frameworks that are relevant in designing behavioral interventions. A glossary at the end of the volume will further facilitate reading by scientists from a diverse range of disciplines.

This monograph is intended not only for established investigators of STDs and HIV infection but also for students of the clinical and social sciences. Despite the growing importance of behavioral interventions in clinical medicine, the training of physicians and nurses in the behavioral sciences continues to be dominated by theories of psychopathology and abnormal personality which operate at the level of the individual. This book provides a complementary, interdisciplinary perspective on health and behavior that cuts across specific disease categories and encourages conceptualization of behavioral interventions at the societal, community, and individual levels. In part because the behavioral research issues and approaches surrounding STDs, including HIV infection, are so timely and highly visible, the monograph also offers graduate students in a wide variety of social science disciplines a relevant model for the potential application of behavioral interventions to health promotion and disease prevention.

The development of safe and effective interventions for prevention and control of STDs, including HIV infection, is one of the most urgent and complex challenges facing scientists today. We hope that this monograph will help the biomedical and behavioral research communities build the mutually reinforcing collaborations needed to respond optimally to this challenge.

The Importance of an Interdisciplinary Approach to Prevention of Sexually Transmitted Diseases

P. F. Sparling and Sevgi O. Aral

Sexually transmitted diseases (STDs) are a serious problem in most parts of the world. Although certain STDs such as gonorrhea and syphilis have been controlled to a significant extent in many industrialized societies, they remain major problems in the developing world and in the United States, particularly among the urban poor and underclasses. The most dramatic problems, of course, concern the recent emergence and spread of human immunodeficiency virus (HIV), but other STDs are more prevalent in most countries and cause serious health problems, particularly for women and infants. Sexually transmitted infections (STIs) caused by human papillomavirus (HPV) and herpes simplex virus (HSV) probably affect over 10% of the population in the United States (7, 9). HPV almost certainly is an important factor in the etiology of cervical carcinoma (4, 5), and HSV results in severe perinatal morbidity. Genital chlamydial infections may affect 5 to 15% of young, sexually active persons and are much more common than gonorrhea (6), despite ready treatment and excellent tools for diagnosis. Chlamydial infections are a major cause of cervicitis and salpingitis and therefore of both maternal and fetal morbidity. Syphilis is increasing rapidly in incidence in the United States, and congenital syphilis, a rare disease only a few years ago, is increasing dramatically in many cities and states. Many "classic" STDs are important not only because of their own particular morbidities but also because they are cofactors for transmission of HIV. For example, chancroid, syphilis, and HSV are causes of genital ulcer disease, which is associated with increased risks for HIV transmission (3).

These persistent, and in some cases worsening, problems are occurring in the face of a modern revolution in our understanding of the molecular biology and immunology of the mechanisms of disease caused by most STD pathogenic microbes. Many of the virulence-related genes from these microorganisms have been cloned and sequenced by recombinant DNA techniques, and the roles of their respective gene products in infection are under intensive study. In some instances, recombinant vaccine candidates are being developed (e.g., the glycoproteins of HSV). For nearly all STDs, we know much more today about pathogenic mechanisms than we did 10 years ago. A variety of new and improved diagnostic tests have been developed for many STDs, in many cases based on successful application of modern monoclonal antibody and recombinant DNA technology. These improved diagnostic tests have revealed a much higher prevalence of asympto-

P. F. Sparling – Department of Medicine, University of North Carolina School of Medicine, Chapel Hill, North Carolina 27599-7005. ***Sevgi O. Aral*** – Behavioral and Prevention Research Branch, Division of STD/HIVP, Centers for Disease Control, Atlanta, Georgia 30333.

matic infections than indicated by symptomatic disease. The recent adoption of the term "sexually transmitted infections" (STIs), as distinct from the by-now conventional term STDs, reflects this new awareness, as well as the concept that all STIs (including HIV) share many common epidemiological features. The power of molecular biology is illustrated particularly well by HIV, for which in only a few years we have witnessed the first isolation of the virus, development of extraordinarily effective diagnostic tests, and partially effective therapies. To a microbiologist, the pace of discovery is truly remarkable. Effective therapies have been introduced and are widely used to treat both HSV and HIV disease, which were formerly untreatable. Virtually all nonviral STDs can be treated effectively. Despite these scientific triumphs, STDs remain formidable problems.

What is wrong? Why have we not controlled these diseases, given our much greater understanding of their pathogenesis and natural history? One answer is that therapy fails to eradicate latent viral infection, and thus therapeutic cures are not yet possible for viruses (HSV, HIV) that cause persistent infection. The impact of present, partially effective antiviral therapies on disease transmission is unknown but probably is minimal. Therapy is valuable for individual patients, decreasing the frequency of recurring episodes of genital herpes and prolonging the lives of individual patients with HIV infection. In terms of the overall incidence and prevalence of infection, however, antiviral therapy probably has minimal impact. Indeed, some models suggest that antiviral therapy for HIV could increase the spread of HIV in the community (1).

A second answer is that antimicrobial therapy is a fundamentally inadequate means of total disease control, even if it does result in radical cure of the individually treated patient. Antimicrobial therapy certainly cures gonorrhea and probably eradicates *Chlamydia trachomatis* and *Treponema pallidum* infections, at least insofar as transmission to another individual is prevented. Nevertheless, gonorrhea continues to be a problem, with a relatively stable overall incidence in the United States and increasing antimicrobial resistance in most of the world. Chlamydial infections are not reportable, but there is little reason to believe that the incidence of infection is declining. Syphilis control is not troubled by significant problems of antimicrobial resistance, but the incidence of early infections and congenital syphilis is increasing dramatically. Use of long-acting penicillin therapy is an effective epidemiological tool for controlling the spread of syphilis among named partners, but recent trends toward increased proportions of anonymous partners (2) have blunted the efficacy of this control strategy. Under ideal circumstances, antimicrobial therapy can help to control the prevalence of certain STDs such as syphilis, but it is a reasonable axiom that antimicrobial therapy cannot eradicate any infectious disease in the absence of an effective vaccine.

In terms of public health control programs, what is needed from the basic scientists are effective vaccines. To date, there is no vaccine for any of the major STIs except hepatitis B, and that is underused. There is hope for vaccines for some of the viral and bacterial STDs based on recent dramatic increases in knowledge about surface antigens and their pathogenic roles in infection, but practical vaccines are at best years distant. STD agents for which possible vaccines are under study include *T. pallidum*, *Neisseria gonorrhoeae*, *C. trachomatis*, HSV, and HIV. A field trial of a gonococcal vaccine was attempted in Korea several years ago, but without evident success. Gonococci as well as other STD pathogens, including HIV, are adept at a variety of defensive strategies, including rapid variations in the structure of certain important surface antigens that enable them to escape from potentially effective immune surveillance (10). Because of the ability of these organisms to adapt so effectively, developing vaccines against them is a real challenge—possible, but difficult. The financial investment in basic research aimed at understanding pathogenic mechanisms and at developing vaccines based on rational principles of pathogenic mechanisms and host immune responses has been considerable, and some observers are understandably anxious that introduction of really effective, vaccine-based control programs should be hastened.

The problems in STD control reflect not only the lack of effective vaccines but also the obvious fact that prevalence of STDs is a product of the sexual and health care-seeking behaviors of individuals and groups of people. Clearly, these behaviors are such that STDs are being very well maintained in the population. The problems in behavior are directly linked to a complex set of social and economic problems and to changes in demography. Some of the social and behavioral factors that contribute to maintenance of STDs in the population were reviewed recently (3) and are discussed elsewhere in this volume.

The effectiveness of existing diagnostic, therapeutic, and preventive techniques for the STDs also reflects a different set of behaviors: those manifested by health care providers. If health care providers do not fully employ existing diagnostic tests or do not utilize the most effective treatment regimens, patients will remain undiagnosed or inadequately treated. If physicians do not ensure that all sexual partners are properly examined and treated, repeat infections of the index patient (and others) certainly will occur. If patients with STDs are not counseled about methods to reduce the risk of future exposure to STD pathogens, they are unlikely to modify the sexual behaviors that put them at risk for acquiring and transmitting STDs.

Few would want to live in a society in which there were serious efforts to legislate sexual behaviors. Absolute control of sexual behaviors undoubtedly is not possible in any society. It might be possible, however, to influence sexual and health care behaviors if only we knew enough about determinants of behavior and factors that lead to appropriate, acceptable, and sustained behavior change. Adoption by individuals of such behavioral changes as the more consistent use of condoms and choice of sexual partners with relatively low risk of infection would reduce rates of STD transmission. The question is, how do we convince people of different sociocultural groups in diverse populations to adopt such changes?

To a biomedical scientist or STD clinician, however, these are domains of knowledge that seem beyond reach, daunting in their complexity, and very difficult to study experimentally. The tools and language of the behavioral scientist are even more arcane to the clinician or molecular biologist than are those of epidemiologists, who study relatively familiar concepts such as definitions and distribution of risk factors in individuals or groups of individuals. Just as epidemiologists and behavioral scientists are confused by the language of molecular biologists, the latter are confused by the language of epidemiologists and behavioral scientists. As professionals, we are not accustomed to working together across the boundaries of various disciplines.

ACTIVITIES OF VARIOUS STD WORKERS

Persons who endeavor to prevent and/or treat STDs have diverse backgrounds, training, and interests. To a considerable extent, these workers are involved with and dependent on the activities of each other, even if their interdependence is not always readily discernible.

Health Care Givers

Health care givers (physicians, nurses, physician's assistants) are concerned with individual patients. They take histories, including a sexual behavior history, and try to determine the relative probability of STDs as a function of signs, symptoms, and behavioral risks. In assessing risk, they clearly draw on the results of epidemiologists who have studied the relationship between behavior and disease probability. They may employ specific diagnostic tests, which are the result of previous work by many groups including microbiologists and molecular biologists. Therapy often is administered, and considerations of type of therapy include not only cost, efficacy, and toxicity but also the likelihood of compliance with the prescribed regimen. Compliance is influenced by both individual and social group actions. Behavior change may be recommended to reduce the risk of acquiring or transmitting infection. Knowledge of which behaviors are most likely to be changed and how to motivate behavior change results from behavioral research.

The health care worker may be involved in clinical investigation, trying to determine, for instance, the association of certain microorganisms with particular syndromes (e.g., HPV and cervical neoplasia, or *C. trachomatis* and prenatal morbidity) or the association of sexual practices with particular infections (e.g., receptive anal intercourse and HIV infection). Such studies involve direct interactions with a variety of collaborators, including microbiologists, biostatisticians, sociologists, and psychologists. Studies of antibiotic efficacy (e.g., for gonorrhea) might involve not only microbiologists, who grow gonococci and test them for antimicrobial susceptibility, but also molecular biologists, who study DNA, including the particular genes that determine gonococcal susceptibility to antimicrobial agents.

Clinical Microbiologists

Laboratory workers also are interconnected with other STD workers. Clinical microbiologists use a variety of antibody tests to detect microbial antigens in patient secretions or, conversely, use microbial antigens to detect antibodies in patient serum or other fluids. They also culture organisms from patient specimens, and the success of these endeavors, particularly culture, is directly related to the quality of specimen obtained by the health care worker. Tests for visualizing organisms directly in patient samples (dark-field examination for *T. pallidum*, Gram stain for *N. gonorrhoeae*) also depend on sample quality.

Molecular Biologists

Molecular biology has invaded all fields of medicine, and STDs are no exception. Researchers who employ this tool are interested in characterizing the fine details of host immune response and microbial structure and function, including particularly the structure and regulation of genes and of proteins involved in pathogenesis of infection. Examples include the gonococcal pilin genes, which have been cloned into foreign hosts (*Escherichia coli*) and sequenced, allowing determination of the extent and mechanisms of variations in the structure of the expressed pilin protein. Although cloning and sequencing of DNA are at first glance far removed from the arena of clinical STD work, the results of such studies bear directly on our clinical understanding of such phenomena as why patients develop gonorrhea multiple times. (The answer, at least in part, relates to the extensive antigenic variability of various surface proteins on gonococci, including pili.) Development of vaccine candidates for virtually all STDs is strongly dependent not only on classical microbial chemistry and immunology but particularly on molecular biology techniques, including DNA cloning, sequencing, and mutagenesis. The laboratory worker employing these powerful tools also depends on the clinical investigators and epidemiologists who have defined the importance of particular microbes in certain clinical situations; without their efforts, the molecular biologists would not know what problems are worth studying.

Epidemiologists

Epidemiologists are crucial to solving many important questions related to STD control; they define particular risks for acquiring STDs (e.g., anal intercourse and increased risk of HIV acquisition). The prevalence of particular risks coupled with the magnitude of risk defines population attributable risk, a crucial consideration in developing strategies to reduce disease incidence. Epidemiologists help to determine distribution of risk factors and to design and perform clinical studies and disease intervention programs. Their tools include not only statistical methods but frequently also the diagnostic and clinical tools developed and used by clinicians and laboratory researchers. Their work also overlaps the domains of the psychologists and sociologists who study individual and group behaviors, particularly regarding forces that influence behaviors that lead to increased risk of acquiring STDs.

Psychologists and Sociologists

Psychologists and sociologists study a spectrum of phenomena that are closely related to design and implementation of STD control programs. Individual psychology is concerned with concepts such as attitude and belief formation and personality development and type. Group psychology, or social psychology, measures individuals in their social environment and includes definitions of norms and expectations, pressures, and group processes and dynamics (power distribution and hierarchies; cooperation; conflict resolution). Sociologists are concerned with broader issues affecting society as a whole, including economic and political processes, social stratification, inequality, power relationships, family structure, and others.

Clearly, the individual health care worker cannot expect success from advising STD patients to adopt safer sexual behaviors without considering the individual and group psychology of the patient or the social context in which the patient lives. Adolescent inner city males are subject to strong peer group pressures and may heed pressure of the group, even if contrary to proffered advice from the health care worker. Advising a woman to use condoms is unlikely to be effective if she lives in a social context in which women are not empowered to make these decisions. On a larger scale, one cannot understand (and therefore cannot control) the STD epidemic in large cities in the developing world without comprehension of mass migrations of male workers without wives; risky sexual behaviors are strongly promoted in these circumstances. The point is clear from these few examples that the fruits of the work of individual health care providers, laboratory workers, and epidemiologists are closely intertwined with and dependent on understanding these related fields. STDs are acquired by social behaviors, and behaviors are influenced by individual and group psychology as well as the social, economic, and even political context in which people live.

INTEGRATION OF DISCIPLINES

There are many problems that confront persons studying STDs that can only be solved by working together across lines that separate various disciplines of professional work.

We must continue to define the associations of particular microorganisms with disease syndromes. Many are already well known, but others, including those related to premature delivery and perinatal morbidity, remain to be fully understood. Some of these clinical problems are complex and multifactorial, and the combined efforts of clinicians, epidemiologists, microbiologists, behavioral scientists, and others are required to achieve satisfactory results. For instance, behaviors that lead to acquisition of agents that cause genital ulcers increase the likelihood of acquiring HIV; HIV infection alters host immunity and changes the clinical expression of agents that cause genital ulcers.

STDs will not be eradicated until really effective vaccines are developed. Despite the apparent slowness of vaccine development programs, there is reason to be optimistic that useful vaccines will be developed and that future control programs will include the use of vaccines. Before vaccines are deployed, however, it will be necessary not only to develop them by the combined efforts of microbiologists, molecular biologists, clinicians, and industry, but also to test them in the field. For the latter, the help of epidemiologists and students of behavior will be required. How can one test a vaccine without knowledge of the quantifiable risk of disease in the population under study?

In the immediate future, control of STDs will depend on development and implementation of programs that employ proper use of diagnostic and therapeutic tools and of methods for reducing risky sexual behaviors. Behavior change is virtually the only tool available to interdict the spread of chronic viral STDs for which no effective therapy or vaccine exists. Strategies to change behavior effectively either in individuals or in high-risk groups such as patients with repeated STD infections are in their infancy, but it is a reasonable hope that the concerted efforts of various types of workers will lead to better methods to reduce risky behaviors.

The unifying concept of the chapters in this volume is that control of STDs is possible only if all workers in the field of STD research (clinicians, microbiologists, molecular biologists, epidemiologists, psychologists, sociologists, and public health administrators) are aware of the multiple overlaps among their disciplines and collaborate effectively. To accomplish this, investigators in the various disciplines must first become aware of the power and limitations of research methods in the respective fields and must communicate effectively with each other. The full power of each arena of investigation, however, will be achieved only if we become more aware of and comfortable with the expertise of our colleagues who study STDs but whose tools are different from our own.

Specialized expertise, ranging from microbiology to cognitive developmental psychology, is necessary for research on the prevention and control of STDs. To maximize our returns from investments in research (i.e., to obtain a whole which is greater than the sum of its parts), we need to realize a truly interactive collaboration among the various disciplines. Our failure to prevent and control the spread of STIs points to the urgent need for developing creative, innovative interventions and prevention and control strategies. Simulation models which have been developed to evaluate the relative effectiveness of various prevention strategies indicate that combined behavioral and clinical strategies would achieve greater effectiveness than either clinical or behavioral strategies alone. Development of interdisciplinary research teams, adoption of interdisciplinary approaches to the definition and investigation of research issues, and the building of a truly interdisciplinary body of scientific knowledge will facilitate the formulation of creative, innovative interventions and prevention and control strategies (8).

This monograph is an attempt at building an interdisciplinary body of scientific knowledge in the area of STDs and AIDS. Each chapter included here has been prepared with the contribution of behavioral and clinical scientists and epidemiologists as coauthors, reviewers, or editors. Many of the chapters have been written by interdisciplinary teams. The communication necessitated by this process has provided a real learning experience for those of us who participated in it. In several instances, it has led to the formulation of new hypotheses and new interpretations of existing data. It is difficult to imagine behavioral scientists contributing to microbiology, or microbiologists contributing to theories of attitude formation.

However, it is obvious that a team of microbiologists or a team of behavioral scientists would be less likely to make major contributions to applied research on the prevention and control of STIs than an interdisciplinary team including microbiologists and behavioral scientists as well as epidemiologists and clinicians.

LITERATURE CITED

1. **Anderson, R. M., S. Gupta, and R. M. May.** 1991. Potential of community-wide chemotherapy or immunotherapy to control the spread of HIV-1. *Nature* (London) **350:**356–362.
2. **Andrus, J. K., D. W. Fleming, D. R. Harger, M. Y. Chin, D. V. Bennett, J. M. Horan, G. Oxman, B. Olson, and L. R. Foster.** 1990. Partner notification: can it control epidemic syphilis? *Ann. Intern. Med.* **112:**539–543.
3. **Aral, S. O., and K. K. Holmes.** 1991. Sexually transmitted diseases in the AIDS era. *Sci. Am.* **264:**62–69.
4. **Barrasso, R., J. De Brux, O. Croissant, and G. Orth.** 1987. High prevalence of papillomavirus associated penile intraepithelial neoplasia in sexual partners of women with cervical intraepithelial neoplasia. *N. Engl. J. Med.* **310:**916–923.
5. **Campion, M. J., A. Singer, P. K. Clarkson, and D. J. McCance.** 1985. Increased risk of cervical neoplasia in consorts of men with penile condylomata acuminata. *Lancet* **ii:**943–946.
6. **Chernesky, M. A., J. B. Mahony, S. Castriciano, M. Mores, I. O. Stewart, S. J. Landis, W. Seidelman, E. J. Sargeant, and C. Leman.** 1986. Detection of *Chlamydia trachomatis* antigens by enzyme immunoassay and immunofluorescence in genital specimens from symptomatic and asymptomatic men and women. *J. Infect. Dis.* **154:**141–148.
7. **Johnson, R. E., A. J. Nahmias, L. S. Magder, F. K. Lee, C. A. Brooks, and C. B. Snowdern.** 1981. A seroepidemiologic survey of the prevalence of herpes simplex virus type 2 infection in the United States. *N. Engl. J. Med.* **321:**7–12.
8. **National Institute of Allergy and Infectious Diseases.** 1990. Report of the NIAID study group on integrated behavioral research for prevention and control of sexually transmitted diseases. *Sex. Transm. Dis.* **7:**200–210.
9. **Pao, C. C., C. Y. Lin, J. S. Maa, C. H. Lai, S. Y. Wu, and Y. K. Soong.** 1990. Detection of human papillomaviruses in cervicovaginal cells using polymerase chain reaction. *J. Infect. Dis.* **161:**113–115.
10. **Sparling, P. F., J. Tsai, and C. N. Cornelissen.** 1990. Gonococci are survivors. *Scand. J. Infect. Dis. Suppl.* **69:**125–136.

Biology, Clinical Manifestations, and Epidemiology of Sexually Transmitted Diseases Including HIV Infection

Implications for Interventions and Behavioral Research

Introduction to the Biology and Natural History of Sexually Transmitted Diseases

Robert B. Jones and Judith N. Wasserheit

It is convenient to classify sexually transmitted diseases (STDs) both by the type of microbiological agents responsible and by the type of syndrome or disease state which they produce (Table 1). The microbiological agents responsible for most STDs are bacteria, protozoa, or viruses. Bacterial and protozoal STDs, such as chlamydia, gonorrhea, syphilis, chancroid, and trichomoniasis, usually cause either a discharge from the lower genital tract (vagina, cervix, or urethra) or genital ulcers. Specific diagnostic tests are available, and treatment is usually curative. They are considered "incident" diseases since they can be cured.

Viral STDs, such as genital herpes or human papillomavirus or immunodeficiency virus infections, are more protean in their manifestations and usually cannot be cured. Moreover, as with some bacterial STDs, they can become latent in the sense that the infection is still in the body but there are no overt manifestations. Viral STDs are considered "prevalent" diseases since individuals who are infected usually remain so.

The distinction between bacterial and protozoal and viral STDs with respect to the potential for effecting a cure is useful in considering prevention and treatment strategies and the design of behavioral research instruments and questions. Prevention of initial infection (primary prevention) is particularly important for the currently incurable viral STDs. In contrast to the curative therapy available for bacterial and protozoal STDs, treatment of viral STDs remains palliative and usually does not completely interrupt transmission. As a result, health care behaviors currently provide fewer intervention opportunities for the viral STDs than for the bacterial ones. Furthermore, because of the persistent nature of viral infections, the time frame(s) used to evaluate risk behaviors for transmission of viral STDs should be longer than that used to evaluate risk behaviors for other STDs. Finally, it is unclear whether the impact on subsequent behavior of a diagnosis of an incurable STD, such as genital herpes, differs from that of a curable infection such as gonorrhea.

Syndromic classification into categories such as discharge syndromes and genital ulcers is clinically helpful in that it narrows diagnostic possibilities and helps explain differences in transmission patterns (Table 2). For example, agents that are associated with a urethral or cervical discharge (chlamydia, gonorrhea) or are

Robert B. Jones – Departments of Medicine, Microbiology, and Immunology, Indiana University School of Medicine, Indianapolis, Indiana 46223. ***Judith N. Wasserheit*** – Sexually Transmitted Diseases Branch, Division of Allergy and Infectious Diseases, National Institute of Allergy and Infectious Diseases, Bethesda, Maryland 20892.

Table 1. Syndromes associated with common STDs

Syndrome	Bacterial	Viral
Discharge		
Vaginal	Gonorrhea, chlamydia	
Urethral	Gonorrhea, chlamydia	
Lower abdominal pain (women)	Gonorrhea, chlamydia	
Genital ulcers		
Painful	Chancroid	Herpes
Painless	Syphilis	
Growths		Papillomavirus (genital warts, genital cancer)
Rash	Syphilis	Hepatitis B HIV
Systemic (variable)	Syphilis, LGV Gonorrhea	HIV Hepatitis B
Swollen lymph nodes	LGV[a], syphilis[a,b], chancroid[a]	Herpes[a], HIV[b]
Rectal bleeding, discharge, pain	Gonorrhea, chlamydia	Herpes

[a] Local (usually groin) nodes involved.
[b] Generalized lymph node enlargement.

concentrated in genital secretions (human immunodeficiency virus [HIV]) are more easily transmitted from men to women than from women to men, while male-to-female and female-to-male transmission rates are very similar for those agents primarily associated with ulcers or other superficial lesions (e.g., early syphilis, papillomaviruses).

Finally, among individuals with a discharge, these gender differences are probably related to differences in duration of exposure to the pathogen in question. If the male partner has one of these STDs, infected semen is deposited in the vagina and remains there following intercourse, while if the female partner is infected, the male's duration of exposure is largely limited to the duration of coitus. The symmetry of transmission of pathogens associated with genital ulcers or warts may be due to the fact that transmission of these pathogens depends on small breaks in the epithelium to establish infection, and such breaks probably occur fairly often in both partners during vigorous intercourse.

In addition, syndromic classification offers an indication of the types of complications that may occur. For example, poor pregnancy outcome (e.g., stillbirth) or acquisition of HIV infection is associated with both discharge syndromes and genital ulcer diseases, while impairment of fertility is more associated with the discharge syndromes.

The only STD for which an effective vaccine is presently available is hepatitis B virus (HBV).

BACTERIAL AND PROTOZOAL STDs

Gonorrhea

Although usually it is easy to diagnose and treat, gonorrhea (commonly called clap) is still a major cause of pelvic inflammatory disease (PID) or upper genital tract infection in women, the consequences of which include infertility, ectopic pregnancy, and chronic pelvic pain. Approximately 50% of all women and between 1 and 3% of men infected with gonorrhea are asymptomatic. Curative single-dose therapy is available, but because many isolates of *Neisseria gonorrhoeae* are resistant to older antibiotics, new, more expensive antibiotics may be required for effective treatment. Reinfections are common.

Signs and symptoms

Infection of the cervix with *N. gonorrhoeae* may be associated with a vaginal discharge in women and painful urination (dysuria). Involvement of the upper genital tract (uterus and fallopian tubes) may cause lower abdominal pain, irregular bleeding, or systemic signs such as fever (110). Approximately 50% of women infected with *N. gonorrhoeae* are symptomatic at any given time, although the symptoms may be relatively mild.

Men with urethral infection (urethritis) usually develop symptoms 3 to 5 days after the infection is acquired. Dysuria and a urethral discharge that stains the underwear are common. Most men with urethritis develop symptoms, although 1 to 3% do not (42, 43). However, many ignore their symptoms and continue sexual activity before seeking medical attention (53). *N. gonorrhoeae* can also infect the rectum, resulting in rectal inflammation (proctitis), manifest by an urge to defecate frequently, painful defecation, and a rectal discharge. Proctitis occurs most often in sexually active homosexual men (92).

Complications

Although *N. gonorrhoeae* has been recovered from the lower genital tract in as many as 90% of women with their first episode of PID (113), it may not always be the cause, and current estimates are that 10 to 20% of women who acquire gonorrhea develop acute PID (53). Acute PID can be cured with treatment, but irreversible scarring and distortion of the fallopian tubes may have already occurred, and infertility and/or ectopic (tubal) pregnancy may result. Gonococcal eye infections (conjunctivitis), which can cause blindness, may occur as a result of maternal-to-infant transmission during passage through an infected birth canal. Routine ocular prophylaxis has reduced but not eliminated this disease in infants in industrialized countries (41, 71). Gonorrhea is also associated with septic abortions, prematurity, and other complications in pregnancy that can adversely affect the fetus (15). Occasionally, men with gonorrhea develop epididymitis, producing pain and swelling on one side of the scrotum (8). In addition, recent data suggest that gonorrhea is a risk factor for HIV transmission (M. Laga et al., Abstr. VI Int. AIDS Conf. 1990, Th.C.97, p. 158).

Microbiology and transmission

Only humans are infected by the causative agent of gonorrhea, *N. gonorrhoeae*. The organism cannot survive long outside of the host, and while transmission occasionally occurs during sexual foreplay or via articles such as sexual toys, the organism most commonly is spread through sexual intercourse. The chance of a

Table 2. Characteristics and transmissibility of common STDs

Characteristic	Gonorrhea	Chlamydia	Syphilis
Incubation period			
Men	3–7 days	7–10 days	21 days
Women	7–60 days	7–? days	21 days
Proportion asymptomatic			
Men	10–20%	50–90%	See text
Women	50–80%	> 90%	See text
Proportion with infected partners			
Men	50–90%	50–70%	30–60%
Women	20–50%	20–40%	30–60%
Consequences			
Short term			
Men	Urethritis	Urethritis	Ulcer, rash, etc.
Women	Epididymitis, salpingitis	Epididymitis, salpingitis	Ulcer, rash, etc.
Long term			
Men	Urethral stricture	None	Cardiovascular and neurological disease
Women	Infertility, ectopic pregnancy	Infertility, ectopic pregnancy	Cardiovascular and neurological disease
Efficacy of treatment	> 90% cure	> 90% cure	> 90% cure
Period of infectiousness	Untreated, variable	Untreated, < 1 yr	Variable
Transmission to infants (perinatal)	0–7%	~ 70%	30–100%

[a] Figures for heterosexuals; higher for homosexuals.

woman who has intercourse with an infected man acquiring gonorrhea is between 50 and 90% and probably depends on the number of exposures (53). The chance of a man acquiring it from a woman after a single exposure is approximately 20% and increases with the number of exposures (48, 54).

Diagnosis and treatment

Gonorrhea in men can be diagnosed most of the time by examining a stained smear of the urethral contents obtained with a swab, although culture is sometimes necessary since the smear is negative in 10% of infected men.

Table 2—*Continued*

Chancroid	Herpes	Papillomavirus	HIV	HBV
3–10 days	7–14 days	2–5 mo	See text	6 wk
3–10 days	7–14 days	2–5 mo	See text	6 wk
See text	75%	95%	95%	50%
See text	75%	95%	95%	50%
~ 60%	Low	80%	25–60%	18–27%[a]
Unknown	Low	80%	Unknown	18–27%[a]
Ulcers	Ulcers	Genital warts	Acute illness, social	Acute hepatitis
Ulcers	Ulcers	Genital warts	Acute illness, social	Acute hepatitis
Local disfiguring lesions	Recurrent disease	Genital cancers	Serious disease, death	Chronic hepatitis, cirrhosis, liver cancer
Local disfiguring lesions	Recurrent disease	Genital cancers	Serious disease, death	Chronic hepatitis, cirrhosis, liver cancer
> 90% cure	Suppressive, not curative	~ 25% cure	Suppressive, not curative	None
~ 30 days	Potentially lifetime	Potentially lifetime	Lifetime	Variable
Low	0–8%	Low	~ 25%	Frequent

Approximately 50% of women with endocervical infection can be diagnosed from a stained smear of the endocervical contents. However, cultures must be obtained for the remaining 50% to confirm the presence of the disease. The sensitivity of culture (ability to identify all individuals infected) approaches 90% (53) and its specificity approaches 100% if proper confirmatory laboratory tests are done.

An important element of gonorrhea control is the availability of single-dose treatment regimens, which facilitate compliance. However, many isolates of *N. gonorrhoeae* are now resistant to penicillin and tetracycline. Other antibiotics, such as ceftriaxone, are effective in single-dose regimens but are more expensive (80).

Prevention

Condoms usually are effective in preventing transmission. Spermicides containing nonoxynol-9 in a contraceptive sponge (96), vaginal suppository (20), or contraceptive gel (75) reduce male-to-female transmission, especially if used in conjunction with a diaphragm or condom (2).

Chlamydia trachomatis Infections

Chlamydia trachomatis infections are the most prevalent of bacterial STDs in the United States, with an estimated 4 million cases occurring each year. There are two biovars of *C. trachomatis* that infect humans: lymphogranuloma venereum (LGV) and trachoma. Most persons infected with the trachoma biovar are asymptomatic, and detection frequently depends on screening tests performed during routine examinations. Treatment is usually curative but requires multiple-dose regimens, and reinfections are frequent. Significant complications resulting from infections with the trachoma biovar include PID, infertility, and ectopic pregnancy in women and eye disease and pneumonia in infants born to infected women. The LGV biovar produces LGV (see below) and proctitis.

Signs and symptoms

Infections with the trachoma biovar. Primary infection of the urogenital tract involves the same sites as those infected by *N. gonorrhoeae*. However, chlamydial infections are less acute and produce milder symptoms (110). Women are usually infected at the endocervix, urethra, or both. Infection of the endocervix may produce no symptoms or physical findings, although inflammation of the cervix (cervicitis) is often present and there may be a discharge (16). The most common symptom of urethritis in a woman is a burning sensation while urinating (124). Chlamydia also causes PID with similar, but more indolent, symptoms than those described for gonorrhea. The onset of symptoms of urethritis in men is usually 7 to 10 days after acquisition of an infection and consists of a burning sensation when urinating and a discharge (124). Symptomatic rectal infections occur most often in homosexual men (92) and clinically are similar to rectal gonococcal infections.

Ocular infections in adults occur as a result of inoculation of the eye with infected genital secretions. The result is inflammation with redness, a foreign body sensation, and a discharge from the eye (35). Neonatal eye disease (inclusion conjunctivitis) is similar to eye disease in adults. Infants with pneumonia caused by *C. trachomatis* typically are listless and have a hacking cough but no fever. Most are not ill enough to require hospitalization. This biovar also causes ocular trachoma (not an STD and not discussed here) in trachoma-endemic areas.

Infections with the LGV biovar. The initial lesion in LGV is typically a small, painless bump, blister, or ulcer which appears 3 to 12 days after exposure and, because of the small size and lack of pain, may go unnoticed. Swollen lymph nodes in the groin or pelvic area occurring 2 to 4 weeks after exposure (88) characterize the second stage of the disease in men. These inguinal (groin) lymph nodes, called buboes, may rupture and exude pus. Fever, chills, sweating, nausea, headache, and muscular and joint pain are characteristic of the disease at this stage. Urethritis may also be present. Unfortunately, many people with these symptoms assume they have the "flu" and do not seek (or receive) proper treatment.

Complications

In the United States, in excess of 20% of cases of acute PID are attributed to chlamydial infections (10, 117). However, chlamydial PID is more likely to be mild and chronic than is gonococcal PID (110). As a result, women with chlamydial PID may not seek medical care, or if they do, their PID may not be diagnosed. Consequently, the first indication of a chlamydial infection may be when a woman has difficulty becoming pregnant or has an ectopic pregnancy (59, 116). Chlamydial infection during pregnancy is associated with prematurity, and chlamydial cervicitis appears to increase a woman's risk of acquiring HIV infection (89; M. Laga et al., Abstr. VI Int. AIDS Conf. 1990, Th.C.97, p. 158). Because chlamydial cervicitis (in contrast to genital ulcer disease) is highly prevalent in industrialized countries, it may prove to be a fairly important risk factor for HIV transmission in that setting.

Approximately 70% of infants born to women infected with *C. trachomatis* acquire the infection at the time of birth (1). Neonatal inclusion conjunctivitis occurs in 20 to 30%, and infant pneumonia occurs in 10 to 20%. In contrast to gonococcal conjunctivitis, chlamydial conjunctivitis usually resolves spontaneously without sequelae. Untreated, the pneumonia lasts for several months and may predispose to respiratory problems later in life (13).

In untreated men, the symptoms of urethritis may wax and wane for weeks to months (107, 108). How often the organism is spontaneously eradicated is not known, but there is a 10 to 20% asymptomatic carriage rate of *C. trachomatis* among sexually active men (61, 90). Chlamydial epididymitis develops in about 5% of infected men (8).

In men with LGV, the initial lesion is usually on the penis, and the inguinal lymph nodes are affected because they are in the lymphatic drainage from the penis. The primary complications of LGV involving these nodes are chronic draining sinuses and scarring. However, in women, the initial lesion may be inside the vagina and the affected lymph nodes deep inside the pelvis. When these break down and drain they can cause abscesses inside the pelvis, rectal strictures, or, because of lymphatic blockage, massive enlargement of the external genitals (88).

Microbiology and transmission

As noted above, the strains infecting humans are classified into the LGV and trachoma biovars, each with multiple serovars or strains. The LGV strains cause LGV and proctitis, while the trachoma strains cause eye, lung, or genital disease. Both LGV and trachoma biovars (not discussed here) are uncommon in the industrialized world but are major problems in some developing countries.

C. trachomatis does not survive for any time outside the host, and transmission is almost always directly from one person to another through sexual intercourse, passage through an infected birth canal, or hand-to-eye carriage of infected secretions. Approximately two-thirds of women and one-third of men with infected partners are themselves infected (Table 1) (6). Recurrent infections are common (5, 6).

Diagnosis and treatment

The most sensitive and specific diagnostic test available is isolation in tissue culture. Estimates on the sensitivity range from 70% to only slightly less than 100%, and the specificity is essentially 100% (6). Other diagnostic tests available are less sensitive and specific than culture but are also easier to perform and less expensive. Treatment of uncomplicated infection is usually effective, although compliance with the required week of therapy is often poor. The technical sophistication required for laboratory diagnosis and the absence of single-dose therapy combine with the indolent nature of chlamydial infections to severely limit the effectiveness of control efforts.

Prevention

When used properly, condoms are effective in preventing sexual transmission of chlamydia. As for gonorrhea, spermicides offer women some protection against infection, although it is far from complete (20, 75). Screening and treatment of infected pregnant women substantially reduces perinatal transmission (97).

Syphilis

Individuals who have acquired syphilis are highly infectious for weeks to months and may have serious adverse sequelae later in life. In addition, they are at increased risk for acquiring and transmitting HIV infection. Women run a risk of serious damage to their fetus if they acquire syphilis while pregnant or become pregnant in the early stages of disease. However, there are excellent screening tests for detecting infection; treatment is highly effective and can be given in a single dose for early infection.

Signs and symptoms

Distinct signs and symptoms characterize the three stages of syphilis, primary, secondary, and tertiary. The initial lesion or chancre usually appears at the site of inoculation approximately 3 weeks after the exposure has occurred. However, depending on the size of the inoculum, it may first appear anytime from a few days to several months later (112). The lesion begins as a dull red spot on the skin, evolves into a bump, and then ulcerates. The ulcer (chancre) characteristically is round with a well-defined margin and a thick, firm base. It is usually painless, in contrast to genital ulcers associated with other STDs. Also, there is usually painless lymphadenopathy (lymph node swelling) in the nodes draining the chancre. In heterosexual men, the initial site of infection is usually on the penis, while in women it is on the external genitals or cervix (81). Perianal chancres are common in homosexual men, and chancres have been noted at other sites such as the mouth, breasts, etc. (112). This stage of the disease is referred to as primary syphilis and, if untreated, lasts for 3 to 6 weeks before resolving spontaneously.

Secondary syphilis begins as a systemic illness in which there is frequently fever, aching of the muscles, headache, weight loss, and fatigue (112). Generalized lymphadenopathy is also frequently seen, and a rash involving the palms and soles of the feet is almost always present. In addition, ulcers may form in the mouth or on mucous areas of the genitals. In moist body folds, particularly in the groin and around the anus, the papules may enlarge to form wartlike structures (81). The onset of secondary syphilis is about 3 to 6 weeks after the first appearance of the chancre. Although they may be ignored, there are almost always some manifestations of secondary syphilis in an infected person in whom the primary disease has not been treated. The manifestations of secondary syphilis also resolve spontaneously after weeks to months and may be followed by a prolonged latent period during which no symptoms are present but laboratory tests can confirm infection.

Complications

The most serious consequences of untreated syphilis occur later in life and are called tertiary syphilis. Between 15 and 40% of untreated patients develop late complications, with cardiovascular problems being most frequent and neurological disorders second (104). Cardiovascular syphilis involves the heart and main vessel leading from it and is usually not recognized until 15 to 30 years after the initial infection (57).

Neurological complications include (i) inflammation of the arteries leading to the brain, resulting in a stroke, which occurs 5 to 12 years after initial infection; (ii) general paresis, which is a combination of dementia and other neurological changes and which occurs 15 to 20 years after initial infection; and (iii) tabes dorsalis, which involves the spinal cord with loss of sensation, especially in the legs, and which occurs 20 to 25 years after the initial infection (47).

The other major complication of syphilis is transmission to a fetus. The outcome of pregnancy in women with syphilis is related to the stage of syphilis. Women with primary or secondary syphilis usually deliver a child that either has syphilis or is premature or stillborn, while women in later stages are more likely to give birth to healthy children (31). Congenital syphilis causes enlargement of the spleen and liver, malformation of the bones, and a variety of different neurological syndromes (101).

There is also a strong association between syphilis and HIV infection, with the implication that syphilis both increases risk of acquisition of HIV and facilitates its transmission (52, 79, 99).

Microbiology and transmission

Humans are the only natural host of the responsible organism, *Treponema pallidum*, which is a spirochete that enters the body through a break in the skin or mucous membrane (81). The incubation period is 10 days to 10 weeks, with an average of 3 weeks. The period of infectiousness ranges from 2 to 4 years, although most transmission occurs during the first year.

As indicated above, primary syphilis is characterized by an ulcer at the site of invasion. Organisms disseminate from this site to virtually every organ in the body to produce secondary syphilis (82). Untreated secondary syphilis resolves spontaneously in 2 to 6 weeks, but approximately 25% of infected individuals will have at least one relapse during the first year and a smaller proportion will relapse during the second year (34, 104). The skin and mucous membrane lesions of primary and secondary syphilis are highly infectious, and infected persons remain infectious as long as relapses occur. Between 30 and 62% of secondary contacts of persons with primary or secondary syphilis become infected (100, 112). Latent syphilis occurs when there is serological evidence of syphilis but no clinical manifestations (81). Once the immune system has brought the infection under control and latency has been established, infected persons generally are not infectious, nor are persons with tertiary disease.

Diagnosis and treatment

Diagnosis of primary syphilis is best made by microscopic identification of the organisms in a fresh sample of fluid obtained from the chancre. Serology to measure serum antibodies is also helpful, since between 70 and 90% of individuals with a chancre will be seropositive (112). Two sequential blood tests are necessary to assess change in antibodies for individuals who have had previous positive syphilis serologies. Spirochetes can also be observed in lesions of secondary syphilis, and serological tests are almost always positive. Treatment for primary and secondary syphilis is generally effective, although it may be less so in HIV-infected persons, particularly those with the central nervous system involvement (9, 58).

Prevention

Condoms have limited effectiveness, since they may not prevent direct contact with infectious lesions located at sites other than the distal penis or inside the vagina.

Chancroid

Chancroid is a major cause of painful genital ulcers in individuals in many parts of the world and appears to greatly facilitate HIV transmission. Definitive diagnosis requires culture, which is relatively difficult and expensive. Treatment is generally effective, and single-dose regimens are available, although antibiotic resistance has become an increasingly important problem.

Signs and symptoms

Approximately 4 to 7 days after exposure, a tender bump surrounded by redness appears. Over the next 1 to 2 days it becomes pus filled and then erodes to form an ulcer. Unlike the ulcer of primary syphilis, this ulcer characteristically is quite painful, with ragged, undermined edges. Multiple ulcers may be present, and these may merge to form large, serpiginous lesions. Approximately 50% of men have a single ulcer, while women tend to have more than one (94). Ulcers in men are usually located near the foreskin, and uncircumcised men are at greater risk of acquiring the disease. In women, the ulcers are usually located around the entrance to the vagina but can be intravaginal, where they may produce few symptoms. Other symptoms that may be present in women include pain on urination or defecation, rectal bleeding, pain with intercourse, and vaginal discharge (94). Painful swollen inguinal lymph nodes (buboes) are present in approximately 50% of patients. The nodes become pus filled and may spontaneously rupture and drain. Fever and fatigue may occur in association with the acute phase of chancroid, but spread to other organs does not occur. Without treatment, the ulcers usually heal in approximately 1 month.

Complications

The primary complications associated with chancroid are local tissue destruction, especially in the groin, and, occasionally, persistent ulcers. Chancroid is strongly associated with augmented transmission of HIV in some settings (77).

Microbiology and transmission

Chancroid is caused by *Haemophilus ducreyi*, which has humans as its only host. It is common in several areas of the world including Southeast Asia, central Africa, and some urban centers in the United States. Women are often asymptomatic, while men are usually symptomatic. Consequently, a few female prostitutes with genital ulcers can transmit the disease to a large number of men, and in epidemic outbreaks, prostitutes have been the major reservoir (11, 94).

Diagnosis and treatment

To obtain an accurate diagnosis, it is necessary to culture the organism and exclude other diseases that may produce similar ulcers and lymphadenopathy. Culture is approximately 80% sensitive when more than one type of culture medium is used (94). *H. ducreyi* has become resistant to many antibiotics (23), and those that remain effective are either relatively expensive or require multiple doses over several days (24). Treatment appears to be effective in most cases, although therapy is more likely to fail in persons with HIV infection than in those without (76).

Prevention

Condoms may be effective in some cases (e.g., penile ulcers) but not all. Their efficacy in preventing transmission has not been adequately evaluated.

Trichomoniasis

Trichomoniasis is a fairly common sexually transmitted protozoan infection that produces vaginal inflammation and discharge in women and (occasionally) mild urethritis in men. In women it increases the risk of acquiring HIV infection and is associated with adverse pregnancy outcome (preterm delivery and low birth weight). Perinatal transmission occurs infrequently. Trichomonas vaginal infections can usually be cured with single-dose therapy if the sex partner(s) is treated simultaneously. Infections are usually self-limited in men but persist until treatment in women. Strains resistant to standard therapy exist and are very difficult to eradicate.

Signs and symptoms

Trichomonas vaginalis infection in women produces primarily vaginal discharge and vulvar itching and irritation (18, 123). There also may be burning on urination, pain with intercourse (93), and, occasionally, lower abdominal pain. The discharge may be malodorous (123) but usually is not. On vaginal examination, a gray or yellow-green discharge is found along with some redness of the vaginal walls. The irritation is more noticeable during or just after menses (18). The majority of infected men are asymptomatic, although they may experience a mild urethral discharge and burning on urination (93).

Complications

Trichomonas infections resolve spontaneously in men over a few weeks with essentially no complications (119). However, in pregnant women they are associated with both low birth weight and preterm delivery (83). In addition, they appear to facilitate acquisition of HIV infection by women (M. Laga et al., Abstr. VI Int. AIDS Conf. 1990, Th.C.97, p. 158). Perinatal transmission occurs in up to 5% of babies born to infected women. Infected neonates usually have vaginitis, although occasionally the urinary tract may be involved (93).

Microbiology and transmission

T. vaginalis, classified as a protozoan, is a motile, single-celled parasite capable of attaching to and infecting the lining of the vagina, urethra, and associated ducts and glands including the prostate (18, 118). It is exclusively a parasite of humans and essentially always transmitted sexually. Chronic infections occasionally occur in men, but most infections in men are self-limited (119), and thus men are infective for relatively short periods. However, chronic persistent infections are common in women (18), and infected women serve as the primary reservoir.

Diagnosis and treatment

Diagnosis depends on demonstration of the organism. The most commonly used technique, direct microscopic examination of vaginal discharge mixed with saline (wet mount), has a sensitivity of 50 to approximately 65% (70, 98) and close to 100% specificity. Pap smears have a similar sensitivity but lower specificity (70). Culture shows a sensitivity approaching 100% (70, 98), but this method is not widely available. Techniques such as fluorescent antibody staining appear promising but are not yet commercially available (70). Treatment is >95% effective in women if the sexual partner is also treated (93) and can be given as a single dose (38), although multiple-dose regimens may be more effective in men (93). The drug used, metronidazole, produces unpleasant side effects with alcohol ingestion. Persistent trichomonas vaginitis resulting from metronidazole-resistant strains is being recognized with increasing frequency (36, 74).

Prevention

Condoms are likely to prevent transmission. Use of spermicides slightly decreases the incidence of infection in women, while the use of oral contraceptives (as opposed to an intrauterine device or tubal ligation) greatly decreases it (3). The basis for this effect of contraceptives on trichomonas infections is not known.

VIRAL STDs

Genital Herpes

Genital herpes is a chronic ulcerative disease with significant medical and psychosocial complications. There are two types: herpes simplex virus type 1 (HSV-1) which is usually associated with the common cold sore or fever blister, and HSV-2, which is usually associated with genital herpes. However, both can infect either site. Perinatal infection may be fatal or produce mental retardation. Drug therapy reduces the frequency and duration of recurrences but is not curative.

Signs and symptoms

Initial infection at a skin or mucosal site results in the formation of vesicles (small blisters) that progress to form shallow painful ulcers. Several small lesions may coalesce to form larger ones (21). Skin ulcers crust over before healing. In primary (initial infection) genital herpes, systemic manifestations such as fever, headache, and fatigue are frequent and begin at about the same time as the skin or mucous membrane lesions appear. Extragenital lesions on the thighs or buttocks also are fairly common, as is associated pharyngeal infection. Cervical infection occurs in approximately one-third of women with external genital lesions. Urethritis occurs in both men and women and can be responsible for pain with urination, as can passage of urine over external ulcers in women. Tender, swollen lymph nodes appear in the majority of patients. Occasionally, meningitis, neurological abnormalities, or disseminated disease will occur and be severe enough to require hospitalization. A primary infection usually lasts about 3 weeks.

Following primary infection, latent infection develops in the sensory nerves that run to the site of the original infection and perhaps in other cells at that site (105). Recurrent episodes are shorter in duration (usually 8 to 12 days) than primary ones, have fewer lesions, and usually do not have associated systemic manifestations. Prodromal symptoms occur in about one-half of the patients just prior to a recurrence. Examples are mild tingling sensations at the site where the lesions will appear or shooting pains in the buttocks, hips, or legs. Approximately 50% of individuals with genital herpes caused by HSV-1 will have one or more recurrences within the first year after primary infection, in contrast to 90% whose primary infection is due to type 2 virus. The median recurrence rate for a 2-year follow-up period is five episodes per year (21). Although there is an impression that recurrence rates become less frequent with time, adequate data are not available to allow definitive conclusions to be drawn.

Complications

The primary complications of genital herpes, other than the psychological and social problems associated with the disease itself, are neonatal infection and possibly facilitation of HIV transmission. Infants may be infected at, or before, birth as a result of either primary or recurrent disease in the mother. Such perinatal infections are often fatal or lead to complications such as severe mental retardation (21, 106). Primary infection, especially early in pregnancy, can cause spontaneous abortion, fetal malformations, or prematurity and is more likely than recurrent disease to result in infant infection. Recurrent disease is not associated with adverse pregnancy outcomes other than infant infection. In recurrent disease, infant infection usually occurs at the time of birth (21, 106). The estimated incidence of neonatal HSV infections is 1 in 2,000 to 1 in 5,000 deliveries per year or approximately 1,000 cases per year in the United States (106).

Several prospective and retrospective studies in homosexual men have demonstrated an association between presence or acquisition of genital herpes and acquisition of HIV infection (reviewed in reference 21). However, two other studies of homosexual men (63, 64) and one of female prostitutes (44) did not find such an association. Thus, the extent to which HSV infection is a risk factor for HIV acquisition or transmission remains to be defined.

Microbiology and transmission

Both HSV-1 and HSV-2 are capable of infecting the genitals, mouth, or throat. However, HSV-1 is more often associated with oral infections and HSV-2 with genital ones (22). Seroprevalence studies indicate that more than 50% of adults have been exposed to HSV-1 and 30% or more have been exposed to HSV-2 (21). Virus is shed and an individual is infective at the time of each recurrence. However, virus is also shed between recurrences in the absence of lesions that are apparent to either the infected person or an examiner (21, 95). Moreover, 73% of women delivering infants who develop neonatal herpes have no history of genital herpes or recognizable lesions at the time of delivery (120). Consequently, people are frequently infected, and infectious, without realizing it. Fortunately, transmission rates appear to be relatively low (78).

Diagnosis and treatment

When typical signs and symptoms are present, clinical diagnosis is relatively easy. In their absence, viral cultures or other tests are required for confirmation. The sensitivity of culture varies according to the stage of the disease but ranges from 90% when vesicles or pustules are present to 30% after crusting has occurred (28).

The antiviral drug acyclovir is effective in shortening the course of primary disease (17) and in suppressing recurrent disease (26, 109). However, it is not curative, and when individuals stop taking it, they usually have recurrences at about the same rate as before they started taking it.

Prevention

Suppressive therapy with acyclovir does not prevent transmission, although it probably reduces it (95). Similarly, depending on the location of the lesions, barrier methods of contraception (especially condoms) would be expected to reduce but not eliminate transmission.

Papillomaviruses

Papillomaviruses are probably the most prevalent STD organisms in the United States. Certain variants or types are responsible for genital warts, while others are highly associated with genital cancer. Removal of associated growths (warts or cancer) sometimes is curative, but recurrences are common. Most infected people are asymptomatic.

Signs and symptoms

Depending on the infecting type and other unknown factors, a genital papillomavirus infection may result in (i) no obvious lesions, (ii) a small papule or bump (flat condylomata), (iii) an exophytic genital wart with spikelike projections (condylomata acuminata), or (iv) eventually a cancer (most often cervical) (21, 84). Most persons with genital or perianal warts have no symptoms and are mainly concerned about the appearance of the warts. In men they are usually located on the penis, scrotum, or urethra, while in women they are located on the labia, introitus, vagina, and cervix. They are found in the perianal area in both sexes (14). Occasionally such warts become large enough to interfere with coitus or bowel movements. The symptoms associated with genital (vulvar, penile, cervical), perianal, or rectal cancers depend on the size and location and are highly variable.

Complications

Although the different papillomavirus types differ in their propensity to cause warts as opposed to genital or rectal cancer, cancer is the most significant complication. Perinatal transmission also occurs, with infection of the infant manifest by warts involving the genital tract or, occasionally, the respiratory tract (68, 84). The latter can involve the throat, larynx, bronchial tree, or lung tissue. These papillomas do not spread to other parts of the body, but the laryngeal ones can obstruct the airway and cause death. Moreover, they are prone to frequent recurrences and require surgical removal with each recurrence. The risk of a child acquiring them has been estimated at approximately 1 in 400 if the mother has genital warts (62).

Microbiology and transmission

Papillomaviruses infect cells in the lower (innermost) layers of the skin or mucous membranes. Over 60 types of papillomaviruses have been identified, of which 20 primarily infect the anal-genital area (86). The virus multiplies in infected cells while they mature and migrate to the surface, where they are shed and infective viral particles are released. However, papillomaviruses induce the cells to multiply in a disorderly fashion, producing a wart, a precancerous growth, or a cancer (86). The true prevalence of human papillomavirus infections is not known. Past estimates in sexually active populations have ranged from approximately 5 to 20% (68, 84). However, new, more sensitive techniques for detection suggest that past studies have greatly underestimated the prevalence, and it may approach 50% in sexually active college women (7) and >80% in prostitutes (14). There are no data on the chance of acquisition after a single exposure, but approximately two-thirds of male sex partners of women with cervical condylomata or early neoplasia have evidence of genital warts (4). The usual incubation period is 3 months, with a range of 3 weeks to 8 months (85). Anal or genital warts may also occur in children as a result of infection at birth, close nonsexual contact within a family, or sexual abuse (84).

Diagnosis and treatment

To date, it has not been possible to grow papillomaviruses in tissue culture. Diagnosis is based on clinical appearance, with biopsy for pathologic study if a lesion is atypical. Treatment consists of removal of lesions through a variety of different surgical or other ablative techniques depending on size and location (14). A high proportion of people who are infected have lesions that are not readily apparent to a clinician. Many of these can be detected by using an optical magnifying device and by the application of acetic acid, which turns infected tissue white. However, normal-appearing skin or mucosa can be infected, and recurrences near the site of previously removed condylomata are extremely common (25, 27). Perhaps 25% of people with genital warts are cured of the viral infection by ablative therapy (14). Papillomavirus DNA can be detected by hybridization techniques on scrapings from the skin or mucosal surfaces. However, such tests do not appear to be very sensitive (7, 14). Detection by polymerase chain amplification is very sensitive (7) but technically difficult and expensive to perform.

Prevention

While condoms probably offer some protection for distal penile and intravaginal lesions, they are unlikely to completely prevent transmission. Careful screening and removal of genital lesions may reduce transmission.

HBV

HBV is one of the most common causes of hepatitis or liver inflammation and is the only one of the hepatitis-associated viruses for which sexual transmission is a major means of spread. Infection occasionally leads to death from acute or chronic liver failure or liver cancer. Once hepatitis develops, there is no effective therapy, although the majority of cases resolve spontaneously. There is an effective vaccine.

Signs and symptoms

HBVs infects liver cells, with overproduction of proteins that compose the coat of the virus. These surface antigens usually can be detected in the serum 2 to 3 months after exposure and 2 to 5 weeks before the onset of symptoms (32, 49). Between one-third and two-thirds of infections are asymptomatic. When present, the initial symptoms are usually nonspecific, such as fever, rash, and painful joints. These are followed by fatigue, nausea, loss of appetite, and frequently pain in the area of the liver. Yellow eyes and skin (jaundice) and dark urine may develop, and abnormal amounts of liver enzymes can be detected in the blood, reflecting liver damage. Over 95% of patients recover completely, usually within 6 to 8 weeks.

Complications

Approximately 1 in 1,000 people with acute HBV infection dies from acute fulminant liver failure (32). This most often occurs when there is superinfection (or sometimes coinfection) of an HBV carrier with the delta agent (50). The latter is an incomplete virus that requires HBV to be infective for cells. Its epidemiology and transmission patterns are almost identical to those of HBV. Ninety to 95% of normal HBV-infected adults clear the HBV from their system. They then are not infective and are themselves immune against reinfection. However, 6 to 10% continue to have virus replication in their liver and circulating virus in their bloodstream. Most are asymptomatic, without evidence of liver disease. However, a small proportion develop chronic active hepatitis leading to cirrhosis and death or develop cancer of the liver, which is also fatal.

Microbiology and transmission

HBVs can be transmitted parenterally (blood to blood), sexually, perinatally, or horizontally. In developed countries, parenteral transmission occurs primarily in intravenous drug users who share needles and in health care workers who may receive needle stick or other injuries. The virus is present in salvia, semen, vaginal fluid, and probably most other body fluids. Sexual transmission is highly associated with numbers of sexual partners, receptive or insertive anal intercourse, or having a regular sexual partner, e.g., spouse, who is infective (56, 66, 73). Between 18 and 27% of susceptible cohabiting spouses of infectious individuals become infected (56, 73). HBV is frequently transmitted perinatally, particularly in areas of the world such as Southeast Asia and Africa, where over 90% of the population has serological evidence of current or past infection (73). Infants who are infected perinatally usually become chronic carriers without having manifestations of acute disease, although they may later develop chronic hepatitis. Horizontal transmission also occurs in household settings in which there is a person with HBV infection and no recognized parenteral or sexual exposure. Objects passed from the mouth of one child to another are an example of how such transmission can occur (72).

Diagnosis and treatment

Only about one-third of infected adults are diagnosed clinically as having viral hepatitis. One-third have mild symptoms without jaundice, while another third are completely asymptomatic (60). Diagnosis of asymptomatic carriers of the virus depends on demonstration of viral antigen in the serum, a test which is 90% sensitive in the acute phase of the disease and approaches 100% sensitivity in chronic carriers (73). However, there are occasional carriers who do not have serum antigen (51). There is no effective therapy for HBV infection.

Prevention

There is a vaccine that provides protective immunity for up to 2 years in 80% of recipients, although by 5 years immunity is low or not detectable in half (37). Despite this vaccine having been available and recommended for use in high-risk groups since 1982, rates of hepatitis B have increased rather than decreased (60). Resistance to use of the vaccine has been attributed to high cost, unfounded fear of acquiring HIV infection from the vaccine, and a failure to effectively target the individuals at highest risk for acquiring hepatitis B. High-titer immunoglobulin is also effective in preventing HBV infection when given after a known high-risk exposure.

HIV

HIV infection produces high morbidity and mortality. Antiviral therapy delays the progression of disease but does not prevent it and is not curative. Once someone is infected, they are infected for life. Transmission is sexual, parenteral (through injection of virus-infected blood or blood products), or from mother to infant during pregnancy or breast-feeding.

Signs and symptoms

The disease is described in terms of three stages. Among adults, the first stage is characterized by an acute mononucleosislike illness 2 to 4 weeks after infection (114). Sore throat, fever, fatigue, headache, and swollen lymph nodes are prominent manifestations. This illness generally lasts 3 to 14 days but is not severe, and many infected individuals will not seek medical care. At this point, the virus usually becomes latent and the infected person becomes asymptomatic. The second stage, AIDS-related complex (ARC), is characterized by fatigue, weight loss, chronic headaches, fever, and lymphadenopathy or sometimes by AIDS-related dementia. The latter is manifest by personality or mood changes, memory loss, or cognitive disorders. The third stage, AIDS, is characterized by the onset of opportunistic infections or cancers.

Complications

There are multiple complications of HIV infection, including ARC, AIDS, and AIDS-related dementia. The duration of the asymptomatic period is highly variable. The mean time to the development of AIDS is 7 to 9 years but may extend to 15 years or longer (46). AIDS itself is a clinical diagnosis based on the presence of one or more of a defined group of opportunistic infections and cancers. The course of disease is highly variable and is determined by the occurrence of infections, cancers, and those symptoms directly attributable to HIV itself, such as generalized wasting and dementia. In addition, infants born to infected women are more likely to be premature and of low birth weight than infants born to uninfected women (40).

Microbiology and transmission

HIV type 1 (HIV-1) is a new (or, at least newly recognized) sexually transmitted agent. A closely related virus, HIV-2, which also causes AIDS has been identified in western Africa, but it is not yet as widely spread as HIV-1 (91). The virus has an affinity for receptors that are present on helper lymphocytes (cells that serve critical regulatory functions in the immune system) and on circulating cells that migrate to the brain. Infection of helper cells by HIV-1 can result in their dysfunction or destruction, rendering the infected person susceptible to the infections and cancers

Table 3. Major risk factors for HIV transmission

Population	Risk factor(s)
Everyone	Multiple sex partners, receipt of blood or blood products (unscreened)
Homosexual men	Receptive anal intercourse, recent partner with AIDS, genital herpes, or syphilis
Heterosexual men	Prostitute contact, genital ulcers in themselves or sexual contacts, presence of a foreskin
Heterosexual women	Genital ulcers, chlamydial or gonococcal cervicitis, trichomonal vaginitis, receptive anal intercourse
Intravenous drug abusers	Needle sharing
Health care workers	Needle stick injuries

associated with AIDS. Infection of cells that migrate to the brain results in inflammation with tissue destruction and neurological or psychiatric disorders such as dementia (46). The virus has a very high spontaneous mutation rate such that a given individual at any one time is infected with a population of viruses rather than with a single virus (39). This may be one reason why disease due to infection with HIV-1 is more rapidly progressive in some individuals than others and perhaps why some individuals appear to be more infectious than others (19). Infection with the virus requires exposure to infected blood or sexual contact with an infected person. Major risk factors for transmission of HIV-1 are identified in Table 3.

The STDs that cause genital ulcers have been identified as risk factors for acquisition of HIV; these include chancroid (77), syphilis (52, 79, 99), and genital herpes (21), although the role of the latter has recently been questioned (44, 63, 67). Nonulcerative STDs such as gonococcal or chlamydial cervicitis and trichomonas vaginitis may also facilitate transmission (89; M. Laga et al., Abstr. VI Int. AIDS Conf. 1990, Th.C.97, p. 158), as may the use of oral contraceptives (89). Receptive anal intercourse is a major risk factor in both men and women (65, 87, 121), as is the presence of a foreskin (being uncircumcised) in men (103).

The virus is transmitted perinatally. Between 22 and 39% of infants born to infected women are themselves infected. Most are diagnosed within the first 2 years of life and die within the subsequent 2 years (12, 40, 102). Breast-feeding has also been implicated in maternal-infant transmission (12).

Diagnosis and treatment

Diagnosis of AIDS is a clinical diagnosis. Diagnosis of HIV infection depends on demonstration of the virus or antibodies against it in blood or other tissues. Measurable antibodies against the virus usually appear within 2 months after acquisition of the infection, and by 6 months 95% of infected individuals have them (55), although in some cases the initial infection may not stimulate an antibody response for several months (122).

One antiviral agent, zidovudine (ZDV or AZT), has been shown to delay disease progression (30, 115) and has been approved for treatment of people with advanced disease. Moreover, the use of ZDV and prophylaxis for selected infections appears to have slowed the overall rate at which people with HIV infection develop AIDS (33). Other antiviral agents are under investigation.

Prevention

Available data suggest that antiviral drugs such as ZDV have no effect on recovery of virus from semen and, thus, presumably on infectiousness (69). When used consistently, latex condoms appear to be effective in preventing transmission of HIV (29, 89). The spermicide nonoxynol-9 has activity in tissue culture against HIV (45), which has led many to advocate its use, especially in association with barrier methods of contraception. However, the extent to which it may actually prevent transmission is not known. Behavior change seems to offer the greatest promise for prevention in the near future.

Acknowledgments. We express our gratitude to Suzanne Steinmetz and Robert E. Hornick for their editorial assistance.

LITERATURE CITED

1. **Alexander, E. R., and H. R. Harrison.** 1983. Role of *Chlamydia trachomatis* in perinatal infection. *Rev. Infect. Dis.* **5:**713–719.
2. **Austin, H., W. C. Louv, and W. J. Alexander.** 1984. A case-control study of 4 spermicides and gonorrhea. *J. Am. Med. Assoc.* **251:**2822–2824.
3. **Barbone, F., H. Austin, W. C. Louv, and W. J. Alexander.** 1990. A follow-up study of methods of contraception, sexual activity, and rates of trichomoniasis, candidiasis, and bacterial vaginosis. *Am. J. Obstet. Gynecol.* **163:**510–514.
4. **Barrasso, R., J. De Brux, O. Croissant, and G. Orth.** 1987. High prevalence of papillomavirus-associated penile intraepithelial neoplasia in sexual partners of women with cervical intraepithelial neoplasia. *N. Engl. J. Med.* **317:**916–923.
5. **Batteiger, B. E., J. Fraiz, W. J. Newhall, B. P. Katz, and R. B. Jones.** 1989. Association of recurrent chlamydial infection with gonorrhea. *J. Infect. Dis.* **159:**661–669.
6. **Batteiger, B. E., and R. B. Jones.** 1987. Chlamydial infections, p. 55–81. *In* H. H. Handsfield (ed.), *Infectious Disease Clinics of North America: Sexually Transmitted Diseases,* vol. 1. W. B. Saunders Co., Philadelphia.
7. **Bauer, H. M., Y. Ting, C. E. Greer, J. C. Chambers, C. J. Tashiro, J. Chimera, A. Reingold, and M. M. Manos.** 1991. Genital human papillomavirus infection in female university students as determined by a PCR-based method. *J. Am. Med. Assoc.* **265:**472–477.
8. **Berger, R. E., E. R. Alexander, G. D. Monda, J. Ansell, G. McCormick, and K. K. Holmes.** 1978. *Chlamydia trachomatis* as a cause of acute "idiopathic" epididymitis. *N. Engl. J. Med.* **298:**301–304.
9. **Berry, C. D., T. M. Hooton, A. C. Collier, and S. A. Lukehart.** 1987. Neurologic relapse after benzathine penicillin therapy for secondary syphilis in a patient with HIV infection. *N. Engl. J. Med.* **316:**1587–1589.
10. **Black, J. R., H. H. Handsfield, and E. W. Hook III.** 1989. Single-dose ofloxacin vs. amoxicillin plus probenecid for treatment of uncomplicated gonococcal infection. *Rev. Infect. Dis.* **11**(Suppl. 5):S1313–S1314.
11. **Blackmore, C. A., K. Limpakarnjanarat, J. G. Rigau-Perez, W. L. Albritton, and J. R. Greenwood.** 1985. An outbreak of chancroid in Orange County, California: descriptive epidemiology and disease-control measures. *J. Infect. Dis.* **151:**840–844.
12. **Blanche, S., C. Rouzioux, M.-L. G. Moscato, F. Veber, M.-J. Mayaux, C. Jacomet, J. Tricoire, A. Deville, M. Vial, G. Firtion, A. deCrepy, D. Douard, M. Robin, C. Courpotin, N. Ciraru-Vigneron, F. Le Deist, and C. Griscelli.** 1989. A prospective study

of infants born to women seropositive for human immunodeficiency virus type 1. *N. Engl. J. Med.* **320:**1643–1648.

13. **Brasfield, D. M., S. Stagno, R. J. Whitley, G. Cloud, G. Cassell, and R. E. Tiller.** 1987. Infant pneumonitis associated with cytomegalovirus, *Chlamydia, Pneumocystis,* and *Ureaplasma*: follow-up. *Pediatrics* **79:**76–83.
14. **Brown, D. R., and K. H. Fife.** 1990. Human papillomavirus infections of the genital tract. *Med. Clin. North Am.* **74:**1455–1485.
15. **Brunham, R. C., K. K. Holmes, and J. E. Embree.** 1990. Sexually transmitted diseases in pregnancy, p. 771–801. *In* K. K. Holmes, P.-A. Mardh, P. F. Sparling, P. J. Wiesner, W. Cates, Jr., S. M. Lemon, and W. E. Stamm (ed.), *Sexually Transmitted Diseases,* 2nd ed. McGraw-Hill Book Co., New York.
16. **Brunham, R. C., J. Paavoonen, C. E. Stevens, N. Kiviat, C. W. Critchlow, and K. K. Holmes.** 1984. Mucopurulent cervicitis: the ignored counterpart in women of urethritis in men. *N. Engl. J. Med.* **311:**1–6.
17. **Bryson, Y. J., M. Dillon, M. Lovett, G. Acuna, S. Taylor, J. D. Cherry, B. L. Johnson, E. Wiesmeier, W. Growdon, T. Creagh-Kirk, and R. Keeney.** 1983. Treatment of first episodes of genital herpes simplex virus infection with oral acyclovir. A randomized double-blind controlled trial in normal subjects. *N. Engl. J. Med.* **308:**916–921.
18. **Catterall, R. D.** 1972. Trichomonal infections of the genital tract. *Med. Clin. North Am.* **56:**1203–1209.
19. **Clumeck, N., H. Taelman, P. Hermans, P. Piot, M. Schoumacher, and S. DeWit.** 1989. A cluster of HIV infection among heterosexual people without apparent risk factors. *N. Engl. J. Med.* **321:**1460–1478.
20. **Cole, C. H., T. G. Lacher, J. C. Bailey, and D. L. Fairclough.** 1980. Vaginal chemoprophylaxis in the reduction of reinfection in women with gonorrhea. Clinical evaluation of the effectiveness of a vaginal contraceptive. *Br. J. Vener. Dis.* **56:**314–318.
21. **Corey, L.** 1990. Genital herpes, p. 391–413. *In* K. K. Holmes, P.-A. Mardh, P. F. Sparling, P. J. Wiesner, W. Cates, Jr., S. M. Lemon, and W. E. Stamm (ed.), *Sexually Transmitted Diseases,* 2nd ed. McGraw-Hill Book Co., New York.
22. **Corey, L., and K. K. Holmes.** 1983. Clinical course of genital herpes simplex infections: current concepts in diagnosis, therapy and prevention. *Ann. Intern. Med.* **98:**973–983.
23. **Dangor, Y., R. C. Ballard, S. D. Miller, and H. J. Koornhof.** 1990. Antimicrobial susceptibility of *Haemophilus ducreyi. Antimicrob. Agents Chemother.* **34:**1303–1307.
24. **Dangor, Y., R. C. Ballard, S. D. Miller, and H. J. Koornhof.** 1990. Treatment of chancroid. *Antimicrob. Agents Chemother.* **34:**1308–1311.
25. **de Villiers, E.-M., D. Wagner, A. Schneider, G. Gross, and H. zur Hausen.** 1987. Human papillomavirus infections in women with and without abnormal cervical cytology. *Lancet* **ii:**703–706.
26. **Douglas, J. M., C. Critchlow, J. Benedetti, G. J. Mertz, J. D. Connor, M. A. Hintz, A. Fahnlander, M. Remington, C. Winter, and L. Corey.** 1984. A double-blind study of oral acyclovir for suppression of recurrences of genital herpes simplex virus infection. *N. Engl. J. Med.* **310:**1551–1556.
27. **Ferenczy, A., M. Mitao, N. Nagai, S. J. Silverstein, and C. P. Crum.** 1985. Latent papillomavirus and recurring genital warts. *N. Engl. J. Med.* **313:**784–788.
28. **Fife, K. H., and L. Cory.** 1990. Herpes simplex virus, p. 941–952. *In* K. K. Holmes, P.-A. Mardh, P. F. Sparling, P. J. Wiesner, W. Cates, Jr., S. M. Lemon, and W. E. Stamm (ed.), *Sexually Transmitted Diseases,* 2nd ed. McGraw-Hill Book Co., New York.
29. **Fischl, M. A., G. M. Dickinson, G. B. Scott, N. Klimas, M. A. Fletcher, and W. Parks.** 1987. Evaluation of heterosexual partners, children, and household contacts of adults with AIDS. *J. Am. Med. Assoc.* **257:**640–644.
30. **Fischl, M. A., D. D. Richman, N. Hansen, A. C. Collier, J. T. Carey, M. F. Para, W. D. Hardy, R. Dolin, W. G. Powderly, J. D. Allan, B. Wong, T. C. Merigan, V. J. McAuliffe, N. E. Hyslop, F. S. Rhame, H. H. Balfour, S. A. Spector, P. Volberding, C. Pettinelli, and J. Anderson.** 1990. The safety and efficacy of zidovudine (AZT) in the

treatment of subjects with mildly symptomatic human immunodeficiency virus type 1 (HIV) infection: a double-blind, placebo-controlled trial. *Ann. Intern. Med.* **112:**727–737.

31. **Fiumara, N. J., W. L. Fleming, J. G. Downing, and F. L. Good.** 1952. The incidence of prenatal syphilis at the Boston City Hospital. *N. Engl. J. Med.* **247:**48–52.
32. **Francis, D. P.** 1983. Selective primary health care: strategies for control of disease in the developing world. III. Hepatitis B virus and its related diseases. *Rev. Infect. Dis.* **5:**322–329.
33. **Gail, M. H., P. S. Rosenberg, and J. J. Goedert.** 1990. Therapy may explain recent deficits in AIDS incidence. *J. Acquired Immune Defic. Syndr.* **3:**296–306.
34. **Gjestland, T.** 1955. The Oslo study of untreated syphilis: an epidemiologic investigation of the natural course of syphilitic infection based on a restudy of the Boeck-Bruusgaard material. *Acta Dermato. Venereol.* **35**(Suppl.)**:**1–368.
35. **Grayston, J. T., and S. Wang.** 1975. New knowledge of chlamydiae and the diseases they cause. *J. Infect. Dis.* **132:**87–105.
36. **Grossman, J. H., III, and R. P. Galask.** 1990. Persistent vaginitis caused by metronidazole-resistant trichomonas. *Obstet. Gynecol.* **76:**521–522.
37. **Hadler, S. C., D. P. Francis, J. E. Maynard, S. E. Thompson, F. N. Judson, D. F. Echenberg, D. G. Ostrow, P. M. O'Malley, K. A. Penley, N. L. Altman, E. Braff, G. F. Shipman, P. J. Coleman, and E. J. Mandell.** 1986. Long-term immunogenicity and efficacy of hepatitis B vaccine in homosexual men. *N. Engl. J. Med.* **315:**209–214.
38. **Hager, W. D., S. T. Brown, S. J. Kraus, G. S. Kleris, G. J. Perkins, and M. Henderson.** 1980. Metronidazole for vaginal trichomoniasis: seven-day vs. single-dose regimens. *J. Am. Med. Assoc.* **244:**1219–1220.
39. **Hahn, B. H., G. M. Shaw, M. E. Taylor, R. R. Redfield, P. D. Markham, S. Z. Salahuddin, F. Wong-Staal, R. C. Gallo, E. S. Parks, and W. P. Parks.** 1986. Genetic variation in HTLV-III/LAV over time in patients with AIDS or at risk for AIDS. *Science* **232:**1548–1553.
40. **Halsey, N. A., R. Boulos, E. Holt, A. Ruff, J. R. Brutus, P. Kissinger, T. C. Quinn, J. S. Coberly, M. Adrien, and C. Boulos.** 1990. Transmission of HIV-1 infections from mothers to infants in Haiti: impact on childhood mortality and malnutrition. *J. Am. Med. Assoc.* **264:**2088–2092.
41. **Hammerschlag, M. R., C. Cummings, P. M. Roblin, T. H. Williams, and I. Delke.** 1989. Efficacy of neonatal ocular prophylaxis for the prevention of chlamydial and gonococcal conjunctivitis. *N. Engl. J. Med.* **320:**769–772.
42. **Handsfield, H. H., T. O. Lipman, J. P. Harnisch, E. Tronco, and K. K. Holmes.** 1974. Asymptomatic gonorrhea in men: diagnosis, natural course, prevalence and significance. *N. Engl. J. Med.* **290:**117.
43. **Harrison, W. O., R. R. Hooper, P. J. Wiesner, A. F. Campbell, W. W. Karney, G. H. Reynolds, O. G. Jones, and K. K. Holmes.** 1979. A trial of minocycline given after exposure to prevent gonorrhea. *N. Engl. J. Med.* **300:**1074.
44. **Hayes, C. G., C. R. Manaloto, V. Basaca-Sevilla, et al.** 1990. Epidemiology of HIV infection among prostitutes in the Philippines. *J. Acquired Immune Defic. Syndr.* **3:**913–920.
45. **Hicks, D. R., L. S. Martin, J. P. Getchell, J. L. Heath, D. P. Francis, J. S. McDougal, J. W. Curran, and B. Voeller.** 1985. Inactivation of HTLV-III/LAV-infected cultures of normal human lymphocytes by nonoxynol-9 in vitro. *Lancet* **ii:**1422–1423. (Letter.)
46. **Hirsch, M. S.** 1990. Clinical manifestations of HIV infection in adults in industrialized countries, p. 331–353. *In* K. K. Holmes, P.-A. Mardh, P. F. Sparling, P. J. Wiesner, W. Cates, Jr., S. M. Lemon, and W. E. Stamm (ed.), *Sexually Transmitted Diseases*, 2nd ed. McGraw-Hill Book Co., New York.
47. **Hobson, D., and F. W. A. Johnson.** 1977. The effect of penicillin on genital strains of *Chlamydia trachomatis* in tissue culture. *J. Antimicrob. Chemother.* **3:**49–56.
48. **Holmes, K. K., D. W. Johnson, and H. J. Trostle.** 1970. An estimate of the risk of men acquiring gonorrhea by sexual contact with infected females. *Am. J. Epidemiol.* **91:**170–174.

49. **Hoofnagle, J. H.** 1981. Serologic markers of hepatitis B virus infection. *Annu. Rev. Med.* **32:**1–11.
50. **Hoofnagle, J. H.** 1989. Type D (delta) hepatitis. *J. Am. Med. Assoc.* **261:**1321–1325.
51. **Hoofnagle, J. H., L. B. Seefe, Z. B. Bales, and H. J. Zimmerman.** 1978. Type B hepatitis after transfusion with blood containing antibody to hepatitis B core antigen. *N. Engl. J. Med.* **298:**1379–1383.
52. **Hook, E. W., III.** 1989. Syphilis and HIV infection. *J. Infect. Dis.* **160:**530–534.
53. **Hook, E. W., III, and H. H. Handsfield.** 1990. Gonococcal infections in the adult, p. 149–165. *In* K. K. Holmes, P.-A. Mardh, P. F. Sparling, P. J. Wiesner, W. Cates, Jr., S. M. Lemon, and W. E. Stamm (ed.), *Sexually Transmitted Diseases,* 2nd ed. McGraw-Hill Book Co., New York.
54. **Hooper, R. R., et al.** 1978. Cohort study of venereal disease. I. The risk of gonorrhea transmission from infected women to men. *Am. J. Epidemiol.* **108:**136–144.
55. **Horsburgh, C. R., J. Jason, I. M. Longini, K. H. Mayer, G. Schochetman, G. W. Rutherford, G. R. Seage, C. Y. Ou, S. D. Holmberg, C. Schable, A. R. Lifson, J. W. Ward, B. L. Evatt, and H. W. Jaffe.** 1989. Duration of human immunodeficiency virus infection before detection of antibody. *Lancet* **ii:**637–639.
56. **Inaba, N., R. Ohkawa, A. Matsuura, J. Kudoh, and H. Takamizawa.** 1979. Sexual transmission of hepatitis B surface antigen. Infection of husbands by HBsAg carrier-state wives. *Br. J. Vener. Dis.* **55:**366–368.
57. **Jackman, J. D., Jr.** 1989. Cardiovascular syphilis. *Am. J. Med.* **87:**425–433.
58. **Johns, D. R., M. Tierney, and D. Felsenstein.** 1987. Alteration in the natural history of neurosyphilis by concurrent infection with the human immunodeficiency virus. *N. Engl. J. Med.* **316:**1569–1572.
59. **Jones, R. B., S. L. Hui, and R. E. Cleary.** 1982. Correlation between serum antichlamydial antibodies and tubal factor as a cause of infertility. *Fertil. Steril.* **38:**553–558.
60. **Kane, M. A., M. J. Alter, S. C. Hadler, and H. S. Margolis.** 1989. Hepatitis B infection in the United States: recent trends and strategies for control. *Am. J. Med.* **87**(Suppl. 3A):11S–13S.
61. **Karam, G. H., D. H. Martin, T. R. Flotte, F. O. Bonnarens, J. R. Joseph, T. F. Mroczkowski, and W. D. Johnson.** 1986. Asymptomatic *Chlamydia trachomatis* infections among sexually active men. *J. Infect. Dis.* **154:**900–903.
62. **Kashima, H. K., K. Shah, and M. Goodstein.** 1990. Recurrent respiratory papillomatosis, p. 889–893. *In* K. K. Holmes, P.-A. Mardh, P. F. Sparling, P. J. Wiesner, W. Cates, Jr., S. M. Lemon, and W. E. Stamm (ed.), *Sexually Transmitted Diseases,* 2nd ed. McGraw-Hill Book Co., New York.
63. **Keet, I. P., F. K. Lee, G. J. van Griensven, J. M. Lange, A. Nahmias, and R. A. Coutinho.** 1990. Herpes simplex virus type 2 and other genital ulcerative infections as a risk factor for HIV-1 acquisition. *Genitourin. Med.* **66:**330–333.
64. **Kingsley, L. A., J. Armstrong, A. Rahman, M. Ho, and C. R. Rinaldo.** 1990. No association between herpes simplex virus type-2 seropositivity or anogenital lesions and HIV seroconversion among homosexual men. *J. Acquired Immune Defic. Syndr.* **3:**773–779.
65. **Kingsley, L. A., R. Kaslow, C. R. Rinaldo, K. Detre, N. Odaka, M. VanRaden, R. Detels, B. F. Polk, J. Chmiel, S. F. Kelsey, D. Ostrow, and B. Visscher.** 1987. Risk factors for seroconversion to human immunodeficiency virus among male homosexuals. *Lancet* **i:**345–348.
66. **Kingsley, L. A., C. R. Rinaldo, Jr., D. W. Lyter, R. O. Valdiserri, S. H. Belle, and M. Ho.** 1990. Sexual transmission efficiency of hepatitis B virus and human immunodeficiency virus among homosexual men. *J. Am. Med. Assoc.* **264:**230–234.
67. **Koutsky, L. A., R. L. Ashley, K. K. Holmes, C. E. Stevens, P. Wolner-Hanssen, and L. Corey.** 1990. The frequency of unrecognized type 2 herpes simplex infection among women. *Sex. Transm. Dis.* **17:**90–94.
68. **Koutsky, L. A., D. A. Galloway, and K. K. Holmes.** 1988. Epidemiology of genital human papillomavirus infection. *Epidemiol. Rev.* **10:**122–163.
69. **Krieger, J. N., R. W. Coombs, A. C. Collier, S. O. Ross, K. Chaloupka, D. K.**

Cummings, V. L. Murphy, and L. Corey. 1991. Recovery of human immunodeficiency virus type 1 from semen: minimal impact of stage of infection and current antiviral chemotherapy. *J. Infect. Dis.* **163:**386–388.

70. **Krieger, J. N., M. R. Tam, C. E. Stevens, I. O. Nielsen, J. Hale, N. B. Kiviat, and K. K. Holmes.** 1988. Diagnosis of trichomoniasis: comparison of conventional wet-mount examination with cytologic studies, cultures, and monoclonal antibody staining of direct specimens. *J. Am. Med. Assoc.* **259:**1223–1227.
71. **Laga, M., F. A. Plummer, P. Piot, P. Datta, W. Namaara, J. O. Ndinya-Achola, H. Nzanze, G. Maitha, A. R. Ronald, H. O. Pamba, and R. C. Brunham.** 1988. Prophylaxis of gonococcal and chlamydial ophthalmia neonatorum: a comparison of silver nitrate and tetracycline. *N. Engl. J. Med.* **318:**653–657.
72. **Leichtner, A. M., J. Leclair, D. A. Goldmann, R. T. Schumacher, and A. J. Katz.** 1981. Horizontal nonparental spread of hepatitis B among children. *Ann. Intern. Med.* **94:**346–349.
73. **Lemon, S. M., and J. E. Newbold.** 1990. Viral hepatitis, p. 449–466. *In* K. K. Holmes, P.-A. Mardh, P. F. Sparling, P. J. Wiesner, W. Cates, Jr., S. M. Lemon, and W. E. Stamm (ed.), *Sexually Transmitted Diseases,* 2nd ed. McGraw-Hill Book Co., New York.
74. **Lossick, J. G.** 1990. Treatment of sexually transmitted vaginosis/vaginitis. *Rev. Infect. Dis.* **12**(Suppl. 6):S665–S681.
75. **Louv, W. C., H. Austin, W. J. Alexander, S. Stagno, and J. Checks.** 1988. A clinical trial of nonoxynol-9 for preventing gonococcal and chlamydial infections. *J. Infect. Dis.* **158:**518–523.
76. **MacDonald, K. S., D. W. Cameron, L. J. D'Costa, J. O. Ndinya-Achola, F. A. Plummer, and A. R. Ronald.** 1989. Evaluation of fleroxacin (RO23-6240) as single oral dose therapy of culture-proven chancroid in Nairobi, Kenya. *Antimicrob. Agents Chemother.* **33:**612–614.
77. **Melbye, M., A. Bayley, J. K. Manuwele, S. A. Clayden, W. A. Blattner, R. Tedder, E. K. Njelesani, K. Mukelabai, F. J. Bowa, A. Levin, R. A. Weiss, and R. J. Biggar.** 1986. Evidence of heterosexual transmission and clinical manifestations of human immunodeficiency virus infection and related conditions in Lusaka, Zambia. *Lancet* **ii:**1113.
78. **Mertz, G. J., R. W. Coombs, R. Ashley, J. Jourden, M. Remington, C. Winter, A. Fahnlander, M. Guinan, H. Ducey, and L. Corey.** 1988. Transmission of genital herpes in couples with one symptomatic and one asymptomatic partner: a prospective study. *J. Infect. Dis.* **157:**1169–1177.
79. **Miotti, P. G., G. Dallabetta, E. Ndovi, G. Liomba, A. J. Saah, and J. Chiphangwi.** 1990. HIV-1 and pregnant women: associated factors, prevalence, estimate of incidence and role in fetal wastage in central Africa. *AIDS* **4:**733–736.
80. **Moran, J. S., and J. Zenilman.** 1990. Therapy for gonococcal infections: options in 1989. *Rev. Infect. Dis.* **12**(Suppl. 6):S633–S644.
81. **Musher, D. M.** 1987. Syphilis, p. 83–95. *In* H. H. Handsfield (ed.), *Infectious Disease Clinics of North America: Sexually Transmitted Diseases,* vol. 1. W. B. Saunders Co., Philadelphia.
82. **Musher, D. M.** 1990. Biology of *Treponema pallidum,* p. 205–211. *In* K. K. Holmes, P.-A. Mardh, P. F. Sparling, P. J. Wiesner, W. Cates, Jr., S. M. Lemon, and W. E. Stamm (ed.), *Sexually Transmitted Diseases,* 2nd ed. McGraw-Hill Book Co., New York.
83. **Nugent, R., D. Martin, M. F. Cotch, and P. Rettig.** 1990. Chlamydial infection and adverse pregnancy outcome: interim results from a multicenter prospective study, p. 344–347. *In* W. R. Bowie, H. D. Caldwell, R. B. Jones, P.-A. Mardh, G. L. Ridgway, J. Schachter, W. E. Stamm, and M. E. Ward (ed.), *Chlamydial Infections: Proceedings of the Seventh International Symposium on Human Chlamydial Infections.* Cambridge University Press, Cambridge.
84. **Oriel, D.** 1990. Genital human papillomavirus infection, p. 433–441. *In* K. K. Holmes, P.-A. Mardh, P. F. Sparling, P. J. Wiesner, W. Cates, Jr., S. M. Lemon, and W. E. Stamm (ed.), *Sexually Transmitted Diseases,* 2nd ed. McGraw-Hill Book Co., New York.
85. **Oriel, J. D.** 1971. Natural history of genital warts. *Br. J. Vener. Dis.* **47:**1–13.

86. **Paavonen, J., L. A. Koutsky, and N. Kiviat.** 1990. Cervical neoplasia and other STD-related genital and anal neoplasias, p. 561–592. *In* K. K. Holmes, P.-A. Mardh, P. F. Sparling, P. J. Wiesner, W. Cates, Jr., S. M. Lemon, and W. E. Stamm (ed.), *Sexually Transmitted Diseases,* 2nd ed. McGraw-Hill Book Co., New York.

87. **Padian, N., L. Marquis, D. P. Francis, R. E. Anderson, G. W. Rutherford, P. M. O'Malley, and W. Winkelstein.** 1987. Male-to-female transmission of human immunodeficiency virus. *J. Am. Med. Assoc.* **258:**788–790.

88. **Perine, P. L., and A. O. Osoba.** 1990. Lymphogranuloma venereum, p. 195–204. *In* K. K. Holmes, P.-A. Mardh, P. F. Sparling, P. J. Wiesner, W. Cates, Jr., S. M. Lemon, and W. E. Stamm (ed.), *Sexually Transmitted Diseases,* 2nd ed. McGraw-Hill Book Co., New York.

89. **Plummer, F. A., J. N. Simonsen, D. W. Cameron, J. O. Ndinya-Achola, J. K. Kreiss, M. N. Gakinya, P. Waiyaki, M. Cheang, P. Piot, A. R. Ronald, and E. N. Ngugi.** 1991. Cofactors in male-female sexual transmission of human immunodeficiency virus type 1. *J. Infect. Dis.* **163:**233–239.

90. **Podgore, J. K., K. K. Holmes, and E. R. Alexander.** 1982. Asymptomatic urethral infections due to *Chlamydia trachomatis* in male U.S. military personnel. *J. Infect. Dis.* **146:**828.

91. **Quinn, T. C.** 1990. Unique aspects of human immunodeficiency virus and related viruses in developing countries, p. 355–369. *In* K. K. Holmes, P.-A. Mardh, P. F. Sparling, P. J. Wiesner, W. Cates, Jr., S. M. Lemon, and W. E. Stamm (ed.), *Sexually Transmitted Diseases,* 2nd ed. McGraw-Hill Book Co., New York.

92. **Quinn, T. C., W. E. Stamm, S. E. Goodell, E. Mkrtichian, J. Benedetti, L. Corey, M. D. Schuffler, and K. K. Holmes.** 1983. The polymicrobial origin of intestinal infections in homosexual men. *N. Engl. J. Med.* **309:**576–582.

93. **Rein, M. F., and M. Muller.** 1990. Trichomonas vaginalis and trichomoniasis, p. 481–492. *In* K. K. Holmes, P.-A. Mardh, P. F. Sparling, P. J. Wiesner, W. Cates, Jr., S. M. Lemon, and W. E. Stamm (ed.), *Sexually Transmitted Diseases,* 2nd ed. McGraw-Hill Book Co., New York.

94. **Ronald, A. R., and W. Albritton.** 1990. Chancroid and *Haemophilus ducreyi,* p. 263–271. *In* K. K. Holmes, P.-A. Mardh, P. F. Sparling, P. J. Wiesner, W. Cates, Jr., S. M. Lemon, and W. E. Stamm (ed.), *Sexually Transmitted Diseases,* 2nd ed. McGraw-Hill Book Co., New York.

95. **Rooney, J. F., J. M. Felser, J. M. Ostrove, and S. E. Straus.** 1986. Acquisition of genital herpes from an asymptomatic sexual partner. *N. Engl. J. Med.* **314:**1561–1564.

96. **Rosenberg, M. J., W. Rojanapithayakorn, P. J. Feldblum, and J. E. Higgins.** 1987. Effect of contraceptive sponge on chlamydial infection, gonorrhea, and candidiasis. A comparative clinical trial. *J. Am. Med. Assoc.* **257:**2308–2312.

97. **Schachter, J., R. L. Sweet, M. Grossman, D. Landers, M. Robbie, and E. Bishop.** 1986. Experience with the routine use of erythromycin for chlamydial infections in pregnancy. *N. Engl. J. Med.* **314:**276–279.

98. **Schmid, G. P., L. C. Matheny, A. A. Zaidi, and S. J. Kraus.** 1989. Evaluation of six media for the growth of *Trichomonas vaginalis* from vaginal secretions. *J. Clin. Microbiol.* **27:**1230–1233.

99. **Schoenbaum, E. E., M. P. Webber, S. Vermund, and H. Gayle.** 1990. HIV antibody in persons screened for syphilis: prevalence in a New York City emergency room and primary care clinics. *Sex. Transm. Dis.* **17:**190–193.

100. **Schroeter, A. L., R. H. Turner, J. B. Lucas, and W. J. Brown.** 1971. Therapy for incubating syphilis: effectiveness of gonorrhea treatment. *J. Am. Med. Assoc.* **218:**711–713.

101. **Schulz, K. F., F. K. Murphy, P. Patamasucon, and A. Z. Meheus.** 1990. Congenital syphilis, p. 821–842. *In* K. K. Holmes, P.-A. Mardh, P. F. Sparling, P. J. Wiesner, W. Cates, Jr., S. M. Lemon, and W. E. Stamm (ed.), *Sexually Transmitted Diseases,* 2nd ed. McGraw-Hill Book Co., New York.

102. **Scott, G. B., C. Hutto, R. W. Makuch, M. T. Mastrucci, T. O'Connor, C. D. Mitchell,**

E. J. Trapido, and W. P. Parks. 1989. Survival in children with perinatally acquired human immunodeficiency virus type I infection. *N. Engl. J. Med.* **321:**1791–1796.

103. **Simonsen, J. N., D. W. Cameron, M. N. Gakinya, J. O. Ndinya-Achola, L. J. D'Costa, P. Karasira, M. Cheang, A. R. Ronald, P. Piot, and F. A. Plummer.** 1988. Human immunodeficiency virus infection among men with sexually transmitted diseases. Experience from a center in Africa. *N. Engl. J. Med.* **319:**274–278.

104. **Sparling, P. F.** 1990. Natural history of syphilis, p. 213–219. *In* K. K. Holmes, P.-A. Mardh, P. F. Sparling, P. J. Wiesner, W. Cates, Jr., S. M. Lemon, and W. E. Stamm (ed.), *Sexually Transmitted Diseases,* 2nd ed. McGraw-Hill Book Co., New York.

105. **Spear, P.** 1990. Biology of the herpesviruses, p. 379–389. *In* K. K. Holmes, P.-A. Mardh, P. F. Sparling, P. J. Wiesner, W. Cates, Jr., S. M. Lemon, and W. E. Stamm (ed.), *Sexually Transmitted Diseases,* 2nd ed. McGraw-Hill Book Co., New York.

106. **Stagno, S., and R. J. Whitley.** 1990. Herpes virus infection in the neonate and children, p. 863–887. *In* K. K. Holmes, P.-A. Mardh, P. F. Sparling, P. J. Wiesner, W. Cates, Jr., S. M. Lemon, and W. E. Stamm (ed.), *Sexually Transmitted Diseases,* 2nd ed. McGraw-Hill Book Co., New York.

107. **Stamm, W. E., and B. Cole.** 1986. Asymptomatic Chlamydia trachomatis urethritis in men. *Sex. Transm. Dis.* **13:**163–165.

108. **Stamm, W. E., L. A. Koutsky, J. K. Benedetti, J. L. Jourden, R. C. Brunham, and K. K. Holmes.** 1984. Chlamydia trachomatis urethral infections in men. Prevalence, risk factors, and clinical manifestations. *Ann. Intern. Med.* **100:**47–51.

109. **Straus, S. E., H. E. Takiff, M. Seidlin, S. Bachrach, L. Lininger, J. J. DiGiovanna, K. A. Western, H. A. Smith, S. N. Lehrman, and T. Creagh-Kirk.** 1984. Suppression of frequently recurring genital herpes. A placebo-controlled double-blind trial of oral acyclovir. *N. Engl. J. Med.* **310:**1545–1550.

110. **Svenssen, L., L. Westrom, K. T. Ripa, and P.-A. Mardh.** 1980. Differences in some clinical and laboratory parameters in acute salpingitis related to culture and serologic findings. *Am. J. Obstet. Gynecol.* **138:**1017–1021.

112. **Thin, R. N.** 1990. Early syphilis in the adult, p. 221–230. *In* K. K. Holmes, P.-A. Mardh, P. F. Sparling, P. J. Wiesner, W. Cates, Jr., S. M. Lemon, and W. E. Stamm (ed.), *Sexually Transmitted Diseases,* 2nd ed. McGraw-Hill Book Co., New York.

113. **Thompson, S. E., and W. D. Hager.** 1977. Acute pelvic inflammatory disease. *Sex. Transm. Dis.* **4:**105–113.

114. **Tindall, B., D. A. Cooper, B. Donovan, and R. Penny.** 1988. Primary human immunodeficiency virus infection: clinical and serologic aspects, p. 329–341. *In* R. C. Moellering, Jr. (ed.), *Infectious Disease Clinics of North America: Medical Management of AIDS,* vol. 2. W. B. Saunders Co., Philadelphia.

115. **Volberding, P. A., S. W. Lagakos, M. A. Koch, C. Pettinelli, M. W. Myers, D. K. Booth, H. H. Balfour, R. C. Reichman, J. A. Bartlett, M. S. Hirsch, R. L. Murphy, W. D. Hardy, R. Soeiro, M. A. Fischl, J. G. Bartlett, T. C. Merigan, N. E. Hyslop, D. D. Richman, F. T. Valentine, and L. Corey.** 1990. Zidovudine in asymptomatic human immunodeficiency virus infection: a controlled trial in persons with fewer than 500 CD4-positive cells per cubic millimeter. *N. Engl. J. Med.* **322:**941–949.

116. **Walters, M. D., C. A. Eddy, R. S. Gibbs, J. Schachter, M. A. Holden, and C. J. Pauerstein.** 1988. Antibodies to Chlamydia trachomatis and risk for tubal pregnancy. *Am. J. Obstet. Gynecol.* **159:**942–946.

117. **Wasserheit, J. N., T. A. Bell, N. B. Kiviat, P. Wolner-Hanssen, V. Zabriskie, B. D. Kirby, E. C. Prince, K. K. Holmes, W. E. Stamm, and D. A. Eschenbach.** 1986. Microbial causes of proven pelvic inflammatory disease and efficacy of clindamycin and tobramycin. *Ann. Intern. Med.* **104:**187–193.

118. **Weatherly, N. F.** 1988. Medical protozoology, p. 950–969. *In* W. K. Joklik, H. P. Willett, D. B. Amos, and C. M. Wilfert (ed.), *Zinsser Microbiology,* 19th ed. Appleton & Lange, Norwalk, Conn.

119. **Weston, T. E. T., and C. S. Nicol.** 1963. Natural history of trichomonal infection in males. *Br. J. Vener. Dis.* **39:**251–257.

120. **Whitley, R. J., L. Corey, A. Arvin, F. D. Lakeman, C. V. Sumaya, P. F. Wright, L. M. Dunkle, R. W. Steele, S.-J. Soong, A. J. Nahmias, C. A. Alford, D. A. Powell, and V. San Joaquin.** 1988. Changing presentation of herpes simplex virus infection in neonates. *J. Infect. Dis.* **158:**109–116.
121. **Winkelstein, W., D. M. Lyman, N. Padian, R. Grant, M. Samuel, J. A. Wiley, R. E. Anderson, W. Lang, J. Riggs, and J. A. Levy.** 1987. Sexual practices and risk of infection by human immunodeficiency virus: the San Francisco men's health study. *J. Am. Med. Assoc.* **257:**321–325.
122. **Wolinsky, S. M., C. R. Rinaldo, S. Kwok, J. J. Sninsky, P. Gupta, D. Imagawa, H. Farzadegan, L. P. Jacobson, K. S. Grovit, M. H. Lee, J. S. Chmiel, H. Ginzburg, R. A. Kaslow, and J. P. Phair.** 1989. Human immunodeficiency virus type I (HIV-I) infection a median of 18 months before a diagnostic Western blot: evidence from a cohort of homosexual men. *Ann. Intern. Med.* **111:**961–972.
123. **Wolner-Hanssen, P., J. N. Krieger, C. E. Stevens, N. B. Kiviat, L. Koutsky, C. Critchlow, T. DeRouen, S. Hillier, and K. K. Holmes.** 1989. Clinical manifestations of vaginal trichomoniasis. *J. Am. Med. Assoc.* **261:**571–576.
124. **Wong, E. S., and W. E. Stamm.** 1983. Urethral infections in men and women. *Annu. Rev. Med.* **34:**337–358.

The Transmission Dynamics of Sexually Transmitted Diseases: the Behavioral Component

Roy M. Anderson

In recent years, a body of theory has emerged pertaining to the transmission dynamics of infectious diseases in human communities (6). It seeks to provide a framework within which biological and epidemiological information about infectious agents may be organized to codify similarities and differences among the important infections of humans and, most importantly, to identify key relationships among the variables that determine the course of infections within an individual host and the epidemiological patterns observed in communities of people.

The majority of this body of theory is concerned with the transmission dynamics of common respiratory infections such as measles and rubella or tropical parasitic infections such as malaria or the filarial and schistosome helminths. However, recently, increased attention has been devoted to sexually transmitted diseases (STDs), in part owing to their growing importance over the past 20 years in many countries and in part owing to the emergence of a new and very lethal infectious agent, the human immunodeficiency virus (HIV), which is the etiological agent of AIDS.

Before the emergence of AIDS as a disease of pandemic significance, theoretical work on the transmission of STDs centered on gonorrhea. The work of Cooke and Yorke (11) on mathematical models of the spread and persistence of gonorrhea provided the impetus for a series of reports in the late 1970s and early 1980s. The monograph by Hethcote and Yorke (14) on the dynamics and control of gonorrhea provides an excellent summary of this body of research and is exemplary for the way models are grounded on data and how the conclusions derived are aimed at public health issues in a way that emphasizes the ideas and not the mathematical details of the model framework. This body of work provided a useful starting point for the development of an understanding of the transmission of HIV via sexual contact (7, 16).

Most STDs possess characteristics that differ somewhat from those of infections such as measles or malaria, which have received the greatest attention in the literature on transmission dynamics. First, for infections such as HIV or hepatitis B, the communities or population at risk from infection tend to be some fraction of the total community (e.g., sexually active adults, intravenous drug users, homosexual or bisexual men, or newborn infants). The groups at risk and the interrelationships

---

Roy M. Anderson – Parasite Epidemiology Research Group, Imperial College, London University, London SW7 2BB, England.

between such groups require careful definition. Second, in contrast with many directly transmitted respiratory viral or bacterial infections, a doubling in host population density does not tend to double the rate at which new infections are produced by infectious persons. Third, the carrier phenomenon, in which certain individuals harbor asymptomatic infection, perhaps for long periods, is important in determining net transmission rates. This is the case for many women infected with gonorrhea and is especially important in the spread of HIV, in which infected persons may be asymptomatic but infectious to their sexual partners for many years. Fourth, many STDs induce little or no acquired immunity, such that if recovery occurs (perhaps resulting from chemotherapeutic treatment), individuals are susceptible to reinfection. In other cases, such as HIV or herpesvirus infection, the infectious agent persists within the host and is able to evade immunological attack that aims to eliminate the infection, perhaps for the entire life of the host. This seems to be the case in the majority of people infected with HIV or the genital herpesvirus. The reasons for persistence are not clearly understood, but genetic variability in the infectious agent population within the host (HIV) or the occupancy of immunologically privileged sites (herpesvirus) are important factors. Fifth, great variability in the course of infection (particularly the incubation period between first infection and the diagnosis of symptoms of disease) is typically observed in groups of infected persons. For certain infections, genetic variability in both host and infectious agent is in part responsible. Sixth, and finally, patterns of STD infections in communities are characterized by great heterogeneity in transmission rates within and between different populations. Such variability is directly related to differences in sexual behavior. This aspect of human behavior appears to be much more heterogeneous in defined populations than the behaviors that influence the transmission of many other types of infectious agents.

In this brief review of the biological and behavioral factors that determine the transmission dynamics of STDs, the focus is on identifying the major components of the transmission rate, how these components vary in human communities, and how each component influences epidemiological patterns. Simple mathematical models are employed to provide a framework for the analyses, but technical details are omitted, with the focus on what theory tells us about the interpretation of observed patterns and what needs to be measured via epidemiological study to facilitate understanding. In this latter context, special attention is given to the behavioral component of transmission.

THE BASIC REPRODUCTIVE RATE OF INFECTION

The basic reproductive rate, R_0, is an important parameter in the epidemiological study of infectious diseases. It defines the average number of secondary infections generated by one primary case in a susceptible population of defined density. This definition depends on the conceptual framework we employ to study a particular infection. For most STDs, it is sensible to divide the host population into compartments, representing susceptible persons, infected persons who are not yet infectious (latent), and infectious persons. Reproductive success or transmission is therefore defined in terms of the generation of secondary cases of infection and not in terms of the number or density of infectious agents transmitted between hosts.

The measurement of reproductive success is fraught with many problems both theoretical and practical. However, it is important to attempt to make such measurements, since the magnitude of reproductive success determines the pattern of infection within a community and the speed with which an infection spreads when introduced into a naive population. The theoretical problems surrounding the definition of R_0 center on the manner in which we define a particular population and the linkages that population has with other groups at risk of infection. To start, we consider a single risk group population of sexually active adults who mix homogeneously (choose sexual partners at random). In these circumstances, R_0 is defined as the product of the average probability that the infection is transmitted per sexual partner contact per unit of time, β, times the average duration of infectiousness of an infected person, D, times the average number of sexual partners per unit of time, c:

$$R_0 = \beta D c \tag{1}$$

For an epidemic to occur, clearly $R_0 > 1$. The measurement of each of the three components that determine the magnitude of R_0 is fraught with difficulties, particularly in relation to what is exactly meant by the term average. Epidemiological data suggest that each component is highly variable between individuals and over time. It is therefore necessary to take into account the underlying distributional properties of each parameter (β, D, and c) if R_0 is to be defined more precisely. Each is considered in turn.

The Transmission Coefficient, β

In equation 1 above, the transmission coefficient is defined per partner contact per unit of time. However, within sexual partnerships or relationships, the number of sex acts per unit of time that enable transmission to occur will vary widely between different individuals. It is straightforward to reformulate the transmission coefficient in terms of the number of sex acts. One assumption is that there is, on average, some constant transmission probability, δ, per sexual act of a defined type and that these probabilities compound independently and randomly. The overall probability for an infected individual to infect a sexual partner then increases with the number of acts, and this Poisson process gives, on average, a transmission probability per partnership per unit of time, β, of approximately $1 - \exp(-\delta n)$ after an average of n contacts in that unit of time. However, this elaboration still omits much behavioral detail. For example, we ideally need to take account of variability in n within the population, variation in the value of δ according to the type of sexual act (i.e., penile-vaginal contact, oral-penile contact, anal sex, etc.), and the distributional properties of, and correlation between, different types of sexual behavior. There is no great difficulty in formulating models with such complexities, but the major need at present is for quantitative data upon which to base the description of the transmission coefficient. In addition, the limited data that are available at present for infections such as HIV fail to show a clear relationship between the number of sex acts per unit of time within a sexual relationship between infected and susceptible partners and the likelihood of transmission (8).

The Infectious Period, *D*

The infectiousness of an infected person is also subject to great variation, with respect to both duration and intensity. For HIV, for example, current evidence suggests that over the long incubation period of HIV infection (an average of around 8 to 10 years in adults), there are two major peaks of infectiousness, one soon after infection and the second as patients develop symptoms of disease (AIDS-related complex or AIDS). If we divide the duration of infectiousness, D, into three phases to denote a first phase of high infectiousness (of duration t_1 with transmission coefficient β_1), a second, longer phase of low infectiousness (of duration t_2 with coefficient β_2), and a third phase of high infectiousness (of duration t_3 with coefficient β_3), then the basic reproductive rate, R_0, becomes

$$R_0 = cD(\beta_1 t_1 + \beta_2 t_2 + \beta_3 t_3) \quad (2)$$

where $D = t_1 + t_2 + t_3$, and β_1 and $\beta_3 > \beta_2$. With regard to the dynamics of transmission, interestingly, the magnitudes of β_1 and t_1 determine the initial rate at which the epidemic increases, while the overall magnitude of R_0 determines the total size of the epidemic (1, 17). Added complexity is introduced if we take into account the facts that the incubation period varies widely between individuals and that the magnitudes of the durations of each infectious phase (the t_is) also vary. If we assume that individuals move from one to the next phase of infectiousness at constant rates, then the overall infectious period distribution is approximately gamma in form (15). Observed distributions of the incubation period (approximately equivalent to the infectious period) of HIV infection are best described by the Weibull distribution, but as yet we have only observed some fraction of the total incubation period distribution (roughly 10 years of observations on the longest running cohort of infected persons for whom points of infection are known). The interpretation of current and future information on the incubation period will be made complicated by the use of the drug zidovudine (AZT), which is thought to slow the rate at which symptoms of disease develop. As for the transmission coefficient, the factor that hinders better description of the infectious period as a component of the basic reproductive rate is the availability of quantitative information.

The Mean Rate of Sexual Partner Change, *c*

If the transmission coefficient is defined as the probability of transmission per partner per unit of time, then the most important measure of sexual behavior is the rate of sexual partner change within the population. Note, however, that other

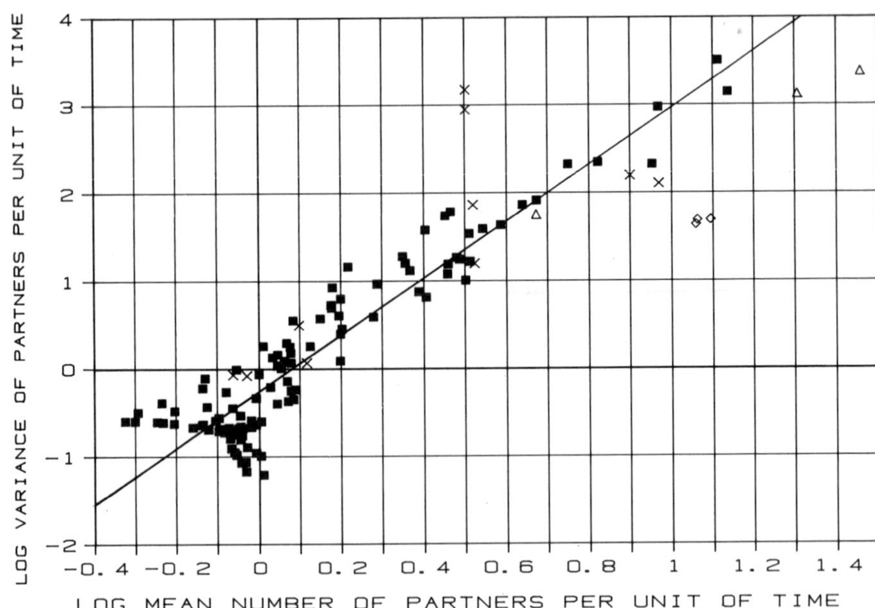

Figure 1. Log-log plot of the variances (σ^2) and means (m) of the distribution of the number of different sexual partners over past time intervals as recorded in a wide variety of published and unpublished surveys of sexual behavior in heterosexual and homosexual communities in developed and developing countries (5). ■, data for heterosexual men and women sampled in population surveys; ×, data for heterosexuals attending STD clinics; △, data for heterosexual men in a sub-Saharan African country; ◇, data for homosexual men. The straight line is the best-fit linear regression.

measures can be incorporated into the transmission coefficient, as described above, such as the mean number of sex acts of a defined type per unit of time. However, in the absence of good data, the rate of partner change is considered in order to illustrate how heterogeneity in sexual behavior within the population influences the measurement and interpretation of R_0.

Rates of sexual partner change depend on many demographic (e.g., age and sex) and social factors. In addition, their magnitudes are likely to be correlated with other behavioral variables such as number of sex acts per unit of time (positively or negatively correlated?) and type of sexual contact (e.g., frequency of anal or oral sex, etc). The large-scale surveys of sexual behavior that are currently under way or nearing completion in a number of countries will help to define the relationships of this variable with other demographic and behavioral factors. An important factor, however, is the high degree of variability in this quantity observed in surveys of sexual behavior. An illustration of this point is presented in Fig. 1, in which means (m) and variances (σ^2) of sex partners per unit of time are plotted on a log-log scale. The data were collated from a wide variety of surveys of particular risk groups including homosexual men and heterosexuals of various ages in developed and developing countries, and various methods of census and survey were employed (5). The graph illustrates three important points. First, the variance in activity (σ^2) is typically greater than the mean rate (m). Second, variability is related to average behavior, and third, this relationship is approximately linear in form on a log-log scale and of power form on untransformed axes. More precisely, the relationship is of the form

$$\sigma^2 = am^b \tag{3}$$

where a and b are constants (estimated by linear regression on a log-log scale). Interestingly, the value of b is approximately 3. Why such a tight relationship holds, despite the variability between the study populations and methods of survey, is unclear at present. However, it is probable that the relationship highlights some as yet unidentified feature of sexual behavior that is common to all societies or communities. Empirically, it simply states that average behavior sets the extremes of behavior, with such extremes being positively related to the average. It would be interesting to examine this relationship for other variables, such as the number of sex acts of a defined type per unit of time, as behavioral data from surveys accumulate.

Clues to what factors underpin the observed association between the mean and the variance can be derived from simple models of sexual behavior, pair formation and dissolution, and mixing between groups with different rates of sexual partner change (1, 10). However, as yet little research has been undertaken to investigate which behavioral rules generate patterns similar to those observed.

With respect to the derivation of R_0, heterogeneity in rates of sexual partner change alters the definition of what is exactly meant by the average rate of sexual partner change. Simple models based on the notion of proportionate mixing (partner choice is random but the net rate of partner change of an individual is weighted by his or her mean rate of partner change per unit of time) suggest that the effective average rate of partner change, c, should be defined as the mean rate, m, plus the variance-to-mean ratio, σ^2/m. Thus, R_0 becomes (7)

$$R_0 = \beta(m + \sigma^2/m)D \tag{4}$$

This interesting result demonstrates that the magnitude of the variability (σ^2) has a significant influence on the magnitude of reproductive success. High variability (with other parameters constant) increases transmission success, since those with high rates of sexual partner change are both more likely to acquire and more likely to transmit the infection. In addition, the highly sexually active core of the population has a major impact on the initial rate at which an epidemic grows and the long-term persistence of the infection within a community. Control measures targeted at the individuals in the right-hand tail of the distribution of sexual partner change rates (see Fig. 2) have a much greater impact on the size of an epidemic than similar measures targeted at the less sexually active groups. The validity of this argument does not simply depend on mathematical analysis but is intuitively obvious from an inspection of observed distributions of rates of sexual partner

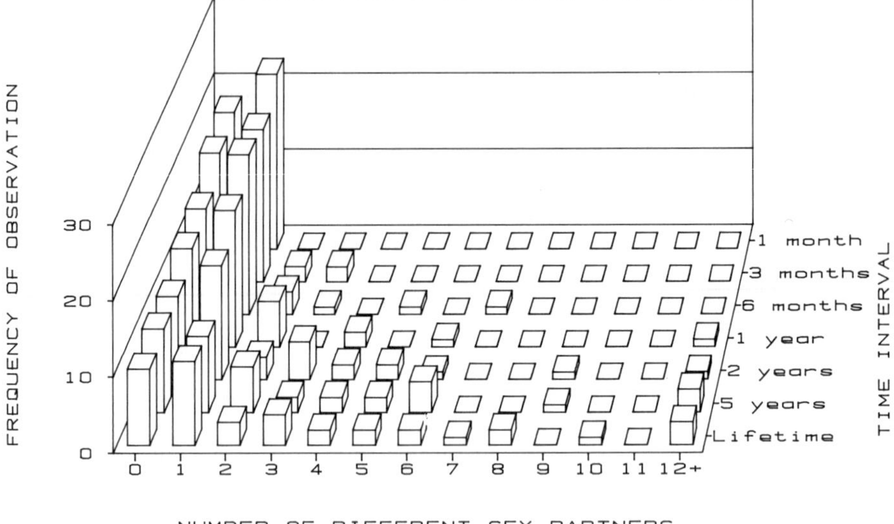

Figure 2. Frequency distributions of claimed number of different sexual partners over various time periods (1 month to lifetime) recorded in a survey of male and female students in 1987 in England (1).

change (Fig. 2). It is usually the case that irrespective of the community surveyed, more than 70% of the total number of sexual partnerships formed in an interval of time are associated with less than 30% of the total population. In the context of the basic reproductive rate, a simple numerical example serves to illustrate the importance of the highly sexually active core of the population and the significance of variability in behavior when compared with average behavior. With respect to HIV transmission, suppose that the probability of transmission per partnership per year is 0.05, that the average duration of infectiousness is 5 years, and that the mean rate of partner change is 1 per year. If the distribution of rates of partner change is random (nonheterogeneous), the variance σ^2 is equal to the mean and the magnitude of R_0 (from, e.g., equation 4) is 0.25. In this case, $R_0 < 1$ and the infection will not persist and no epidemic will occur. Alternatively, if sexual behavior is highly heterogeneous, such that the variance is four times greater than the mean ($\sigma^2 = 4$), the value of R_0 is 1.25 and hence an epidemic will occur.

Aside from determining whether or not an epidemic will occur (or whether the infection will persist in the population), the degree of heterogeneity in behavior will also determine the prevalence of infection within a community. A simple way to illustrate this point is to consider a closed epidemic in a population of fixed size not subject to births, deaths, immigration, or emigration. In such circumstances, it is possible to estimate the fraction infected over the entire epidemic after the introduction of the infection as a function of the magnitude of R_0 and the mean and the variance of the rate of sexual partner change. For the purpose of illustration, we

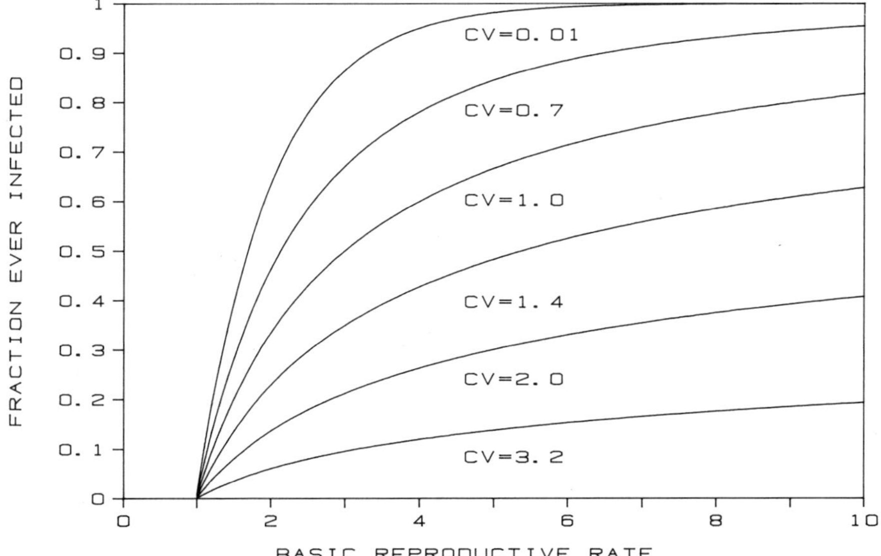

Figure 3. Relationships between the fraction ever infected with HIV in an epidemic in a closed population and the coefficient of variation (cv) of the rate of acquisition of new sexual partners predicted by a simple model of the transmission dynamics of the virus (17).

employ the coefficient of variation, cv, which is defined as the standard deviation, σ, divided by the mean, m (cv $= \sigma/m$). As illustrated in Fig. 3, the magnitude of cv (other parameters being constant, except for the magnitude of R_0) has a major influence on the fraction infected. If variability in sexual activity is high, the fraction infected is low and vice versa. Thus, paradoxically, high variability enhances the likelihood of an epidemic occurring but results in a smaller fraction infected than a comparable situation with low variability in sexual activity.

The preceding discussion has skipped over much detail, particularly that concerned with the pattern of mixing between sexual activity classes (stratified on the basis of the rate of sexual partner change). However, before turning to this issue, it is important to note that precise quantitative information on rates of sexual partner change and their distribution within a population greatly facilitates the interpretation and analysis of the epidemiology of sexually transmitted infections. There are, of course, many problems surrounding the collection of such data and in ascertaining the veracity of responses recorded in any survey. However, before leaving the topic of rates of sexual partner change, note that this measure of sexual behavior is only one component of a much more complicated picture in which frequency and type of activity within a partnership and partnership duration all have a significant influence on the transmission success of an infection. Much more work is required in this area, both in the terms of the definition of R_0 and in the acquisition of representative data.

Mixing Patterns between Risk Groups

So far, I have ignored the complexities arising from the patterns of mixing between different strata of the population. In consideration of this problem much depends on the criteria employed to stratify the population. These criteria could be spatial location, broadly defined risk groups (such as homosexual men, intravenous drug users, heterosexuals, etc.), age, ethnicity, or sexual activity. For the purposes of illustration, we choose sexual activity and the variable, rate of sexual partner change per unit of time. The central question of importance in determining transmission success concerns the frequency with which an individual in a specific group forms a sexual partnership with individuals in his or her own group and other groups. In other words, we ideally need to know who mixes with whom. To proceed with the problem, we need to define a mixing matrix whose elements, p_{ij}, define the probability that a person in group i forms a sexual relationship with someone in group j. By group, we refer to a class of people with a defined rate of sexual partner change (or a defined range of rates). If we divide the frequency distribution of sexual partner change rates (or a defined range of rates) (Fig. 2) into n groups (with constant or variable intervals on the horizontal axis), then the mixing matrix contains n^2 elements. In other words, with respect to data, we require a lot of information to be able to insert numerical values for each element of the matrix. Before proceeding to give an example of such a matrix, it is necessary to distinguish between a *mixing* matrix and a *contact* matrix. The former defines the proportion of the partnerships formed by individuals in a particular group with those in the same and other groups, while the contact matrix defines the number of partnerships formed by individuals in their own and other groups. There are clearly a set of constants for the elements of the mixing matrix and, concomitantly, for the elements of the contact matrix. Formally, for the mixing matrix, these are as follows:

$$\Sigma p_{ij} = 1 \tag{5}$$

$$1 > p_{ij} > 0 \tag{6}$$

$$p_{ij} P_i c_i = p_{ji} P_j c_j \tag{7}$$

where c_i is the mean rate of second partner change in group i and P_i is the proportion of the population in group i (Fig. 2). In verbal terms, equation 5 states that the sum of the proportion of partnerships formed in each group must equal unity, equation 6 states that the proportion must be between 0 and 1, and equation 7 states that the total number of partnerships formed by people in group i with people in group j must equal the total number of partnerships formed by people in group j with people in group i. This latter constant is of obvious importance, since it defines the need to match demand with supply.

In reality, the demand and supply problem is a very dynamic one since the number of individuals (or proportions) in each group may change through time, particularly for a lethal disease such as AIDS in which mortality will be greatest in those groups with the highest rates of sexual partner change (owing to their increased likelihood of acquiring infection early in the course of the epidemic compared with individuals in lower-activity groups). In these circumstances, the mixing matrix defines the ideal choice of partner, while the contact matrix defines what actually occurs once demand is matched with supply. It will often be the case that demand exceeds supply, and in these circumstances, it is necessary to define (in theoretical work) or measure (in behavioral study) what actually takes place to balance the equation. For example, if demand for sexual partners exceeds supply (say because of high mortality in the highly active groups), does the demand remain unsatisfied or does activity rise to meet the demand? More subtly, we ideally need to know precisely how each individual activity class changes its contacts with regard to alterations in the elements of the mixing (i.e., ideal preference) matrix, changes in mean rates of sexual partner formation within a class, and the concomitant changes in the distribution of the population between classes. These are complex issues, and behavioral scientists and epidemiologists have not begun to address how to measure and define the behavioral rules that operate in given societies in response to awareness of infection and, in particular, to a lethal infection such as AIDS. In the context of behavioral changes, perhaps induced by factors such as age or education about disease, very little is understood at present concerning who precisely changes behavior. For example, with respect to rates of sexual partner change, is a decline in the overall mean for the population associated with a decline in the variance in activity or are changes more likely to occur among individuals with low, as opposed to high, rates of partner change? In other words, to fully understand the likely impact of a change in average sexual behavior on disease transmission, it is necessary to understand precisely who changes behavior and how the elements of the mixing matrix alter in response to a decline in average activity.

As in many areas of scientific study, theory has outstripped data availability, and hence our understanding of the significance of the mixing matrix to the dynamics of STD transmission tends to rely on assumptions that are free from the constraints of empirical observation. However, this observation does not detract from the significance of these assumptions, and by way of an illustration, I will comment briefly on how their structure affects transmission success.

As soon as we define a mixing matrix and stratify the population according to the variable that delineates the elements of the matrix (i.e., rate of sexual partner change), it is necessary to alter our definition of the basic reproductive rate to take into account transmission success within and between groups.

Stratification of the population by risk group (i.e., according to the rate of sexual partner change) results in a change in the definition of the basic reproductive rate, R_0. For a heterogeneous population made up of n subgroups, a natural extension is to define a basic reproductive rate matrix with the element $R(0)_{ij}$ representing the number of secondary cases of infection generated in group i by one case in group j. Given our earlier definition of the basic reproductive rate, it is also necessary to specify that all members of group i are susceptible to infection. In these circumstances, $R(0)_{ij}$ is defined as

$$R(0)_{ij} = c_j p_{ij} \beta D \tag{8}$$

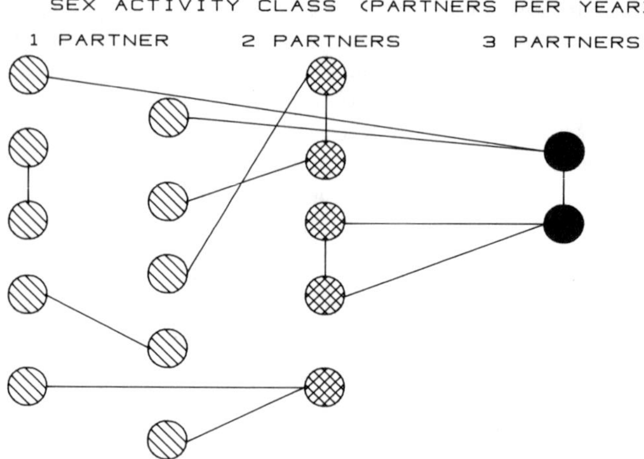

Figure 4. Simple schematic illustration of a sexual partner choice network in which 17 individuals are distributed into three sexual activity classes (partners per year) (2).

It is assumed that the duration of infectiousness, D, and the transmission coefficient, β, are the same for all groups. The term p_{ij} denotes the elements of the mixing matrix. If only a fraction of group i are susceptible, S_i, then the effective reproductive rate, R_{ij}, is given by

$$R_{ij} = c_j p_{ji} \beta D S_i \tag{9}$$

If the infection attains an endemic equilibrium state, then $R_{ij} = 1$.

Equation 8 makes clear the possibility that the disease could persist in the total population if only certain of the values of $R(0)_{ij}$ exceed unity in value. In other words, a few groups could maintain the infection in the total population, whereas in their absence the infection would die out. This idea is analogous to the notion of a core group of highly sexually active individuals maintaining infection within a community.

Equation 8 also makes clear that to decipher the relative contribution of the different sexual activity groups within the population to the net transmission success of the infection, it is necessary to define the elements of the mixing matrix. Very little behavioral research has been directed toward the question of who mixes with whom. To define a mixing network, it is necessary to ask questions not only about numbers of different sexual partners over a defined period but also about who those partners were in order to ascertain their rates of sexual partner change by additional interviews. Such follow-up studies are difficult to do in practice owing to the understandable reluctance of participants in behavioral surveys to identify their sexual partners. In the absence of good data, we can construct a hypothetical network of sexual partnerships and illustrate how the elements of the mixing matrix are calculated. The network is presented in Fig. 4, and the corresponding

Table 1. Mixing matrix, p_{ij}, derived from the sexual partner network presented in Fig. 4[a]

j	No. of different partners per year (c_i) where i is:		
	1	2	3
p_{ij}			
1	0.4	0.4	0.2
2	0.4	0.4	0.2
3	0.33	0.33	0.33
$R(0)_{ij}$			
1	0.64	0.64	0.32
2	1.28	1.28	0.64
3	1.58	1.58	1.58

[a] With an average duration of infectiousness, D, of 8 years and a transmission coefficient, β, of 0.2 per partner per year, this basic reproductive rate matrix, $R(0)_{ij}$, is derived from equation 9 in the main text.

mixing matrix and values c_i and $R(0)_{ij}$ are recorded in Table 1. Note that only certain elements of the $R(0)_{ij}$ matrix exceed unity in value, and hence the infection is maintained within the total community by the more sexually active individuals in this hypothetical example.

A further aspect of importance with respect to mixing matrices or the structure of sexual partner networks concerns the assessment of the degree of within- and between-group mixing. In the limit where individuals only choose sexual partners within their own activity class, the mixing matrix reduces to a simple structure with the values of unity down the diagonal of the matrix. This is the extreme of assortative mixing (i.e., like with like). At the other limit, of disassortative mixing (like with unlike), an individual only chooses partners from groups other than his or her own, and the matrix has zero values down the diagonal. A special case is that of random mixing (usually referred to as proportionate mixing), in which partners are chosen in proportion to the total number of partnerships available in each group (including their own) without a preference for a particular group. As yet, we have little information on where sexual partner networks within human communities fall on the spectrum of assortativeness. However, as indicated in a later section, the precise location has a very significant impact on the rate and degree of spread of a sexually transmitted infection. Despite the obvious difficulties in data collection, this area should be a priority in behavioral research concerned with disease transmission.

TRANSMISSION DYNAMICS

In this section, the importance of various behavioral factors to the dynamics of STD transmission is outlined. By way of an example, the epidemiology of HIV infection and the disease AIDS is considered, but the principles illustrated are relevant to most other sexually transmitted infections.

The Simple Epidemic

Following the introduction of an infection into a susceptible population (subject to constant rates of recruitment and loss from the sexually active adults), provided the basic reproductive rate, R_0, exceeds unity in value, an epidemic will occur as illustrated in Fig. 5A. This figure records the spread of HIV in a homogeneously mixing sexually active homosexual male population of 1,000 at time $t = 0$ (the infectious period, D, was set at 8 years, and the transmission coefficient, β, was set at 0.1 per partner per year). The period from introduction of the infection ($t = 0$) to the peak of the epidemic is set by the magnitude of R_0 (see equation 1). The lag between the rise in cases of infection and cases of AIDS is determined by the average incubation period of the disease (in this example, the incubation period was assumed to be equal to the infectious period, D). If the effective mean rate of sexual partner change, c, is halved in value, as portrayed in Fig. 5B, the epidemic moves on a much slower time scale and peaks at around years 40 to 50 ($R_0 = 3.12$) instead of years 15 to 20, as seen in Fig. 5A ($R_0 = 6.25$). The major points to note in both panels are the long-drawn-out time scale of the epidemic, the attainment of a stable endemic state (Fig. 5A) following the initial epidemic, and the decline in the incidences of infection and disease as the epidemic moves from its peak to the endemic state. This decline occurs irrespective of any changes in sexual behavior resulting from education or other public health measures. Seroprevalence (the proportion infected with HIV) saturates at the peak of the epidemic, at some level less than unity (not all individuals acquire infection even in a homogeneously mixing population), the precise value being positively correlated with the magnitude of R_0 (Fig. 3). In infections such as gonorrhea, with much shorter infectious and incubation periods than HIV, the time scale of the epidemic would be much more rapid than those recorded in Fig. 5.

Heterogeneity in Sexual Activity

Once heterogeneity in sexual activity (i.e., the rate of sexual partner change) is taken into account, the spread of infection can be monitored in different activity classes. An illustration of this is recorded in Fig. 6, where model simulations record the spread of HIV in a community of homosexual men via reference to HIV seroprevalence in the total population (Fig. 6A) and in six different sexual activity classes (Fig. 6B). Classes 6 to 1 represent individuals with mean rates of partner change per annum of 0 to 2, 2 to 5, 5 to 10, 10 to 20, 20 to 50, and 50-plus, respectively. Note that once the infection attains an endemic equilibrium (around year 40), the overall seroprevalence is between 25 and 30%. However, within the different activity classes, it ranges from close to 100% (in class 1) to less than 5% (in class 6). Since the distribution of sexual activity was assumed to be highly

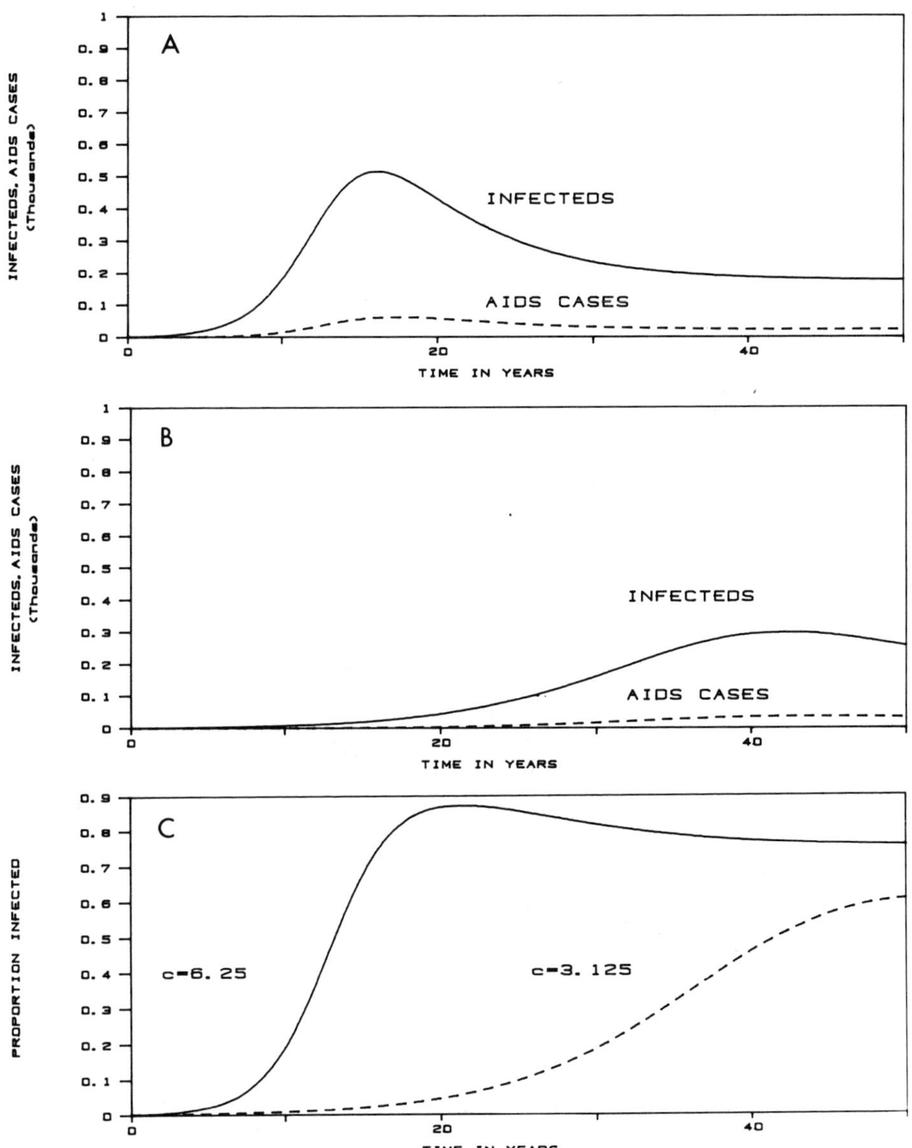

Figure 5. Predictions of a simple, homogeneous mixing model of an AIDS epidemic in a population of 1,000 homosexual men subject to constant rates of immigration and loss from the sexually active age classes (parameter values: $\beta = 0.1$; $D = 8$ years; $c = 6.25$ year^{-1} in panel A [$R_0 = 5.0$]; $c = 3.125$ year^{-1} in panel B [$R_0 = 2.5$]). Panels A and B record changes through time, after the introduction of HIV at time $t = 0$, of the number of persons infected with HIV and the number with AIDS at time t. Panel C records changes in the proportion infected with HIV for two values of the effective mean rate of sexual partner change ($c = 6.25$ year^{-1}, $c = 3.125$ year^{-1}).

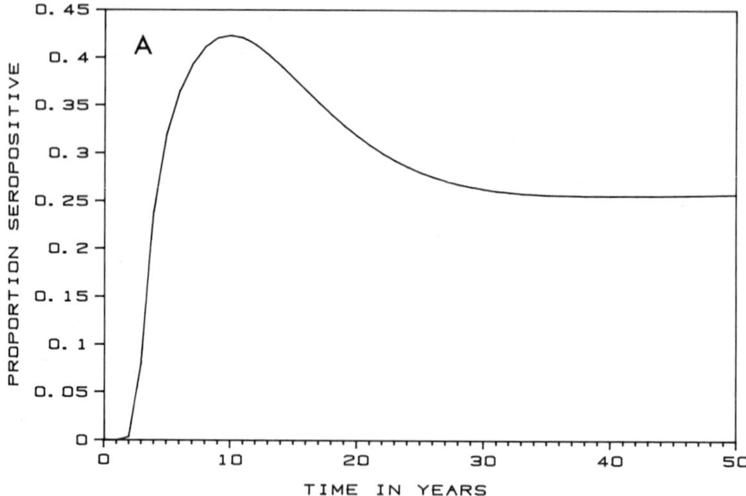

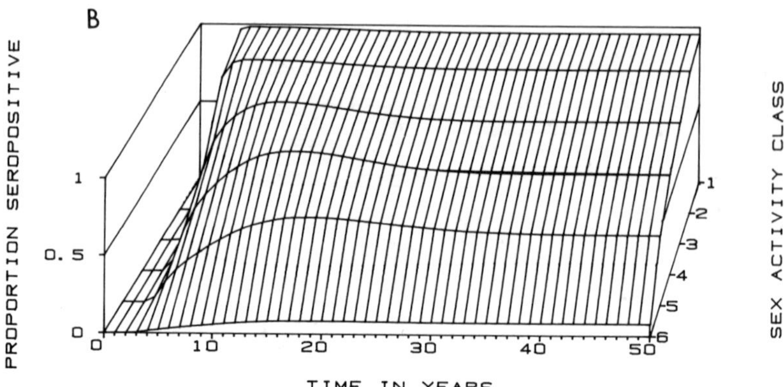

Figure 6. Heterogeneity in sexual activity. Predicted changes in HIV seropositivity (proportion infected) through time in a population divided into six sexual activity classes (see text for details), with class 1 representing high activity and class 6 representing low activity. Panel A records changes in the proportion infected in the total sexually active population, and panel B records changes in each of the activity classes (see references 3 and 13 for details). The calculations were based on the assumption of proportionate mixing.

heterogeneous (as observed, see Fig. 2), in that the majority have few partners and a few have many, the majority of the population are uninfected while most of the highly sexually active individuals acquire infection and the subsequent disease. Furthermore, the infection spreads very rapidly in the high-activity classes and more slowly in the low-activity classes. The precise differences in the time to peak

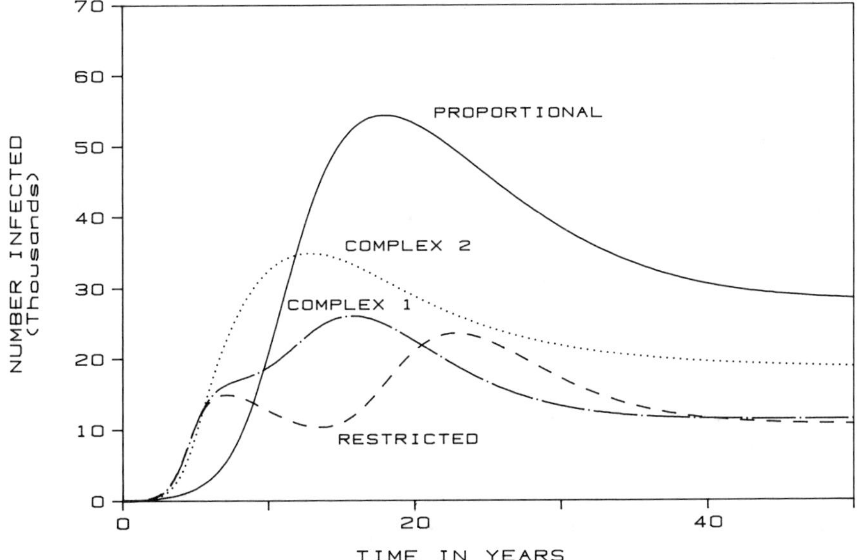

Figure 7. Influence of the structure of the mixing matrix on the predicted temporal changes in the number of HIV-infected individuals at time *t* in a population of homosexual men. The different trajectories denote different mixing assumptions (see text for details; see also references 4 and 13).

infection between the classes depend, to a significant extent, on the nature of the sexual contact network (i.e., whether it is assortative or disassortative).

Who Mixes with Whom

The structure of the mixing matrix (which captures the details of the partner network) has a major influence on the shape of the epidemic. This point is illustrated in Fig. 7, which records simulations of an HIV epidemic in a male homosexual community under various assumptions concerning the structure of the mixing matrix (all other parameters were held constant in the four simulations) (13, 15). The mixing patterns represented in the four simulations were as follows. Proportional mixing denotes choice of partners in proportion to their representation in the population by sexual activity class, weighted by their activity level. Restricted mixing represents no contact between classes, with groups 1 and 2 seeded with the infection. Complex 1 represents very high within-group contact and very low between-group contact. In complex 2, there is high within-group mixing in the highest-activity class and low within-group mixing in the lower-activity class. Both the examples labeled complex are intermediary between the extremes of proportional and restricted mixing. Note that highly assortative mixing can induce multiple peaks in the epidemic as the infection slowly moves (owing to

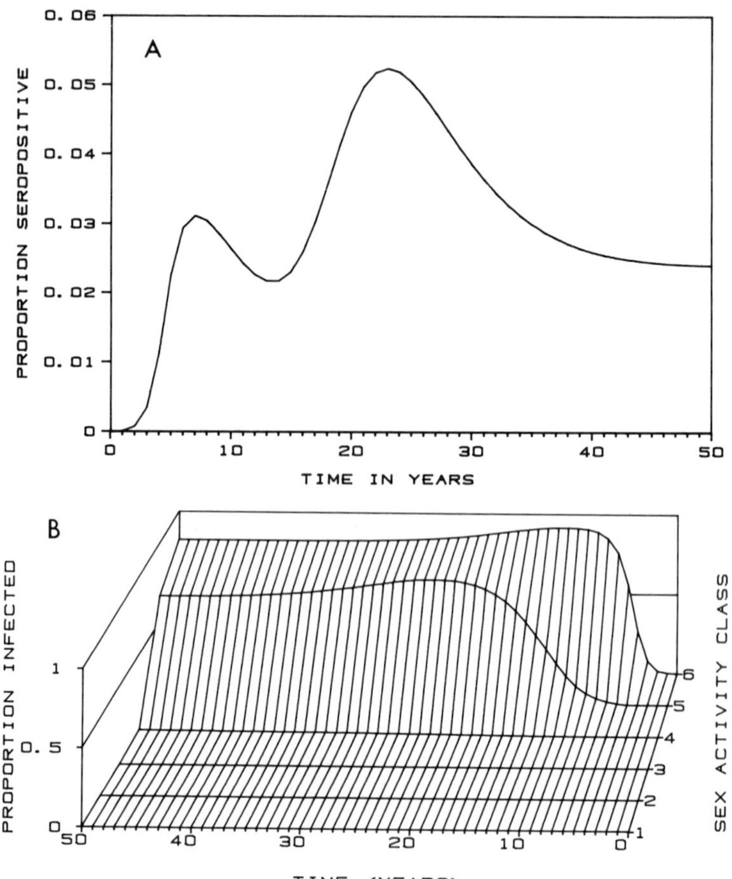

Figure 8. Similar to Fig. 6, but the calculations are based on the assumption of restricted mixing with only the two highest-activity classes (1 and 2) seeded with infection. Panel A records temporal changes in seroprevalence in the total population, and panel B records changes in sexual activity classes (13).

limited between-class contact) from the high- to the lower-activity classes. Similar principles apply to transmission within and between major at-risk groupings such as homosexual men, intravenous drug users, and heterosexuals. The point to note in this context is that an observed decline in the incidence of infection or disease may not necessarily indicate that the worst of the epidemic is over if mixing between classes is highly assortative.

A further point of interest relating to mixing matrices concerns the spread of infection within activity classes. In proportional mixing, the pattern of movement through the six sexual activity classes (defined in the preceding section) is as portrayed in Fig. 6. If mixing is highly assortative (= restricted), a rather different

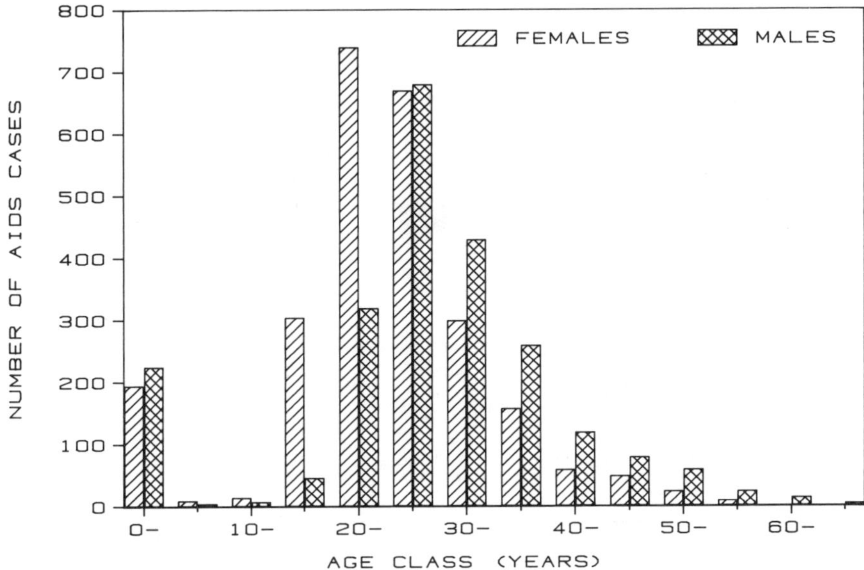

Figure 9. Age and sex distribution of AIDS cases reported in Uganda by the end of July 1988 (9).

pattern emerges, as illustrated in Fig. 8. Note that the initial rise in the prevalence of infection is largely determined by the high rate of within-class mixing in the highest-activity classes.

Age-Dependent Sexual Activity

In the preceding section, our mixing matrix was designed to mirror contact between different sexual activity classes. Similar principles apply if we stratify the population by age and sex to take into account different rates of sexual contact between and within age classes. A good example of the influence of who mixes with whom by age is provided by recent work on the potential demographic impact of AIDS in heterosexual populations in developing countries (8). In many societies in Africa, for example, men tend on average to form sexual partnerships with women of a younger age than themselves. This has a major impact on the distribution of infection and disease within a population and a major demographic impact on the population (Fig. 9). In this example, the age distribution of reported cases of AIDS in Uganda is recorded for men and women. Note that the distribution is skewed to the younger age classes of sexually active women by comparison with that in men. This pattern of infection, presumably related to patterns of age-dependent sexual activity, has a significant impact on the spread and demographic impact of infection, as illustrated in Fig. 10. In this graph, two

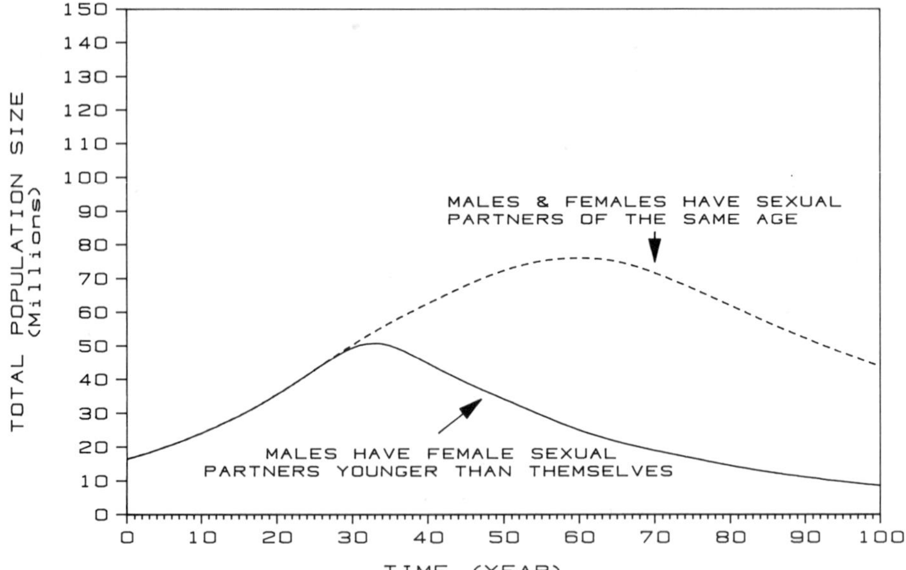

Figure 10. Influence of sexual partner choice by age group on the predicted course of an HIV epidemic in a heterosexual population in a developing country (8). The two trajectories record changes in population size from the point of introduction of HIV at time $t = 0$, in a population of 16 million at the point of introduction of the virus, with a 3.5% annual population growth rate in the absence of infection. In the top trajectory, men and women only choose partners in their own age class, while in the bottom trajectory, men form sexual partnerships with women younger than themselves (all other parameters are the same in the two simulations). ——, complex age choice; – – – –, restricted age choice.

simulations are recorded of the spread of AIDS in a hypothetical heterosexual population (of 16 million at time $t = 0$, when HIV is introduced). In one example, men and women are assumed to only form sexual partnerships with individuals in their own age class; in the other, men form partnerships with women in younger age classes than their own. Note that the latter case results in a greater demographic impact as measured by changes in total population size.

Age-related changes in sexual activity can also have a major impact on the pattern of an epidemic. This point is illustrated in Fig. 11 by reference to simulations of the spread of HIV in a heterosexual population in a developing country. Three simulations are recorded of changes through time in HIV seroprevalence following the introduction of infection. Case 1 represents the assumption that individuals only choose sexual partners in their own age class, with the mean rate of partner change fixed at 3.4 year^{-1} for all age classes. Case 2 represents male preference for women of a younger age than themselves, with a fixed mean of 3.4 year^{-1} for all age classes. Case 3 represents restricted mixing within age classes but

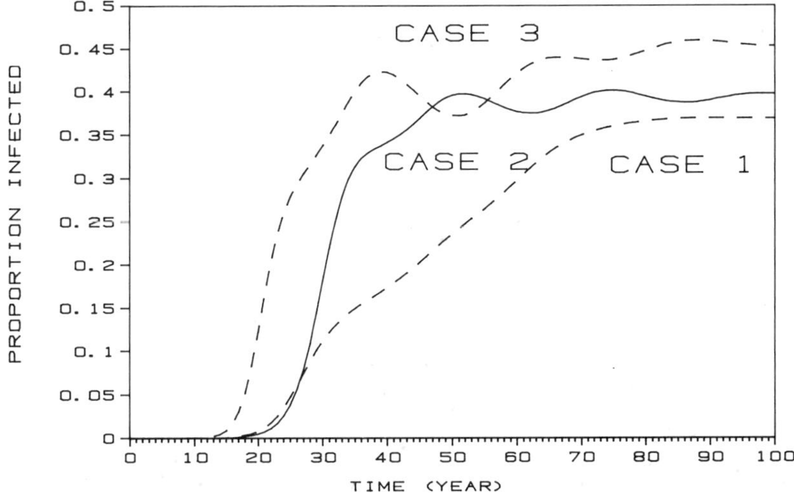

Figure 11. Predicted changes in the proportion of a heterosexual population infected with HIV in a developing country after the introduction of infection at time $t = 0$. The three simulations record changes under different assumptions concerning mixing by age group and the age-dependent rate of sexual partner change (see text for details; see reference 4).

with the mean rate of partner change set at a higher level in younger men and women by comparison with older individuals. In the latter case, the mean across all age classes was again set at 3.4 year^{-1}. Note how the trajectory arising from the assumptions of case 3 differs from that of case 1. This is entirely due to age dependency in the rate of sexual partner change, since all other parameters in the model remained the same in each simulation (4).

Changes in Behavior

Public health measures, and particularly education about safer sex practices, can have a significant influence on the spread of an STD. The recent reduction in the incidence of HIV infection in male homosexual and bisexual populations in the United States and Western Europe has been attributed to such changes. These include reductions in rates of partner change, reductions in the frequency of high-risk sexual activities between partners (e.g., anal sex), and increased use of condoms. As noted in an earlier section, reductions in incidence are to be expected in the absence of such changes, as the infection spreads through the different sexual activity classes and saturation occurs. However, behavioral studies do suggest that significant changes in behavior have occurred within certain communities in recent years (12).

Temporal changes in sexual activity have a significant effect on the shape of an epidemic curve, but their precise influence depends not simply on the average

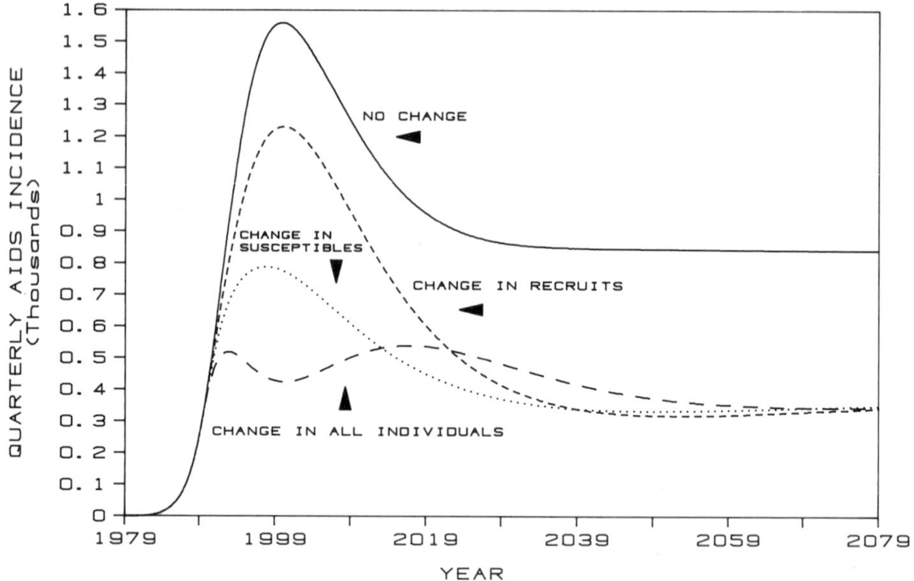

Figure 12. Influence of changes in sexual behavior (rates of sexual partner change) on the predicted time course of the AIDS epidemic in male homosexuals in England and Wales (3). The four simulations show the predicted impact of no change from a mean rate of partner change of 8.7 year^{-1} and of a change from 8.7 year^{-1} to 5.0 year^{-1}, in 1989 and thereafter, in which change is assumed to affect (i) recruits to the sexually active population only, (ii) susceptible individuals only, and (iii) all individuals in the population.

reduction in activity (say, the mean rate of partner change) but also on who changes behavior. It matters whether the reduction in the mean results from changes among highly active individuals, new recruits to the sexually active population, infected persons, or susceptible persons. An illustration of this point is presented in Fig. 12, which records simulations of an HIV epidemic in a male homosexual population initiated in 1979. Four trajectories are recorded. In the first, labeled no change, the mean rate of partner change remains unaltered at 8.7 year^{-1} over the entire period of the simulation. The remaining simulations record temporal changes in AIDS incidence when behavior alters from a mean rate of partner change of 8.7 year^{-1} in 1979 to one of 5.0 year^{-1} in 1989 onward, in recruits to the sexually active population, in susceptible persons and in all recruits, and in all susceptible persons and infected individuals. The change was distributed in proportion to the activity of a given class prior to the alteration in the mean rate of partner change in 1989. Note that the pattern of the epidemic is very dependent on who changes behavior. These types of mathematical epidemiological studies help to identify the most important groups to which education should be targeted. They also suggest that behavioral studies of changes in sexual activity should not focus simply on average values but should try and identify which groups are responding to education and which are not.

DISCUSSION

In the preceding sections of this chapter, simple and complex mathematical models of STD transmission have been employed to identify the relative influences of different behavioral components on the rate at which individuals acquire infection. The approach has been similar to that employed by experimental scientists, in which one factor is varied while others are held constant. The aim has been to make clear the contribution of each factor, without getting too confused by the all-too-apparent complexity of human sexual behavior.

These studies highlight the importance of acquiring detailed quantitative information on a variety of behaviors, including rates of sexual partner change (stratified by age, sex, ethnicity, etc.), networks of sexual contact, and the details of who changes behavior in response to public health measures. The practical problems that surround the acquisition of such information and the methodological issues that must be fully researched before too much reliance is placed on numerical scores obtained via interviews or questionnaire completion are fully appreciated. However, these problems are more a reflection of the need for more research than arguments to deflect researchers from addressing the quantification of behavior relevant to disease transmission. If unambiguous interpretation of an epidemiological pattern is required, then there is no shortcut to the acquisition of precise data on sexual behavior. A good illustration of this point is provided by Fig. 7, in which the influence of sexual partner contact networks on the incidence of HIV infection is recorded. In the restricted mixing example, the decline in infection after the first peak could be interpreted at the time of observation as an encouraging sign of the abatement of the epidemic. However, this interpretation is false, since a larger peak occurs in the future as a consequence of the movement of infection from a small high-risk group to a much larger lower-risk group. Many other examples could be presented in which the quantitative details of behavior significantly influence how we interpret different patterns of infection and disease.

Aside from the issue of quantification, a further factor that often concerns behavioral researchers is the great heterogeneity in sexual activity recorded in defined communities. Variability is not a hindrance to interpretation or the design of policy. Its pattern is often predictable, as illustrated in Fig. 1, in which a linear relationship is recorded (on a log-log scale) between the mean and the variance of the rate of sexual partner acquisition. Furthermore, the description of the variability can help to target public health measures and education at the groups in which it will have the greatest impact on the overall pattern of infection and disease. There is much scope for future research in this area.

In conclusion, I hope that this brief review will help to clarify the reason why epidemiologists are interested in the quantitative detail of human sexual behavior. In the furtherance of such research, the pressing need at present is for greater collaboration between behavioral scientists and epidemiologists in which both attempt to understand the aims, methodologies, strengths, and weaknesses of each other's discipline.

Acknowledgments. I thank the Medical Research Council and the Overseas Development Agency for research grant support.

LITERATURE CITED

1. **Anderson, R. M.** 1988. The epidemiology of HIV infection: variable incubation plus infectious periods and heterogeneity in sexual activity. *J. R. Statist. Soc. A* **151:**66–93.
2. **Anderson, R. M.** 1989. Mathematical and statistical studies of the epidemiology of HIV. *AIDS* **3:**333–346.
3. **Anderson, R. M., S. P. Blythe, S. Gupta, and E. Konings.** 1989. The transmission dynamics of the human immunodeficiency virus type 1 in the male homosexual community in the United Kingdom: the influences of changes in sexual behaviour. *Philos. Trans. R. Soc. Lond. B* **325:**45–98.
4. **Anderson, R. M., S. Gupta, and W. Ng.** 1990. The significance of sexual partner contact networks for the transmission dynamics of HIV. *J. Acquired Immune Defic. Syndr.* **3:**417–429.
5. **Anderson, R. M., and R. M. May.** 1988. Epidemiological parameters of HIV transmission. *Nature* (London) **333:**514–519.
6. **Anderson, R. M., and R. M. May.** 1991. *Infectious Diseases of Humans: Dynamics and Control.* Oxford University Press, Oxford.
7. **Anderson, R. M., G. F. Medley, R. M. May, and A. M. Johnson.** 1986. A preliminary study of the transmission dynamics of the human immunodeficiency virus (HIV), the causative agent of AIDS. *IMA J. Math. Appl. Med. Biol.* **3:**229–263.
8. **Anderson, R. M., T. W. Ng, M. C. Boily, and R. M. May.** 1990. The influence of different sexual contact patterns between age classes on the predicted demographic impact of AIDS in developing countries. *N.Y. Acad. Med. Sci.* **569:**240–274.
9. **Berkley, S., S. Okware, and W. Naamora.** 1989. Surveillance for AIDS in Uganda. *AIDS* **3:**79–85.
10. **Blythe, S. P., and C. Castillo-Chavez.** 1990. Scaling of sexual activity. *Nature* (London) **344:**202.
11. **Cooke, K. L., and J. A. Yorke.** 1973. Some equations modeling growth processes and gonorrhea epidemics. *Math. Biosci.* **16:**75–101.
12. **Ekstrand, M. L., and T. J. Coates.** 1990. Maintenance of safer sexual behaviors and predictors of risky sex: the San Francisco men's health study. *Am. J. Public Health* **80:**973–977.
13. **Gupta, S., R. M. Anderson, and R. M. May.** 1988. Epidemiological parameters of HIV transmission. *AIDS* **3:**514–519.
14. **Hethcote, H. W., and J. A. Yorke.** 1984. Gonorrhea transmission dynamics and control. *Lecture Notes in Biomathematics,* no. 56. Springer-Verlag, Berlin.
15. **Jacquez, J. A., C. P. Simon, J. Koopman, L. Sattenspiel, and T. Perry.** 1988. Modelling and analysing HIV transmission: the effect of contact patterns. *Math. Biosci.* **92:**119–199.
16. **May, R. M., and R. M. Anderson.** 1987. Transmission dynamics and HIV infection. *Nature* (London) **326:**137–142.
17. **May, R. M., and R. M. Anderson.** 1988. The transmission dynamics of the human immunodeficiency virus (HIV). *Philos. Trans. R. Soc. Lond. B* **321:**565–607.

Epidemiology of Sexually Transmitted Diseases in Developing Countries

Robert C. Brunham and Allan R. Ronald

Our knowledge of the epidemiology of sexually transmitted diseases (STDs) in developing societies is sparse. Most hypotheses depend on very few observations from small samples in geographically disparate regions. Extrapolation from this knowledge base to the entire developing world is foolhardy, and even general principles must be stated with reservations. Nonetheless, general principles appear to be emerging. These principles will be highlighted in this chapter. Part of the reason for the paucity of knowledge in this area is the fact that sexually transmitted infections have not been assigned sufficient priority in most developing countries to reflect their role as a major cause of acute and chronic ill health or economic cost secondary to years of productive life lost. In fact, STDs are ranked among the top five illness categories in patients seeking health services in some African countries (31). More regional information on the prevalence and incidence of individual STDs is urgently required to permit national health priorities to be established and resources to be allocated appropriately. Human and financial resources must be deployed strategically to plan, implement, and evaluate STD control programs.

The transmission dynamics and reservoir characteristics of STDs are sufficiently similar to benefit from a common conceptual approach. Understanding the forces that sustain STD transmission allows the rational design of cost-effective control programs. This chapter describes a general model of STD epidemiology. The model partially explains the higher impact that STDs have on health and productivity in developing countries compared with industrialized countries. At our present level of understanding, there is no convincing evidence that the virulence or infectivity of common STD pathogens geographically varies to any significant extent or that differences in these parameters account for any observed global epidemiological differences. Also, no studies support the hypothesis that host differences resulting from genetics or other inborn factors are responsible for any major differences in STD epidemiology. Most observations support the hypothesis that the epidemiology of STDs is similar in all societies, with differences in prevalence and incidence primarily resulting from known determinants of STD epidemiology, including the existence and effectiveness of STD control programs, the availability of diagnosis and treatment services, the demography of the population, sexual behavior, sexual mixing, and the size of the high-frequency

---

Robert C. Brunham – Department of Medical Microbiology, University of Manitoba, Winnipeg, Manitoba, Canada R3E 0W3. ***Allan R. Ronald*** – Section of Infectious Diseases, St. Boniface General Hospital, Winnipeg, Manitoba, Canada R2H 2A6.

Table 1. Major STD microbial agents and their impact

STD	Acute disease	Pregnancy-associated disease	Chronic disease
Bacterial			
Neisseria gonorrhoeae	Urethritis Cervicitis Salpingitis	Prematurity Septic abortion Ophthalmia Postpartum endometritis	Infertility Ectopic pregnancy
Chlamydia trachomatis	Urethritis Cervicitis Salpingitis	Ophthalmia Pneumonia Postpartum endometritis Prematurity (?)	Infertility Ectopic pregnancy
Treponema pallidum	Primary and secondary syphilis	Spontaneous abortion Stillbirth Congenital syphilis	Neurosyphilis Cardiovascular syphilis Gumma
Haemophilus ducreyi	Genital ulcer	None known	None known
Viral			
HIV	Mononucleosis syndrome	Prematurity Stillbirth Perinatal HIV	AIDS
HPV	Genital warts	Laryngeal papillomatosis	Genital cancer
HSV-2	Genital ulcer	Congenital and neonatal HSV Prematurity	Recurrent genital herpes
HBV	Acute hepatitis	Perinatal HBV	Chronic hepatitis Cirrhosis Hepatoma Vasculitis

transmitter core groups. Much of this chapter focuses on discussing reservoir and transmission characteristics.

MAJOR STD PATHOGENS AND THE DISEASES THEY CAUSE

Many microbial agents can be transmitted sexually; however, a smaller subset of agents are of greater importance because of higher prevalence and more frequent rates of complications and sequelae. The STDs that are of greatest public health significance are described in Table 1. These pathogens share the following common characteristics. They infect only humans, and no reservoir of infection external to human populations exists. STD microorganisms are able to survive outside the human host for only short periods (minutes to hours) and require direct contact between persons for efficient transmission. They infect the reproductive tract as their primary site, and thus, transmission occurs principally during sexual intercourse or during birth. As a consequence, STDs are restricted in human populations to sexually active individuals or to infants born to infected mothers. Although STDs are well known to produce acute disease such as genital ulceration or discharge, less clearly understood are their contributions to adverse pregnancy outcomes, poor neonatal health, and chronic diseases such as infertility and genital cancers. AIDS, caused by human immunodeficiency virus (HIV), highlights the role that an STD can play in producing chronic disease. The reproductive and chronic disease sequelae are the most costly and socially damaging effect of STDs.

STD EPIDEMIOLOGY AND RISK FACTORS

STDs share characteristics that cause their epidemiology to be unique compared with that of other infectious diseases. For instance, many STD infections are subclinical, and asymptomatic spreaders are important in transmission. STD infection tends to persist for relatively long periods in an infected host. Reinfection of some hosts frequently occurs. A subset of individuals play a disproportionate role in the transmission of STDs and in maintaining endemicity in a population. STD microorganisms have elaborate pathogenic mechanisms that permit persistence or reinfection in the face of an immune response.

The epidemiology of STDs reflects patterns of sexual behavior and networks of sexual mixing. A large number of individual and societal risk factors have been identified for STDs. STD rates are generally found to be higher in men, in urban residents, in nonmarried persons, and in young adults, and these are also the groups in which sex partner change rates are presumed to be the highest. Clearly, the number of different sexual partners is the major determinant of STD rates. Sexual behavior across societies is extraordinarily heterogeneous. Unfortunately, from the perspective of behavioral intervention, little is known regarding sexual behavior, and this is especially true in developing countries.

Young age is a particularly important variable in STD epidemiology in developing countries because sexual partner change rates are age dependent. The absolute and relative proportions of the population between the ages of 15 and 30 years are greater in developing than in industrialized countries (Fig. 1). This large segment of the population contributes greatly to the increased incidence of sexually transmitted infections seen in developing countries. Closely associated with the young mean age of populations in developing countries are higher birth rates. This is especially true in sub-Saharan Africa, where birth rates have remained unchanged (48 births per 1,000 population per year) since 1950, in striking difference to the remainder of the world, where birth rates have declined (5). Whether pregnancy can facilitate STD transmission, perhaps by representing a state of hypersusceptibility to infection, is unknown, although STDs seem to be the greatest problem in regions where birth rates are highest. Of greater certainty, pregnancy augments the impact of STDs through adverse reproductive outcomes

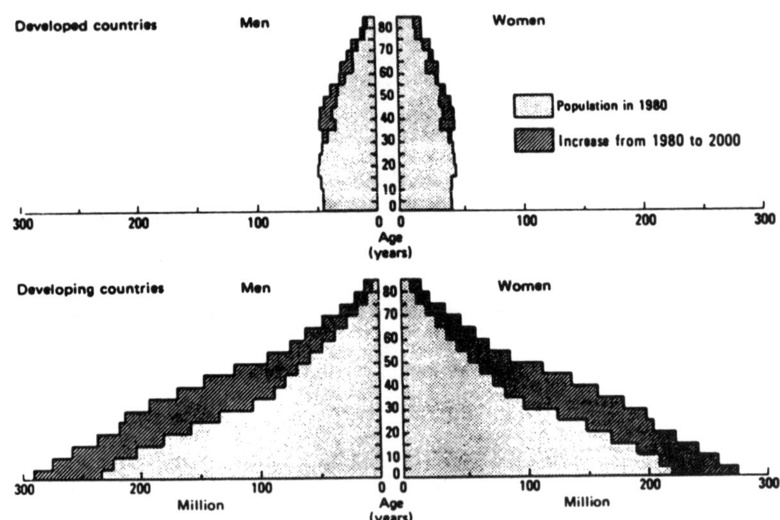

Figure 1. Population pyramid for developed and developing countries according to age and sex for 1980 and projected to the year 2000 (from reference 58). Total population in developed countries in 1980 was 1.1 billion and is expected to reach 1.3 billion in 2000; total population in developing countries was 3.3 billion in 1980 and is expected to reach 4.8 billion by 2000.

and poor infant health. We have reported the considerable impact that STDs have on stillbirth, prematurity, puerperal pelvic infection, and ophthalmia neonatorum rates in one hospital in Nairobi, Kenya (Table 2) (13, 25, 45, 56). Additionally, tubal infertility as a proportion of total infertility is highest in Africa (Fig. 2) (7). This may represent the sequela of tubal infection with *Chlamydia trachomatis*, *Neisseria gonorrhoeae*, or both.

Urbanization is a major social trend in developing countries. Although STDs

Table 2. Effect of STDs on reproduction (Nairobi, Kenya)[a]

Effect	Incidence (%)	*N. gonorrhoeae* (6%)	*C. trachomatis* (7–21%)	*T. pallidum* (3%)	HIV (3%)
Stillbirth	2	—[b]	—	5.3	2.7
Prematurity	5	2.9	—	—	2.1
Postpartum PID	20	4.4	1.7	—	—
Ophthalmia neonatorum	23	42	31	—	—

[a] Associations are expressed as odds ratios except for ophthalmia neonatorum rates, which are expressed as etiological percentages. Incidence refers to the occurrence of pregnancy and puerperal morbidity in cohorts of women studied at Pumwani Maternity Hospital in Nairobi, Kenya. The percentages in parentheses under specific pathogens refer to the observed prevalence rates of infection in the above group of women. Results are abstracted from references 13, 25, 45, and 56.

[b] —, no positive association observed.

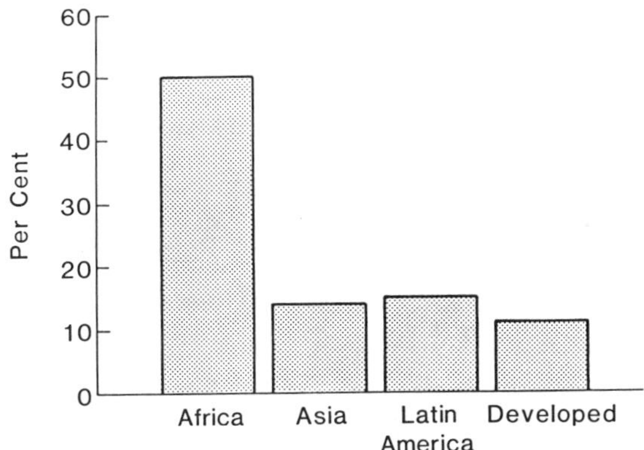

Figure 2. Proportion of infertility attributable to post-PID residua (bilateral tubal occlusion or pelvic adhesions) from a standardized study of over 5,800 couples from four different geographical areas of the world (data from reference 7).

are classically thought of as density-independent infectious diseases, it is apparent that STD incidence and prevalence rates are higher in urban than in rural areas. For instance, the Rwandan HIV Seroprevalence Study Group reported a 13.7-fold-higher seropositivity rate among urban dwellers (17.8%) than among rural residents (1.3%) (49). STDs often maintain stable low endemicity in rural settings (49) but exhibit rapid changes in the urban environment (35, 42). The urban environment exerts a profound destabilizing influence on STD transmission rates, resulting in higher infection rates, perhaps by fostering casual sexual relationships through long working hours, relative isolation from the family, and geographical and social mobility. More attention needs to be paid to the effects that urban development programs have on creating conditions suitable for STD (and other infectious disease) transmission in the developing world.

THE RESERVOIR CONCEPT AND DYNAMICS: STD TRANSMISSION

Because STDs only infect humans, human populations are the reservoir. To be sustained in the population, an STD must infect a host who on average transmits infection to at least one susceptible person. The reproductive rate, R_0, is defined by this number and obviously must be greater than 1 for the infection to persist in the population. R_0 is determined by three interacting variables: β, a measure of infectivity; c, a measure of sexual mixing between susceptible persons and transmitters; and D, a measure of the duration of infectivity (4).

$$R_0 = \beta c D$$

Approximate measures of β and D, together with an estimate of the rate of sex partner change necessary to sustain STD endemicity ($c = 1/\beta D$), are illustrated in Table 3. Each STD seems to require a different and critical threshold of sex partner change rate to persist in the population. The true reservoir of an STD is that subset

Table 3. Estimates of key epidemiological parameters necessary to sustain transmission of five different STDs ($c = 1/\beta D$)[a]

Agent	Duration of infectiousness (D) (yr)	Transmission efficiency (β)	Sex partner change rate/yr (c)
Neisseria gonorrhoeae			
No control	0.5	0.5	4
Control	0.15	0.5	13
Chlamydia trachomatis	1.25	0.2	4
Treponema pallidum			
No control	0.5	0.3	7
Control	0.25	0.3	13
HIV			
African parameters	2	0.1	5
American parameters	8	0.01	13
Haemophilus ducreyi	0.08	0.8	15

[a] Sources for some of these data are found in references 59 (*N. gonorrhoeae*), 27 (*C. trachomatis*), 52 (*T. pallidum*), 1 and 6 (HIV), and 43 (*H. ducreyi*).

of the population in which the infection is present and that sustains sex partner change rates greater than the critical threshold.

A cardinal distinction between STD epidemics and other infectious disease epidemics is the importance of heterogeneity in the ecology of STD infection. To understand the epidemiology of most other infectious diseases, we assume that a population mixes in a homogeneous pattern and that the net transmission rate is directly proportional to the number of susceptible persons and the number of infective persons. However, with STDs we know that sexual mixing is heterogeneous and that only sexually active persons can be STD transmitters. Maternal-fetal or neonatal transmission, while resulting in significant disease, contributes little to the population survival of STD pathogens. The probability distribution of sexual partner change rates is highly skewed, and it seems very likely that the highly sexually active individuals in the tail of the distribution are responsible for maintaining transmission within the community as a whole. Table 3 shows the relatively high annualized rates of sex partner change that are necessary to sustain STD transmission. These high rates are found only in small segments of the sexually active proportion of the population, and these segments form core groups for STD transmission (59). Core groups are characterized by high prevalence and incidence of STDs; they are the reservoir for infection and are the source of infection to others inside and outside the core group. STD transmission outside the core group is, by definition, not sustainable because sexual partner change rates are not high enough.

The structure of core groups seems much different in developing countries than in industrialized countries. In North America, core group members are often distinguished by young age, inner city residence, low socioeconomic status, poor access to medical care, illicit drug use, and nonwhite ethnicity (17). In many developing countries, prostitutes and their male clients are the core groups. Prostitutes are named as source contacts by up to 80% of men with urethritis in some parts of the Third World compared with less than 20% in Europe and North America (31). Prostitutes are even more frequently named as source contacts of men with chancroid. Prostitutes and their clients are probably the important reservoir of STDs in the developing world. This is illustrated by the findings in one well-studied group of prostitutes in the Nairobi Pumwani district in Nairobi, Kenya. These women in a lower social stratum have an extraordinarily high prevalence of gonococcal infection and other STDs (10). Point prevalence surveys show that 65% are infected with *N. gonorrhoeae,* with a mean time to reinfection of 21 days. Other STDs, including those caused by HIV, *C. trachomatis,* and *Haemophilus ducreyi,* also have high prevalence rates (54). Because these women have three to five sexual partners per day, they expose up to 1,000 clients per year. Obviously, the impact that these individuals can have on community persistence of STDs is substantial.

These women also have a high prevalence of concurrent STDs, with 36% having two or more STDs (10). Concurrent STDs are important confounders of STD epidemiology. For several STDs, transmission is amplified in the presence of a second STD. This is best illustrated by the amplifying influence of genital ulcer disease on HIV transmission (6). Spread of antimicrobial resistance among STD pathogens may also be promoted by concurrent infection. The *tetM* resistance gene may have spread through STD microorganisms such as genital mycoplasmas and *N. gonorrhoeae* because of this occurrence (32). The β-lactamase plasmids of *N. gonorrhoeae* and *H. ducreyi* also appear to have been spread across bacterial species by concurrent infection (28, 29).

EPIDEMIOLOGY OF INDIVIDUAL STDS

Neisseria gonorrhoeae

N. gonorrhoeae remains a major health problem in many areas of the developing world. Control strategies that are clearly effective in industrialized countries are impractical for most areas of the developing world and hence are virtually absent. Consequently, *N. gonorrhoeae* prevalence rates are often an order of magnitude greater in developing countries. Best estimates of the population prevalence of *N. gonorrhoeae* infection are obtained from point prevalence surveys of nonsymptomatic women attending antenatal clinics. Results of 19 studies collected from three areas of the developing world are shown in Fig. 3 (57). Rates are highest in Africa (mean, ~10%), intermediate in Latin American countries (mean, ~5%), and lowest in Asian countries (mean, ~3%). These prevalence rates are 3- to 10-fold higher than those observed in comparable populations in industrialized countries.

The spectrum of gonococcal disease is similar in developing countries as

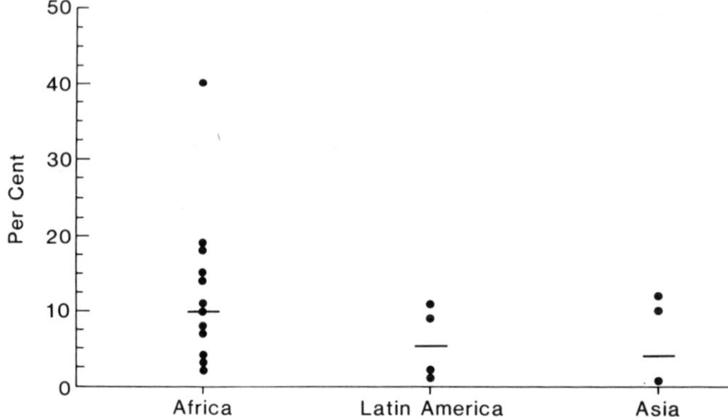

Figure 3. Results of 19 studies from three geographical areas of the world reporting point prevalence estimates of cervical *N. gonorrhoeae* infection among asymptomatic pregnant women attending antenatal clinics (data from reference 57).

elsewhere, although disseminated gonococcal infection may occur less frequently. Acute salpingitis is the most common severe complication of gonococcal infection and is a leading cause of admission to gynecologic wards in many areas of Africa. Etiological studies of pelvic inflammatory disease (PID) in three African studies showed that isolation rates of *N. gonorrhoeae* varied between 23 and 50% (24, 38, 48). The major impact of gonococcal salpingitis is permanent tubal damage resulting in ectopic pregnancy or tubal infertility. A recent seroepidemiological study from Zimbabwe concluded that both *N. gonorrhoeae* and *C. trachomatis* were important causes of post-PID tubal occlusion in this African country (11). In a prospective treatment trial of acute PID in an STD clinic in Nairobi, Kenya, we found that 5 (33%) of 15 women with gonococcal PID had bilateral tubal obstruction at follow-up despite antimicrobial treatment (24). Clearly, gonococcal infection continues to produce profound reproductive disability for women in developing countries.

Although gonococcal prevalence rates are high among pregnant women in many areas of the developing world, infection is seldom detected unless complications arise. Paradoxically, the most common complications that occur during pregnancy are seldom attributed to gonococcal infection. For instance, infected pregnant women have a threefold excess of premature birth and more than a fourfold excess of postpartum PID, but these are not commonly recognized as due to *N. gonorrhoeae* (or other STDs) (13, 45). Infected pregnant women commonly transmit *N. gonorrhoeae* to their newborns during birth. Over 40% of exposed newborns acquire gonococcal ophthalmia neonatorum in the absence of Credé's prophylaxis (25). Credé's prophylaxis reduces transmission rates by about 95% (26). Tragically, it is all too common to see that in those areas with the highest prevalence of maternal gonorrhea, Credé's prophylaxis is not used.

The reservoir for gonococcal infection has not been accurately ascertained.

Urban prostitutes are a readily identifiable and frequently named source of infection for up to 80% of men with urethritis in Nairobi, Kenya (10). This may be typical for many developing countries. As described previously, these women can have an extraordinary prevalence and incidence of gonococcal infection. Presumably, the control of gonococcal infection in these women would substantially reduce the community-wide burden of gonococcal disease.

N. gonorrhoeae strains from many areas of the developing world are more frequently resistant to antimicrobial agents than are strains from industrialized countries. It also appears likely that global dissemination of antibiotic-resistant strains of *N. gonorrhoeae* also commonly arises in developing countries, as was seen with β-lactamase plasmid-containing strains of gonococci (40). Antimicrobial resistance makes the treatment of gonococcal infection even more difficult and expensive, often putting it out of the reach of developing countries' health care budgets. Intervention targeted to high-frequency transmitters of *N. gonorrhoeae* and chemoprophylaxis of neonates may be the best first steps for developing countries to take in the control of *N. gonorrhoeae*.

Chlamydia trachomatis

In industrialized countries, *C. trachomatis* infections often outnumber *N. gonorrhoeae* infections. This is attributed to the effectiveness of gonococcal control programs and the absence of chlamydial control programs. In developing countries, the prevalence and incidence of *C. trachomatis* are unknown. Trachoma caused by ocular chlamydial infection is common in many areas of the developing world but is epidemiologically and microbiologically distinct from sexually transmitted chlamydial infection, which is the subject of this review (3). Limited data suggest that *C. trachomatis* infections are at least as common as gonococcal infections. Studies in pregnant women show that 2 to 23% of women are culture positive (57). Rates are higher in areas where gonococcal infection rates are higher. *C. trachomatis* is associated with a similar spectrum of disease in developing and industrialized countries. Infection in pregnant women is associated with postpartum endometritis and with neonatal conjunctivitis and pneumonia (9, 25, 26, 45). Credé's prophylaxis at birth is not as effective in preventing infant infection, in distinction to its effect on gonococcal infection (26).

C. trachomatis causes 12 to 21% of the cases of acute PID in developing countries (57). This estimate likely underrepresents its true contribution to salpingitis because many (perhaps most) cases are subclinical or present atypically. In fact, seroepidemiological studies suggest that *C. trachomatis* is as important a cause of tubal infertility and ectopic pregnancy in developing countries as it is in industrialized countries (11). In this regard, it is important to note that tubal infertility is most common in areas of the developing world where *C. trachomatis* and other STDs are known to be common (30). *C. trachomatis* is an important cause of postpartum PID, and since most cases of tubal infertility in Africa are cases of secondary infertility (7), puerperal ascension of chlamydial infection may be the major pathophysiologic pathway leading to tubal infection and tubal obstruction.

Control of chlamydial infection will be difficult because of the dominant role of subclinical infection in transmission and disease rates. Nonetheless, *C. trachomatis* infections are reliably treated with inexpensive, easily available drugs (tetracycline, erythromycin, and sulfonamides). Clinicians need to recognize the clinical manifestations of chlamydial infection and use these drugs more appropriately. Laboratory resources for diagnosis of chlamydial infection will likely remain beyond the reach of most developing countries. The role of a prostitute reservoir in sustaining *C. trachomatis* transmission is unknown and requires study.

Treponema pallidum

Syphilis is emerging in many developing countries as an important public health problem. The control of the endemic treponematoses during the 1950s may have reduced cross-reactive protective immunity to *Treponema pallidum* and facilitated its current rapid spread. Serological tests are difficult to interpret in some countries because of previous serological experience with endemic treponematoses. However, until recently, syphilis has been the classic example of an STD that can readily be controlled with public health initiatives. Its resurgence among some heterosexual urban populations in the United States is particularly discouraging.

The seroprevalence of syphilis as determined by the treponemal hemagglutination test or the reagin tests (VDRL or rapid plasma reagin) in prenatal patients is available from a number of developing countries and varies up to 30% (18). A seroincidence study of syphilis in Swaziland gave an estimate of 1.4% per annum (16).

Syphilis accounts for a small amount of the total genital ulcer disease in most developing countries and is usually less common than chancroid. In case series, the contribution of *T. pallidum* to the etiology of ulcers is 5 to 10% (14, 44). Fewer patients with genital ulcers resulting from syphilis are treated with effective regimens in developing countries, and as a result, secondary syphilis seems to be more common, although no good data are available. Presumably, many patients, particularly women, infected with *T. pallidum* progress to latent syphilis with risk of infection to the newborn during subsequent pregnancies.

Tertiary syphilis does not appear to be a major public health problem despite the rising incidence of infectious syphilis. This may be due to the widespread use of antimicrobial agents for a variety of illnesses in developing countries. It also may be too early in the current epidemic of syphilis to assume that a rapidly increasing incidence of tertiary disease will not occur. The effects on reproduction are already evident, with about 20 to 30% of pregnancies in mothers with untreated syphilis resulting in a stillborn, 10 to 20% of live-born babies dying in the neonatal period, and 20 to 30% of those who live surviving with active congenital syphilis (47).

Congenital syphilis is now a major pediatric disease burden in many countries. During the past 10 years, the mortality rate for fetal and infant deaths resulting from syphilis was as high as 30 to 60 per 1,000 pregnancies (18). Almost an equivalent number of infants are born live with congenital syphilis and carry serious stigmata because of intrauterine infection. In Swaziland, 13% of 283 deliveries had serological evidence of active syphilis, and the perinatal infant mortality was 22% (16). Maternal programs for screening and treating syphilis and neonatal programs for early recognition and treatment are essential. Despite public health policies in many countries that identify prenatal screening as an important priority, logistical difficulties resulting from lack of supervised prenatal care, reinfections during pregnancy, inadequacies of laboratory screening and reporting, and lack of long-acting penicillins often thwart these programs. An early pregnancy screening program failed to reduce congenital syphilis very significantly in Swaziland, and additional measures were required, including routine prophylactic penicillin at delivery (16). A recognition of the ongoing increase in congenital syphilis and the need to integrate effective diagnosis and treatment activities into maternal and child programs is increasingly evident.

Studies in industrialized countries suggest that positive serology for syphilis is an independent risk factor for HIV seropositivity. Also, *T. pallidum* infection may have altered clinical features and a greater tendency to recur in HIV-immunosuppressed individuals. No studies have as yet been reported from developing countries on the interaction between HIV and *T. pallidum*.

Haemophilis ducreyi

Chancroid (genital ulcer disease) was considered a nasty, painful, inconsequential STD until it was identified as a significant risk factor for the transmission of HIV. The only known clinical manifestations are genital ulcers and inguinal lymphadenitis. After decades of little research interest, *H. ducreyi*, the etiological agent of chancroid, is now being investigated in at least a dozen laboratories.

Since World War II, chancroid has largely become a disease of tropical regions. Disease introduction and outbreaks in industrialized countries have been readily controlled in most instances through widespread treatment of prostitutes, contact tracing, and the effective early treatment of ulcerating lesions. Ongoing epidemics in industrialized countries, such as the one currently ongoing in New York City, appear to require a focus of infection among high-frequency transmitters who are, for the most part, inaccessible to control initiatives (51).

The epidemiology of chancroid has not been well studied in developing countries. Difficulties with diagnosis because of the requirement of sophisticated techniques for culture and the nonspecificity of clinical findings have made it impossible to do satisfactory field studies without laboratory support. *H. ducreyi* cultures are available in a very few areas.

Genital ulcer disease is common throughout the tropics, but it appears to be much less frequent in societies in which male circumcision is widely practiced (43). In many urban cities in eastern and southern Africa, genital ulcers account for between 10 and 30% of illness in men attending STD clinics. On pelvic examination, between 5 and 40% of prostitutes have genital ulcers (10, 44, 54). Most of these are due to *H. ducreyi*. These women usually continue to sell sex and do not seek care for their ulcers. The major reservoir for *H. ducreyi* is assumed to be women with ulcers. The only study in developing countries that has investigated *H. ducreyi* epidemiology found that all source contacts of men with chancroid had ulcers (43). This suggests that asymptomatic carriage of *H. ducreyi* in the absence of ulcers is not a major source of new infections. Also, most secondary contacts were infected and most had genital ulcers. Further studies are needed to delineate the infectious pool and determine its control.

H. ducreyi readily acquires stable plasmid-mediated antimicrobial resistance to numerous agents including the penicillins, tetracycline, trimethoprim, sulfamethoxazole, kanamycin, chloramphenicol, and streptomycin (29). Multiple resistance is very prevalent in most developing countries, and as a result, the options for effective treatment are few. This increases the difficulty of achieving control through early diagnosis with inexpensive regimens. Only erythromycin and perhaps the new fluoroquinolones are currently proved to be effective oral treatment, with cure rates of 95% or more (50). Ceftriaxone and perhaps spectinomycin are effective by single-dose intramuscular injection.

Prospective studies suggest that infection with HIV type 1 (HIV-1) increases the prevalence of genital ulcer disease in prostitutes, leads to more invasive destructive genital lesions, and portends a suboptimal response to therapy, with a marked increase in single-dose failures (22). If these observations are confirmed, chancroid can be anticipated to increase rapidly in populations in which the seroprevalence of HIV infection is increased. Also, the contribution of chancroid to the spread of retroviruses is only now being fully understood. The interaction between *H. ducreyi* and HIV-1 appears to be synergistic, with each enabling the other to be transmitted more efficiently (46).

Granuloma Inguinale and Lymphogranuloma Venereum

Both granuloma inguinale, resulting from *Calymmatobacterium granulomatis*, and lymphogranuloma venereum (LGV), resulting from *C. trachomatis* serovars L1, L2, and L3, are poorly understood sexually transmitted infections, largely confined to the developing world. The reasons for this geographical isolation are unknown. Our knowledge is restricted to clinical description and uncontrolled treatment studies. The epidemiology of these etiological agents is unknown. Most studies suggest that granuloma inguinale is a very focal disease with limited capability for spread. Repeated exposure appears to be necessary, and the incubation period appears to be long. LGV is reported 3 to 10 times more commonly in men, owing to its clinical features. The ratio of symptomatic to asymptomatic infection is not known. The cervix is presumed to be the usual site of infection in women and may remain infected for long periods (39). Effective strategies for control are also uncertain and have not been well evaluated. Little significant research has been done during the past 20 years on either granuloma inguinale or LGV or the pathogens responsible.

Our ignorance about these diseases underlines the low priority given to investigating illnesses rarely seen in Western countries. Diseases confined to areas of the world in which research is a low priority remain poorly understood, with few prospects for control. Granuloma inguinale and LGV have presumably been recognized clinically because of their dermatologic clinical presentations. Other STD pathogens largely confined to developing countries almost certainly exist but have not been recognized. Only as research is done, identifying etiological agents of various syndromes within this milieu, will these elusive pathogens and the illnesses associated with them be characterized. Only then can control strategies be implemented. Presumably, the epidemic of HIV might have progressed much further before receiving its present public attention, research priority, and funds if its spread had been confined to developing countries.

HIV

The rapid spread of HIV-1 in both industrialized and developing countries has been described in detail in numerous publications. The risk behaviors that account for differences in seroincidence within various groups are still being investigated, and more information is required to understand the varying epidemiology of HIV-1 throughout the world.

Few studies have been done in developing countries on risk behavior or risk factors for the male homosexual spread of HIV-1. No studies to date have suggested any significant global differences from Western countries.

The enigma of explosive heterosexual transmission in developing countries is an area of major concern. It is now accepted that penile-vaginal intercourse is the most common means of HIV transmission for both men and women in most developing countries; other routes of transmission seem minor in comparison. Factors that increase risk of HIV-1 transmission and promote high seroincidence with rapid increases in the seroprevalence of HIV are still poorly understood. Only in developing countries has heterosexual transmission led to sustained seroincidences of 1 to 3% annually over the last 5 years. This has occurred in a number of countries in central, southern, and eastern Africa. As a result of this rapid increase, seroprevalence in many urban regions is now in excess of 20% among sexually active women and men or among women presenting for prenatal care. Prostitutes have a seroprevalence of 50 to 90% in these same countries. The impact of this burden of HIV disease is only beginning to be felt in most of the developing world. A rapid increase in AIDS is now occurring.

Heterosexual spread of HIV-1 is occurring in Western societies. However, the statistical risk of transmission appears in most instances to be small with any single episode of penile-vaginal intercourse regardless of which partner is infected. Studies on male-to-female transmission suggest that the risk is less than 0.1% per episode of intercourse and that the cumulative risk is about 5% or less each year. European and American studies report that risk factors for increased transmission include anal-receptive intercourse, more advanced illness in the male partner, and a history of other sexually transmitted infections (36). Transmission from women to men through penile-vaginal intercourse may be substantially less likely. No risk factors have yet been identified in Western countries for male infection following heterosexual intercourse.

Preliminary studies all support the hypothesis that concomitant STDs, particularly genital ulcers, are a major risk factor for acquisition of infection by women, presumably acting as a portal of entry and egress for the virus (6, 19, 20, 53). More recent evidence suggests that *Trichomonas vaginalis* vaginitis and perhaps other STDs are also risk factors for HIV acquisition (41). Among men, the lack of circumcision is associated with an increased risk of HIV-1 in both cross-sectional and prospective studies as well as in two geoepidemiological surveys (6, 33, 53). Among women, cervical ectopy appears to be associated with an increased risk of HIV-1.

The identification of risk factors permits the development of strategies that will have an impact on HIV transmission and are additive with education and information programs already ongoing in developing countries.

Additional epidemiological observations with regard to both AIDS and HIV infection in many developing countries include the concentration of infection in urban areas, the increasing infection rate among individuals with more advanced education, and the high rates among individuals who belong to various mobile groups such as long-distance truck drivers. Although prostitutes are implicated as an initial focus from which HIV is widely disseminated, as has occurred in Nairobi, this is less evident in other populations. We need more information not only on the epidemiology of the virus but also on the epidemiology of behaviors that lead to infection. Well-designed prospective studies to delineate the direction of the epidemic and the factors that permit its occurrence should be a priority in all countries.

Human Papillomavirus

Little is known regarding the epidemiology of human papillomavirus (HPV) infections in developing countries. Cervical cancer, the late sequela of infection with oncogenic HPVs, however, is a common cause of cancer death in the developing world. In Kenya, cervical cancer is the most common fatal cancer in women. Oncogenic HPV type 16 was identified in 35% of cervical cancer samples from women in Kenya and Brazil (12). Because HIV-induced immunosuppression facilitates HPV-induced neoplasia (37), it is speculated that HPV-related cancers will continue to increase in incidence in developing countries, especially in areas where HIV rates are highest. Studies of the epidemiology of HPV infection and of HPV-associated neoplasia are an important priority.

Genital Herpes

The epidemiology of herpes simplex virus (HSV) in Western societies has been reviewed in detail (8). Genital tract infection with either HSV type 1 (HSV-1) or HSV-2 can produce genital herpes, but over 75% of illness is due to HSV-2 (8). Seroepidemiological studies with sensitive type-specific antibodies have only recently been available. Both cross-sectional and prospective studies have defined the seroincidence, association with clinical illness, and risk factors for both HSV-1 and HSV-2. Prospective studies suggest that primary infection with HSV-1 provides some immunity to subsequent HSV-2 infection, modifies the initial illness, and reduces the risk of recurrence of HSV-2 (8). The seroprevalence rate for HSV-1 increases rapidly during childhood and more slowly during adult life (2). Lower annual family income and less education, the so-called "crowding" factors, are associated with increased HSV-1 seroprevalence in childhood (2). However, a number of factors, including duration of sexual exposure and history of other STDs, increase HSV-1 seroincidence in early adult life (2).

HSV-2 is primarily spread sexually. Among U.S. college students, the seroprevalence is less than 1% on entry and rises to about 5% by the fourth year of college (2). A continuing rise occurs subsequently, with 15 to 30% of adult women and 10 to 20% of adult men infected with HSV-2 (15, 23). However, less than 25% of individuals with antibody have a history of genital herpes (15, 23). A higher seroincidence of HSV-2 infection is found in individuals with a history of other STDs, multiple sex partners, and a longer duration of sexual exposure (2, 15). However, seroprevalence is unrelated to socioeconomic or educational parameters (2).

Very few studies have been done in developing countries. The seroprevalence of HSV-1 antibodies increases rapidly during childhood and reaches a level of 70 to 90% by adult life (8). In this setting, with considerable preexisting immunity, HSV-2 disease may be a much less important genital pathogen. However, in Thailand, routine cytologic screening of cervical scrapings showed a rapid increase in HSV inclusions from 0.02 to 0.7% over 7 years (54). Seroepidemiological studies need to be done in developing countries to identify both prevalence and incidence and correlate those with clinical disease and sexual behavior.

In studies from Nairobi, consecutive genital ulcers were investigated by culture. HSV was responsible for 5% of ulcers in both men and women (14, 44).

Genital ulcers caused by HSV appear to be a risk factor for acquisition of HIV in homosexual men in Western societies (19). Also, the immunosuppressive effect of HIV has increased the severity of HSV infection. Further studies should determine the burden of clinical illness caused by genital herpes in developing countries, develop strategies for control, and identify its relationship to other diseases, particularly HIV.

Hepatitis B Virus

The epidemiology of hepatitis B virus (HBV) in industrialized countries has changed significantly during the past 10 years. Screening of blood and blood products, combined with immunization, has almost ended transmission of HBV to recipients of blood transfusions and has markedly reduced the occupational risks of health professions. The "safer sex" education programs among the male homosexual community have reduced the risk of acquisition of HBV among homosexual men. As a result, heterosexual spread of HBV has become the single most important route of HBV spread in Western countries, accounting for 25 to 50% of new cases. In Vienna, Austria, among 107 heterosexual promiscuous individuals without other known risk behaviors, 28% had markers for HBV as compared with only 5.9% of controls (A. Stary, C. Vitouch, and W. Kopp, Int. Union. Vener. Dis., abstr. p. 36, Royal Society of Medicine, London, 1990).

Few data have been collected prospectively to determine the contribution of heterosexual spread of HBV to its spread in developing societies. Seroprevalence of infection is very high among prepubertal children, and the virus appears to be spread efficiently between family members. A recent study from Peru found that 67% of 467 prostitutes compared with 10% of 510 controls were positive for an HBV marker (21). However, only 6 of 306 prostitutes were hepatitis B surface antigen positive. These data suggest that despite a much higher rate of infection, sexually acquired HBV did not lead to a substantial increase in antigen carriage. As a result, only a small number (1.7%) of these prostitutes were infectious for their clients (21). Nonetheless, because of the potentially large number of exposed clients, prostitutes may be an important reservoir for heterosexually transmitted HBV in the developing world.

The risk factors that increase heterosexual spread of HBV have not been adequately studied. In a study from Uganda, a history of an STD was a significant risk factor for HBV markers (20). The efficacy of male-to-female and female-to-male transmission is unknown. The role of mucosal lesions, sexual practices, promiscuity, and the serological status or stage of illness of the infected partner each need to be determined in prospective studies. An HBV vaccine will likely be very cost-effective in industrialized societies in reducing the heterosexual spread of HBV. Epidemiological studies in developing societies to identify the role of heterosexual transmission and the role of any risk factors in HBV transmission are an urgent priority. The impact of HIV prevention activities on HBV epidemiology also needs to be determined. Until further information is available, immunization of individuals at increased risk should be included in any strategy to reduce the risk of HBV transmission.

CONCLUSION

Core groups of high-frequency transmitters have emerged as the dominant concept in STD epidemiology. They are the source of most STD infections for the remainder of the community since only they maintain R_0 greater than 1, they sustain high STD transmission rates because of rapid sex partner change rates and high concurrent infection rates, and they may be the major pool for the origin of antimicrobial-resistant organisms. In developing countries, prostitutes and their clients are readily identifiable as a core group. Because of their multiplier effect on transmission, keeping core group members free of STDs by appropriate diagnosis and treatment and reducing their potential for STD transmission by provision of condoms will have a maximum impact on STD rates for the entire community (34). Focusing control efforts on core groups and the implementation of syphilis screening for pregnant women and Credé's prophylaxis for the newborn are likely the most practical strategies for reducing STDs in the developing world.

LITERATURE CITED

1. **Anderson, R. M., and R. M. May.** 1988. Epidemiological parameters of HIV transmission. *Nature* (London) **333:**514–519.
2. **Breinig, M. K., L. A. Kingsley, J. A. Armstrong, D. J. Freeman, and M. Ho.** 1990. Epidemiology of genital herpes in Pittsburgh: serologic, sexual and racial correlates of apparent and inapparent herpes simplex infections. *J. Infect. Dis.* **162:**299–305.
3. **Brunham, R. C., M. Laga, J. N. Simonsen, D. W. Cameron, P. Peeling, J. McDowell, U. Pamba, J. O. Ndinya-Achola, G. Maitha, and F. Plummer.** 1990. The prevalence of *Chlamydia trachomatis* infection among mothers of children with trachoma. *Am. J. Epidemiol.* **132:**946–952.
4. **Brunham, R. C., and F. A. Plummer.** 1991. A general model of sexually transmitted disease epidemiology and its implications for control. *Med. Clin. North Am.* **74:**1339–1352.
5. **Caldwell, J. C., and P. Caldwell.** 1990. High fertility in sub-Saharan Africa. *Sci. Am.* **May:**118–125.
6. **Cameron, D. W., L. J. D'Costa, G. M. Maitha, M. Cheang, P. Piot, J. N. Simonsen, A. R. Ronald, M. N. Gakinya, J. O. Ndinya-Achola, R. C. Brunham, and F. A. Plummer.** 1989. Female to male transmission of human immunodeficiency virus type 1: risk factors for seroconversion in men. *Lancet* **i:**403–407.
7. **Cates, W., T. M. M. Farley, and P. J. Rowe.** 1985. Worldwide patterns of infertility: is Africa different? *Lancet* **ii:**596–598.
8. **Corey, L., and P. G. Spear.** 1986. Infections with herpes simplex virus. *N. Engl. J. Med.* **314:**686–691, 749–757.
9. **Datta, P., M. Laga, F. A. Plummer, J. O. Ndinya-Achola, P. Piot, G. Maitha, A. R. Ronald, and R. C. Brunham.** 1988. Infection and disease after perinatal exposure to *Chlamydia trachomatis* in Nairobi, Kenya. *J. Infect. Dis.* **158:**524–528.
10. **D'Costa, L. J., F. A. Plummer, I. Bowman, L. Fransen, P. Piot, A. R. Ronald, and H. Nsanze.** 1985. Prostitutes are a major reservoir of sexually transmitted diseases in Nairobi, Kenya. *Sex. Transm. Dis.* **12:**64–67.
11. **DeMuylder, X., M. Laga, C. Tennstedt, E. VanDyck, G. N. M. Aelbers, and P. Piot.** 1990. The role of *Neisseria gonorrhoeae* and *Chlamydia trachomatis* in pelvic inflammatory disease and its sequelae in Zimbabwe. *J. Infect. Dis.* **162:**501–505.
12. **Durst, M., L. Gissmann, H. Ikenberg, and H. zur Hausen.** 1983. A papillomavirus DNA from a cervical carcinoma and its prevalence in cancer biopsy samples from different geographic regions. *Proc. Natl. Acad. Sci. USA* **80:**3812–3815.
13. **Elliott, B., R. C. Brunham, M. Laga, J. O. Ndinya-Achola, G. Maitha, M. Cheang, and F. A. Plummer.** 1990. Maternal gonococcal infection as a preventable risk factor for low birth weight. *J. Infect. Dis.* **161:**531–536.
14. **Fast, M. V., L. J. D'Costa, H. Nsanze, P. Piot, J. Curran, P. Karasira, N. Mirza, I. W. Maclean, and A. R. Ronald.** 1984. The clinical diagnosis of genital ulcer disease in men in the tropics. *Sex. Transm. Dis.* **11:**72–76.
15. **Gibson, J. J., C. A. Hornung, G. R. Alexander, F. K. Lee, W. A. Potts, and A. J. Nahmias.** 1990. A cross sectional study of herpes simplex virus type 1 and 2 in college students: occurrence and determinants of infection. *J. Infect. Dis.* **162:**306–312.
16. **Guinness, L. F., S. Sibandaze, E. McGrath, and A. C. Cornelis.** 1988. Influence of antenatal screening on perinatal mortality caused by syphilis in Swaziland. *Gentiourin. Med.* **64:**294–297.
17. **Handsfield, H. H., R. J. Rice, M. C. Roberts, and K. K. Holmes.** 1989. Localized outbreak of penicillinase-producing *Neisseria gonorrhoeae*. Paradigm for introduction and spread of gonorrhea in a community. *J. Am. Med. Assoc.* **261:**2357–2361.
18. **Hira, S. K., and R. S. Hira.** 1987. Congenital syphilis, p. 113–127. *In* A. O. Osoba (ed.), *Sexually Transmitted Diseases in the Tropics. Bailliere's Clinical Tropical Medicine and Communicable Diseases,* vol. 2. Bailliere's, London.
19. **Holmberg, S. D., J. A. Stewart, and A. R. Gerber.** 1988. Prior herpes simples virus type 2 infections as a risk facter for HIV infection. *J. Am. Med. Assoc.* **259:**1048–1050.
20. **Hudson, C. P., A. J. M. Hennis, P. Kataaha, G. Lloyd, T. Moore, G. M. Sotehall, R.**

Whetstone, T. Wreghitt, and A. Karpas. 1988. Risk factors for the spread of AIDS in rural Africa: evidence from a comparative seroepidemiological survey of AIDS, hepatitis B and syphilis in southwestern Uganda. *AIDS* **2:**255–260.

21. **Hyams, K. C., I. A. Phillips, A. Tejada, O. Li, P. Hermoza, F. Lopez, P. Alva, G. Chauca, S. Sanchez, and F. S. Wignall.** 1990. Hepatitis B in a highly active prostitute population. Evidence for a low risk of chronic antigenemia. *J. Infect. Dis.* **162:**295–298.
22. **Jessamine, P. G., F. A. Plummer, J. O. Ndinya-Achola, M. A. Wainberg, I. Wamola, L. J. D'Costa, D. W. Cameron, J. N. Simonsen, P. Plourde, and A. R. Ronald.** 1990. Human immunodeficiency virus, genital ulcers and the male foreskin synergism in HIV-1 transmission. *Scand. J. Infect. Dis.* **69**(Suppl.)**:**181–186.
23. **Johnson, R. E., A. J. Nahmios, L. S. Maepes, F. K. Lee, C. A. Brooks, and C. B. Snowden.** 1989. A seroepidemiologic survey of the prevalence of herpes simples virus type 2 infection in the U.S. *N. Engl. J. Med.* **321:**7–12.
24. **Kosseim, M., A. Ronald, F. A. Plummer, L. D'Costa, and R. C. Brunham.** 1991. Treatment of acute pelvic inflammatory disease in the ambulatory setting: trial of cefoxitin and doxycycline versus ampicillin-sulbactam. *Antimicrob. Agents Chemother.* **35:**1651–1656.
25. **Laga, M., F. A. Plummer, H. Nsanze, W. Namaara, R. C. Brunham, J. O. Ndinya-Achola, G. Maitha, A. R. Ronald, L. J. D'Costa, V. Bhullar, J. Y. Mati, L. Fransen, M. Cheang, and P. Piot.** 1986. Epidemiology of ophthalmia neonatorum in Kenya. *Lancet* **ii:**1145–1149.
26. **Laga, M., F. A. Plummer, P. Piot, P. Datta, W. Namaara, J. O. Ndinya-Achola, H. Nsanze, G. Maitha, A. R. Ronald, H. O. Pamba, and R. C. Brunham.** 1988. Prophylaxis of gonococcal and chlamydia ophthalmia neonatorum. A comparison of silver nitrate and tetracycline. *N. Engl. J. Med.* **318:**653–657.
27. **Lycke, E., G. B. Lowhagen, G. Hallgagen, G. Johannison, and K. Ramstedt.** 1980. The risk of transmission of genital *Chlamydia trachomatis* infection is less than that of genital *Neisseria gonorrhoeae* infection. *Sex. Transm. Dis.* **7:**6–10.
28. **McNicol, P. J., W. L. Albritton, and A. R. Ronald.** 1986. Transfer of plasmid-mediated ampicillin resistance from *Haemophilus* to *Neisseria gonorrhoeae* requires an intervening organism. *Sex. Transm. Dis.* **13:**145–150.
29. **McNicol, P. J., and A. R. Ronald.** 1984. The plasmids of *Haemophilus ducreyi*. *J. Antimicrob. Chemother.* **14:**561–563.
30. **Meheus, A., J. Reniers, M. Collet, E. Frost, A. LeClerc, R. Gan, and B. Ivanoff.** 1988. *Chlamydia trachomatis* in women with acute salpingitis and infertility in Central Africa, p. 241–244. *In* D. Oriel, J. Ridgway, J. Schachter, D. Taylor-Robinson, and M. Ward (ed.), *Chlamydial Infections*. Cambridge University Press, Cambridge.
31. **Meheus, A., K. F. Schulz, and W. Cates.** 1990. Development of prevention and control programs for sexually transmitted diseases in developing countries, p. 1041–1046. *In* K. K. Holmes, P.-A. Mardh, P. F. Sparling, P. J. Weisner, W. Cates, S. M. Lemon, and W. E. Stamm (ed.), *Sexually Transmitted Diseases*. McGraw-Hill Book Co., New York.
32. **Morse, S. A., S. R. Johnson, J. W. Biddle, and M. C. Roberts.** 1986. High-level tetracycline resistance in *Neisseria gonorrhoeae* is the result of acquisition of streptococcal TetM determinant. *Antimicrob. Agents Chemother.* **30:**664–670.
33. **Moses, S., J. E. Bradley, N. J. D. Nagelkerke, A. R. Ronald, J. O. Ndinya-Achola, and F. A. Plummer.** 1990. Geographical patterns of male circumcision practices in Africa: association with HIV seroprevalence. *Int. J. Epidemiol.* **19:**693–697.
34. **Ngugi, E. N., J. N. Simonsen, M. Bosire, A. R. Ronald, F. A. Plummer, D. W. Cameron, P. Waiyaki, and J. O. Ndinya-Achola.** 1988. Prevention of transmission of human immunodeficiency virus in Africa: effectiveness of condom promotion and health education among prostitutes. *Lancet* **i:**887–890.
35. **Nzilambi, N., K. M. DeCock, D. N. Forthal, H. Francis, R. W. Ryder, C. Malebe, J. Getchell, M. Laga, P. Piot, and J. B. McCormick.** 1988. The prevalence of infection with human immunodeficiency virus over a ten-year period in rural Zaire. *N. Engl. J. Med.* **318:**276–279.
36. **Padian, N., S. L. Marquis, D. P. Francis, R. E. Anderson, G. W. Rutherford, P. M.**

O'Malley, and W. Wienstein. 1987. Male to female transmission of human immunodeficiency virus. *J. Am. Med. Assoc.* **258:**788–790.

37. **Palefsky, J. M., J. Gonzales, R. M. Greenblatt, D. K. Ahn, and H. Hollander.** 1990. Anal intraepithelial neoplasia and anal papillomavirus infection among homosexual males with group IV HIV disease. *J. Am. Med. Assoc.* **263:**2911–2916.
38. **Perine, P. L., M. E. Duncan, D. W. Krause, and S. Aevoke.** 1980. Pelvic inflammatory disease and puerperal sepsis in Ethiopia. I. Etiology. *Am. J. Obstet. Gynecol.* **138:**969–973.
39. **Perine, P. L., and A. O. Osoba.** 1990. Lymphogranuloma venereum, p. 195–204. *In* K. K. Holmes, P.-A. Mardh, P. F. Sparling, P. J. Weisner, W. Cates, S. M. Lemon, and W. E. Stamm (ed.), *Sexually Transmitted Disease*. McGraw-Hill Book Co., New York.
40. **Perine, P. L., W. Schalla, M. Siegal, C. Thornsberry, J. Biddle, K. H. Wong, and S. E. Thompson.** 1977. Evidence for two distinct types of penicillinase-producing Neisseria gonorrhoeae. *Lancet* **ii:**993–995.
41. **Piot, P., F. A. Plummer, F. S. Mhalu, J. L. Lamboray, J. Chin, and J. M. Mann.** 1988. AIDS: an international perspective. *Science* **239:**573–579.
42. **Piot, P., F. A. Plummer, M. A. Rey, E. Ngugi, C. Rouzioux, J. O. Ndinya-Achola, G. Vercauteren, L. J. D'Costa, M. Laga, H. Nsanze, L. Fransen, G. Haase, D. Van der Growen, R. C. Brunham, A. R. Ronald, and F. Brun-Vezinet.** 1987. Retrospective seroepidemiology of AIDS virus infection in Nairobi populations. *J. Infect. Dis.* **155:**1108–1112.
43. **Plummer, F. A., L. J. D'Costa, H. Nsanze, J. Dylewski, P. Karasira, and A. R. Ronald.** 1983. Epidemiology of chancroid and *Haemophilus ducreyi* in Nairobi. *Lancet* **ii:**1293–1295.
44. **Plummer, F. A., L. J. D'Costa, H. Nsanze, P. Karasira, I. W. Maclean, and A. R. Ronald.** 1985. Clinical and microbiologic studies of genital ulcers in Kenyan women. *Sex. Transm. Dis.* **12:**193–197.
45. **Plummer, F. A., M. Laga, R. C. Brunham, P. Piot, A. R. Ronald, V. Bhullar, J. Y. Mati, J. O. Ndinya-Achola, M. Cheang, and H. Nsanze.** 1987. Postpartum upper genital tract infections in Nairobi, Kenya: epidemiology, etiology and risk factors. *J. Infect. Dis.* **156:**92–98.
46. **Plummer, F. A., M. A. Wainberg, P. Plourde, P. Jessamine, L. J. D'Costa, I. A. Wamola, and A. R. Ronald.** 1990. Detection of human immunodeficiency virus-1 (HIV-1) in genital ulcer exudate of HIV-1 infected men by culture and gene amplification. *J. Infect. Dis.* **161:**810–811.
47. **Ratnam, A. V., T. K. Chattergee, and R. C. Mulenga.** 1980. Sexually transmitted diseases in pregnant women. *Med. J. Zambia* **14:**75–81.
48. **Ratnam, A. V., S. N. Din, and T. K. Chattergee.** 1980. Gonococcal infection in women with pelvic inflammatory disease in Lusaka, Zambia. *Am. J. Obstet. Gynecol.* **138:**965–968.
49. **Rwandan HIV Seroprevalence Study Group.** 1989. Nationwide community-based serological survey of HIV-1 and other human retrovirus infections in a central African country. *Lancet* **i:**941–943.
50. **Schmid, G. P.** 1990. Treatment of chancroid. *Rev. Infect. Dis.* **12**(Suppl. 6)**:**S580–S582.
51. **Schmid, G. P., L. L. Sanders, Jr., J. H. Blount, and E. R. Alexander.** 1987. Chancroid in the U.S.: establishment of an old disease. *J. Am. Med. Assoc.* **258:**3265–3268.
52. **Schroeter, A. C., R. H. Turner, J. B. Lucas, and W. J. Brown.** 1971. Therapy for incubating syphilis: effectiveness of gonorrhoea treatment. *J. Am. Med. Assoc.* **218:**711–713.
53. **Simonsen, J. N., D. W. Cameron, M. N. Gakiny, J. O. Ndinya-Achola, L. J. D'Costa, P. Karasira, A. R. Ronald, P. Piot, and F. A. Plummer.** 1988. Human immunodeficiency virus infection in men with sexually transmitted diseases. *N. Engl. J. Med.* **319:**274–278.
54. **Simonsen, J. N., F. A. Plummer, E. N. Ngugi, C. Black, J. K. Kreiss, M. N. Gakinya, P. Waiyaki, L. J. D'Costa, J. O. Ndinya-Achola, P. Piot, and A. Ronald.** 1990. HIV infection among lower socioeconomic strata prostitutes in Nairobi. *AIDS* **4:**139–144.
55. **Srinannoboons, S.** 1979. Cytologic study of herpes simplex infection and dysplasia in the female genital tract. *J. Med. Assoc. Thai.* **62:**201–206.
56. **Temmerman, M., F. A. Plummer, N. B. Mirza, S. Fusallah, J. O. Ndinya-Achola, I. A.**

Wamola, N. Nagelkerke, R. C. Brunham, and P. Piot. 1990. Infection with human immunodeficiency virus (HIV) as a risk factor for adverse obstetrical outcome. *AIDS* **4:**1087–1093.

57. **Wasserheit, J. N.** 1989. The significance and scope of reproductive tract infections among Third World women. *Int. J. Gynecol. Obstet. Suppl.* **3:**145–168.
58. **WHO Expert Committee on Venereal Diseases and Treponematoses.** 1986. *Sixth Report.* Technical report series no. 736, p. 13. World Health Organization, Geneva.
59. **Yorke, J. A., H. W. Heathcoate, and A. Nold.** 1978. Dynamics and control of the transmission of gonorrhea. *Sex. Transm. Dis.* **5:**51–57.

Behavioral Risk Factors for Sexually Transmitted Diseases Including HIV Infection

Risk Factors for Acquisition of Sexually Transmitted Diseases and Development of Complications

Nancy S. Padian, Stephen C. Shiboski, and Penelope J. Hitchcock

Interventions that prevent the spread of sexually transmitted infections (STIs) are based on breaking chains of acquisition and transmission of infection. To accomplish this, one must understand the constellation of causal factors that link the chain. Thus, the first objective of epidemiological research on the prevention and control of sexually transmitted diseases (STDs) is to define the spectrum and prevalence of risk factors associated with all points in the natural history of disease. A natural history time line from initial exposure to the development of adverse sequelae is depicted in Fig. 1. For example, with human papillomavirus (HPV) infection, the time line consists of (i) exposure, (ii) infection, (iii) disease (abnormal epithelial growth resulting in warts or condylomata), and (iv) long-term sequelae (progression to severe dysplasia or carcinoma in situ and [rarely] progression to invasive carcinoma). Risk factors that predict each step in this process may be viewed either as increasing risk (e.g., receptive anal intercourse increases risk of acquiring human immunodeficiency virus [HIV] or hepatitis B virus infection) or as protective (e.g., condom use). This chapter examines the identification and assessment of such factors and is divided into two parts. The first part outlines the types of associations between risk factors and disease outcomes. The second part explores classification schemes for identifying risk factors.

TYPES AND MEASURES OF ASSOCIATION

Causal Associations

Absolute criteria for assessing the causal contribution of a risk factor would require that the factor is both necessary and sufficient to produce the outcome. However, because we cannot identify risk factors that are both necessary and sufficient for the occurrence of most diseases, more pragmatic and epidemiologically valid criteria to assess causality have been developed. In epidemiological studies, causality is defined in a probabilistic sense (5); that is, a risk factor is causally related to an outcome if its presence or absence affects the probability that the outcome will occur. Criteria for assessing the causal contributions of factors have been discussed at length by many epidemiologists (e.g., see reference 25) and

Nancy S. Padian and Stephen C. Shiboski – Department of Epidemiology and Biostatistics, University of California, San Francisco, San Francisco General Hospital, San Francisco, California 94110. *Penelope J. Hitchcock* – Sexually Transmitted Diseases Branch, National Institute of Allergy and Infectious Diseases, Bethesda, Maryland 20892.

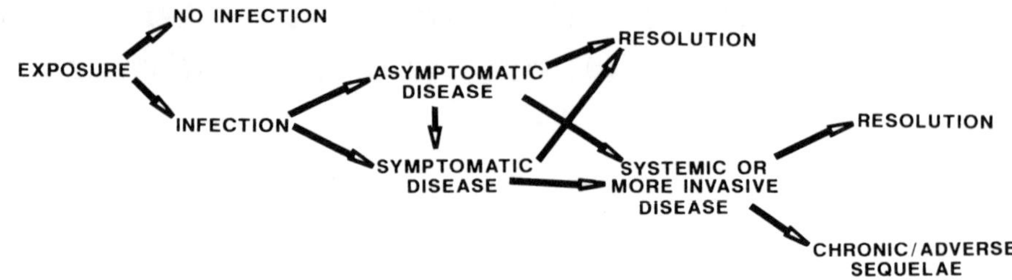

Figure 1. Natural history time line.

are summarized in Table 1. Of these criteria, only temporality would truly be considered by all epidemiologists as a sine qua non for a causal factor.

Risk Factors and Risk Markers

Risk factors (or independent variables) are those factors directly associated with the dependent variable or outcome (infection, disease, or long-term sequelae) that meet most of the criteria outlined in Table 1. They are identified from studies of populations in which affected individuals have the risk factor more often than unaffected individuals. Thus, risk factors represent population profiles and are affected by the composition of the population or sample under study. Because of the aggregate nature of risk factors, there will often be some individuals who have the outcome but apparently lack risk factors, just as there will often be individuals with risk factors who remain without the outcome. This is due not only to individual variation but also to an incomplete understanding of the entire network of causal risk factors.

Sometimes populations rather than individuals can be selected as the unit of analysis. In this kind of ecological research design, risk factors are defined by their overall prevalence, and populations are compared according to the prevalence of the risk factor and the prevalence of the outcome. The associations that result from these analyses may differ from analyses of individuals using the same risk factors and outcomes. This is often the case in examinations of social and demographic risk factors in which associations that occur on a population level are not necessarily the same as those observed from comparisons among individuals. This phenomenon is discussed more fully by Aral et al. (this volume).

Independent variables that are correlated with the risk factor under study but do not appear to directly cause the outcome of interest have been referred to as risk markers or risk indicators (4, 19, 27). Risk markers are related to the outcome because they are associated with other risk factors. Thus, they may be surrogate markers for the risk factor. For example, the use of alcohol during sexual intercourse may decrease the likelihood that condoms will be used. Alcohol is associated with transmission even though its primary effect is not direct. Sometimes, however, the distinction between direct and indirect associations is not so simple.

Table 1. Criteria for assessing causal contributions of associated factors

Criterion	Definition
Consistency	Observation that has been repeatedly observed in a variety of studies under different circumstances and times
Strength	Magnitude of the measure of association (e.g., relative risk)
Specificity	Correspondence of exposure with only one particular form of disease or particular site at which it occurs
Temporality	Exposure must occur before the effect
Coherence	Corroboration between the observed association, biological plausibility, and other known facts
Dose response	Biological gradient in which increased amounts of exposure are associated with increased risk or severity of the outcome

Causal pathways are actually cascades of factors operating together to produce an outcome. A variety of pathways may lead to the same outcome, although for STDs they all must ultimately include the presence of one or more etiological agents. A good example of the domino effect of risk factors is found in studies of transmission subsequent to exposure to an infected individual. Sociocultural and demographic factors influence intentions to practice certain sexual behaviors that can in turn result in exposure of vaginal or anal epithelium to the etiological agent. It can be difficult to differentiate between risk factors and risk markers in this scenario.

In fact, both types of variables are often on a continuum and in many cases differ only in their proximity on the causal pathway to the final mechanism that produces transmission, disease, or progression (Fig. 1). However, as stated above, causal mechanisms, necessary risk factors, and complete causal pathways are rarely, if ever, known. Of course, some factors, including many sociodemographic variables, are more clearly indirect because they almost influence other recognized risk factors. Nevertheless, what is labeled as a risk factor may be associated with an effect that is produced by an unidentified or unmeasurable but more direct causal influence.

In addition, as stated above, the goal in identifying risk factors is to prescribe interventions, and the distinction between risk factor and risk marker, or between direct and indirect associations, does not necessarily facilitate this task. When identifying objectives for intervention programs, it may be easier to target risk markers that are less directly associated with the outcome than to target a more proximal risk factor. For example, number of sexual partners is a marker for the increased risk of encountering an infected partner. This risk is also influenced by the existing prevalence of infection in the population and by patterns of partner recruitment but is most directly and proximately determined by the specific choice of an infected partner. For an incurable, often subclinical STI, such as HIV infection, it may be easier to decrease the average number of partners than to specifically identify and avoid infected partners.

Measures of Association

The importance of a risk factor is usually determined in part by the strength of its effect, as measured by its ability to predict the likelihood of the outcome. This strength is often assessed by a statistical measure such as the relative risk of disease among those with the risk factor compared with the risk of disease among those without the risk factor. Such statistical measures of association provide one of the most important tools of epidemiological research. However, because spurious statistical associations can occur by chance or as a result of bias (e.g., assessing risk in an unrepresentative sample) or confounding (discussed below), statistical techniques should be used in conjunction with other criteria in Table 1.

Because independent variables are associated with each other as well as with the outcome of interest, the examination of one risk factor is affected by other variables that may confound (enhance, attenuate, or entirely mask) the independent association of any one factor alone. In some cases, the effect of such factors can be controlled for in the analysis, as in the example described below. However, sometimes it is better to select only one variable or to devise a composite factor such as an overall risk index. In any analysis, the selection of risk factors and the interpretation of results depend on the particular hypothesis and mechanism of effect under study and on the distribution of independent variables in the particular sample. Identifying risk factors that measure exposures of interest, factors to control for, or factors to eliminate is contingent on the specific research question.

The reputed association between age at first intercourse (the exposure) and cervical dysplasia or in situ cervical neoplasia is an example of confounding. Age at first intercourse appears to be associated with cervical dysplasia largely because it is correlated with the total number of sexual partners; the measure of association between the risk factor (age at first intercourse) and cervical dysplasia decreases when number of sexual partners is considered in the analysis (12). On the other hand, if early age of first intercourse could be shown to "condition" an individual to have a large number of lifetime sexual partners, early intercourse could be viewed not as a confounder but as an indirect or less proximate behavioral risk factor that is part of the causal pathway leading to dysplasia.

Another important consideration in addition to the strength of the association of the factor with the outcome (e.g., the magnitude of the relative risk) is the prevalence of the risk factor in the population. Although the effect of a risk factor may be very strong, few individuals may actually have the risk factor. For example, receptive anal intercourse increases the likelihood of male-to-female transmission of HIV (20), but if receptive anal intercourse is practiced by only a small percentage of the female population, then despite its strength as a risk factor, it may not be the highest priority for an intervention. Population-attributable risk is a useful measure that combines estimates of the relative risk for a risk factor with information about its prevalence in the population. Although the prevalence of the risk factor is best measured in population-based surveys, it can also be estimated in studies specifically designed to measure relative risks (6).

TAXONOMY OF RISK FACTORS

Classification Schemes

STDs, like other infectious diseases, are unique to epidemiology because two categories of parameters can be specified: those necessary for pathogen transmission and those necessary for the development of disease. One way to classify risk factors is within the theoretical framework of models based on these parameters. This results in a functional classification that groups risk factors by their role in transmission or in the disease process. Parameters related to transmission in this type of model include number of partners, characteristics of the partner, number of contact episodes per partner, the probability that the partner is infected, the probability of transmission given exposure (or infectivity), and the duration of infectiousness (1, 16). One such model is described in detail by Anderson (this volume).

Models have been used to make predictions about epidemics and to specify factors that determine the rate of transmission or the process leading from initial infection to disease. Application of these same models to the development of sequelae is less well understood. However, many of the same model parameters can apply. The complex of behavioral and biomedical factors related to the probability of transmission is analogous to factors that predict the likelihood of sequelae. For example, number of partners and contact episodes may not only determine risk of transmission of infection but also have a bearing on progression to sequelae through repeat infections or disease episodes. In addition, the duration of untreated infection has a direct bearing on the probability of the progression of infection to disease and to its sequelae.

A shortcoming in such epidemic models is that they generally fail to account adequately for the historical context in which they operate. Use of the same model can result in disparate predictions in different social and cultural environments. For example, depending on norms of sexual behavior, factors that affect the efficiency of transmission of infection per contact may differ, because use of condoms or types of sexual practices are affected by norms. Likewise, the duration of infectiousness differs depending on the availability, acceptability, and quality of health care, which are also mediated by sociocultural norms. Thus, the historical sociocultural framework provides a class of variables that, while not included as model parameters, are crucial for understanding both the acquisition of infection and disease and the development of sequelae.

There are other ways to classify risk factors and markers. One system (24) defines a triumvirate of factors related to (i) the agent and infectiousness, including the size or dose of the infectious inoculum, (ii) the host and susceptibility, and (iii) environmental factors.

Another system elaborates on a list of factors by grouping highly correlated factors (3). Typical categories in this system include (i) demographic factors such as socioeconomic status, religion, age, gender, race or ethnic background, marital status, place of residence; (ii) sexual practices, including contraceptive behaviors;

(iii) health care-seeking behavior, including access to health care and compliance with therapy; (iv) behavioral factors such as drug use and smoking; (v) hygienic practices such as douching and tampon use; and (vi) biological factors such as immune competence and integrity of mucosal linings.

In addition to understanding the mechanism of transmission, it is also important to specify which factors are subject to change and may be targeted as modifiable risk factors and objectives for interventions. Thus, another classification scheme focuses on the development of interventions (27). Behavioral and social factors are generally more modifiable than biological factors, although treatment regimens, chemotherapeutic prophylaxis, and vaccine development may be directed toward biological factors. Modifiable factors are also generally subject to individual influences. Factors that are ecological and operate on a population level, such as many demographic, cultural, and social factors, are more difficult to modify.

Although these systems are useful (and are not necessarily mutually exclusive), we will explore types of risk factors using a theoretical model based upon that presented by Anderson (this volume). Table 2 summarizes the model parameters we will use to identify risk factors. Risk factors are classified as biological or behavioral-sociological and by whether they are associated with transmission or long-term sequelae. Each parameter in Table 2 is discussed below.

Table 2. Model parameters (classes of risk factors and markers) that predict the spread of STDs[a]

Parameter	Type of factor[b]		Outcome[c]	
	Biological	Behavioral-sociological	Transmission	Sequelae
No. of partners		X	X	x
Probability that partner is infected (prevalence of infection)	NA[d]	NA[d]	X	x
No. of contacts per partner		X	X	x
Characteristics of sexual partner and patterns of partner selection		X	X	x
Infectivity and probability of sequelae	X	X	X	X
Duration of infection	X	X	X	X
Sociocultural factors	X	X	X	X

[a] X, definite association; x, tentative association, only insofar as repeat infections are related to development of sequelae.
[b] Type of factor refers to classes of risk factors that are either biological or behavioral and/or sociological (including demographic factors).
[c] Outcome refers to whether the parameter applies to transmission or initial infection or to disease or long-term sequelae.
[d] NA, not applicable. Prevalence of infection is assessed on a population level. An individual cannot have risk factors that influence this parameter; thus, classifying types of factors is irrelevant.

Measurement of Number of Partners, Probability that a Random Partner Is Infected, and Number of Contacts

Number of sexual partners is measured as a rate—the number of new partners per unit time. However, in addition to the absolute number of partners per individual, the variability in number of partners within a population is also a critical variable (2). Thus, if only a few people in a population are having a large number of sexual partners while most others are relatively monogamous, the spread of STDs will be quite different than if most people are having multiple partners, even if the average number of partners in each community is identical. In addition to absolute number and variations in number of sexual partners, the temporal grouping (simultaneous versus single encounter [serial monogamy]) of partners is also crucial. The effect of this selection pattern varies depending on the particular pathogen. For diseases such as syphilis or gonorrhea, which have relatively short periods of infectiousness (the period in which the pathogen can be transmitted from person to person), having multiple partners during a brief period results in greater risk of dissemination of infection than having serial monogamous partners. For chronic viral infections that are sexually transmitted (such as HIV) and that have long periods of infectiousness, this is less important. For diseases such as genital herpes that have long periods of quiescent infection interrupted by periodic shedding, simultaneous partners would have more of an effect only during periods in which the virus is shed.

The probability that a randomly selected partner is infected is determined by the prevalence of infection within a community. This is the one parameter that operates on a population level; an individual cannot change the prevalence of infection in the population from which the partner is selected, although as stated earlier, patterns of partner selection can be modified by individuals, which in turn will affect the incidence of new infection.

Number of sexual partners and number of contacts with each partner are two parameters that are mediated entirely by individual behavioral factors and thus are clearly subject to intervention. Of course, the key factor is to determine the number of contacts that occurred after infection of the index case. The date of this event can rarely be determined; thus, contact counts are subject to error, a fact that needs to be accounted for in any data analysis (21). Types of sexual contact and the use of prophylaxis are also important to consider.

Interactions among Number of Partners, Probability that a Random Partner Is Infected (Prevalence of Infection), Number of Contacts, and Infectivity

Greater numbers of partners increase the chance of contact with an infected partner. However, the number of partners is less important in communities characterized by a high prevalence of infection (such as the 50% prevalence of HIV in homosexual communities in San Francisco [28]) than in communities characterized by a lower prevalence of infection. In San Francisco, there is a good chance that one random partner will be infected with HIV, whereas in other communities with a lower population prevalence of infection, it would on average take a larger number of partners to encounter one partner who is infected.

The per contact probability of infection (efficiency of transmission or infectivity, discussed below) also affects the relative contribution of number of partners and number of contacts per partner to the spread of infection. Assuming a constant prevalence of infection in a community with a homogeneous infectivity rate, a low infectivity rate suggests that repeated contacts with an infected partner would be more important than the number of partners; whereas when the infectivity rate is high, transmission could occur after any episode of intercourse, and thus the number of partners would have a greater effect (18).

Sexual Partner Characteristics

Partner selection processes are dictated by many individual behavioral factors. One important characteristic of a potential sexual partner is his or her level of sexual activity.

Core group transmission

Surveys have shown that most individuals have fewer than 10 sexual partners over a lifetime (8) and that STD epidemics are driven by small groups of sexually active individuals with many partners. A recent survey of young adults in Canada (15) revealed that these sexually active individuals not only have a larger number of partners, but also practice behaviors that may increase the likelihood of transmission, e.g., they use condoms less frequently and have more anal intercourse (associated with HIV transmission [20]). Groups of individuals who have unprotected sex with numbers of partners sufficiently large to sustain the spread of an STI are referred to as core groups of high-frequency transmitters (13). The probability that a random partner is infected depends not only on the number of partners and the overall prevalence of infection in the population but also on the probability that a particular partner is a member of a core group in which there are high levels of infection. Thus, a critical parameter in modeling the epidemic spread of STDs is how partners are selected (qualitative aspects of partner selection [7]).

The existence of core groups has been confirmed by studies (e.g., see references 22 and 23) in which the role of residential proximity was examined with respect to partner choice. In an STD epidemic, the core, like the eye of a hurricane, can actually be plotted (by residence) on a map. Like any other group of people, the core does not represent a closed population, and the mixing between core and noncore members can mediate transmission of STDs to a larger group of partners. Although the core is often responsible for seeding epidemics, it is also the magnet to which epidemics in the general population migrate. For example, Hansfield et al. (11) documented the presence of a penicillinase-producing strain of *Neisseria gonorrhoeae* in STD clinic populations in Seattle. The initial incidence was characterized by cases in whites (men had higher infection rates than women). After a time, infection by the strain was limited to densely populated inner city areas, inhabited by black men and women of low socioeconomic class, and often involved patients using illicit drugs and practicing prostitution or having sex with prostitutes. In this epidemic and others, core groups have comprised minority groups living in urban areas characterized by a high prevalence of drug use and prostitution. Another example is that of AIDS in the United States, which first achieved high incidence among white homosexual men. Here too, the core group now includes inner city populations similar to that described in Seattle (11, 14).

Patterns of partner selection

Although researchers have been able to identify core groups, it is difficult for individuals to identify core group members when they select sexual partners. Often the place where the partners meet (e.g., a bar or park) provides a clue if such places are known to be frequented by core members (22). Partners may attempt to elicit information about history of STDs or the practice of certain sexual behaviors. As the length of the presexual relationship grows, the likelihood that reliable information can be gathered usually increases. Mixing among ethnic, social, and risk groups (e.g., commercial sex workers or intravenous drug users [IVDUs]) provides some estimates as to the permeability of boundaries between the core and other groups. Examples of this kind of assessment are the studies of IVDUs and their sexual partners. The extent to which IVDUs choose non-IVDU sexual partners will, in part, determine the speed with which the HIV epidemic will spread within heterosexual communities.

Probability of Transmission or Progression

Infectivity rate and likelihood of transmission

The infectivity rate is the probability that transmission will occur after one exposure to an infected partner (i.e., the probability of infection per contact). Risk factors in this category consist of biological variables including factors related to the pathogen, infectiousness of the source (i.e., the amount of the inoculation presented to an exposed partner), and the susceptibility of the host (exposed partner). Because these biological factors reflect the pathophysiologic mechanisms of transmission, they are often thought of as the necessary risk factors that are part of the final common pathway in transmission events. The infectiousness of the source is determined by whether the source is shedding infectious organisms at the time of the sexual encounter and, if so, by the number of organisms being shed in relation to the number of organisms necessary to establish infection in a partner. In general, for most communicable diseases, including most STIs, the number of organisms shed increases steadily during the incubation period, peaks during the early stages of acute symptoms (for example, during the stage of urethral discharge in the male or cervical discharge in the female with gonorrhea), decreases as the host immune response begins to suppress the infection, persists for various periods at low levels during the phase of chronic infection and recovery, and then, depending on the STI, may or may not eventually be completely eliminated from the body. During the most acute phase of symptoms, the presence of a profuse discharge or an open sore could be viewed as a mechanism that increases efficiency of transmission to another person should the infected individual choose to have sexual contact during the stage of acute symptoms.

Factors related to host susceptibility include genetic factors, immunological status, coinfection with other organisms, nonspecific defense mechanisms such as those related to the normal flora, and anatomical features due to age. Studies of the pathophysiologic mechanism of transmission help to elucidate virulence factors unique to the pathogen. For example, if *Chlamydia trachomatis* is an intracellular parasite that binds to and enters the columnar epithelium, then the presence of columnar cells on the ectocervix (cervical ectopy) could increase the likelihood of transmission (26). Behaviors associated with the presence of cervical ectopy in an exposed woman, such as oral contraceptive use or early sexual debut, could also be associated with transmission.

This parameter also includes behavioral risk factors and risk markers. Sexual practices such as oral or anal intercourse and sexual intercourse during menstruation, use of barriers (such as condoms), circumcision, and hygienic practices such as douching or tampon use and perhaps even smoking fall into this category. Likewise, drug and alcohol use influences the likelihood that behaviors associated with transmission will occur. Similarly, psychological factors such as motivation, cognitive abilities, and individual past experiences also affect the likelihood of behaviors that will or will not be practiced that might influence transmission. Demographic and sociocultural factors such as age, race, and socioeconomic status also affect the likelihood of transmission, because these frame the sociocultural context in which the behavior occurs. Several of these factors are discussed in more detail in later chapters.

Probability of disease and of sequelae

As summarized in Fig. 1, infection may or may not lead to disease or to long-term sequelae. Many factors that are associated with the probability of transmission have also been associated with the probability of developing severe disease and subsequent sequelae. For example, oral contraceptives have been associated with an increased risk of acquiring cervical chlamydial infection (several studies) but with a decreased risk of symptomatic pelvic inflammatory disease among women with cervical chlamydial infection. Smoking has not only been associated with increased risk of infection with HPV, it is also associated with the risk of cervical and anal neoplasia (10, 17). Douching is often advocated to decrease the risk of acquiring and transmitting an STD; however, in conjunction with cervical chlamydial infection, douching has been associated with increased likelihood of pelvic inflammatory disease and future ectopic pregnancies (9, 29). However, perhaps the most important behavioral factor that determines the probability of developing severe disease and sequelae is health care-seeking behavior, which interacts with the availability of and access to good health care. For example, the probability of severe damage to the fallopian tubes is directly correlated with the severity of inflammation of the tubes when treatment is begun, which in turn is directly related to the delay from onset of abdominal pain until treatment is begun. Thus, a patient who promptly seeks treatment after onset of abdominal pain has reduced her risk of tubal damage. Similarly, women with cervical HPV infection who obtain regular Pap smears will receive treatment when dysplasia is first detected and will be at low risk for cervical cancer. Other behavioral risk factors for progression of infection to disease or to subsequent sequelae, especially sexual behaviors, have not been clearly delineated. Nevertheless, one would expect a similar interplay among biological, behavioral, and possibly psychosocial factors that affect the likelihood of the development of long-term sequelae.

Duration of Infection or Infectiousness

The duration of infection is the amount of time an infectious organism is viable in the host before it is eliminated by the natural resolution of the infection, which may or may not include the effects of treatment or specific immune function. It is important for transmission because, in general, the longer an infection persists, the longer an infected individual is able to transmit infection to susceptible partners. It is important for progression because the longer the time of infection, the greater the likelihood an infection will spread to other anatomical sites, thereby increasing the severity of the disease and the likelihood of the development of sequelae. The duration of infectiousness may differ from the duration of infection, if the pathogen is shed in a transmissible form only transiently (e.g., most cases of hepatitis B) or intermittently (e.g., herpes simplex virus infection). Furthermore, as discussed above, the level of infectiousness may vary with the stage of infection. This may also be true for HIV, which (in some studies) appears to be most infectious during the first few weeks after acquisition of infection and during the late stages, with onset of immunosuppression and of symptomatic disease.

As with factors associated with the probability of transmission or sequelae, biological and behavioral factors interact to affect the duration of infection. For example, the specific or nonspecific immune status of both the infected individual and the exposed individual can affect the duration of infection. With many STIs, previous infection produces only partial immunity or no immunity to reinfection. Antimicrobial sensitivity is also important. If the organism is resistant, treatment may fail and the infection can persist.

Behavioral factors that affect the duration of infection include health care-seeking behaviors and access to health care as well as compliance with therapy required to cure the infection. In addition to clinical care, health care can be thought of in a more generic sense to include public health programs such as screening, availability of treatment guidelines, and programs for vaccine distribution, partner notification, and behavior change.

In addition to social and cultural factors associated with participation in these programs, the type of infection or disease may also dictate the most likely entrance into the health care delivery system. Screening programs may be more important for pathogens that commonly cause asymptomatic infections, whereas clinical services that treat symptomatic patients may be more important for pathogens that typically cause symptomatic infections (19). *C. trachomatis* can cause asymptomatic infection in both men and women; consequently, infected individuals may be sexually active carriers and transmitters of infectious organisms. Screening programs, therefore, are viewed as very important in chlamydia control. In contrast, gonorrhea produces symptoms in a high proportion of men, and services that provide treatment for symptomatic men and notify their exposed partners are particularly important for gonorrhea control. Genital ulcer disease caused by *Haemophilus ducreyi* is also likely to be symptomatic. Obviously, the success of efforts to improve health care-seeking behavior for STDs depends not only on social, cultural, and psychological factors that affect acceptance and compliance, but also on programs that screen or diagnose and treat symptomatic infection. Location of the clinic, cost of services, quality of care, and perceived risk also affect access to health care. These factors are described in detail in this book.

Sociocultural Context

Sociocultural factors include biological and behavioral factors with the most indirect effect because although they may be measured on an individual basis, they are generally defined on a population level (i.e., social, cultural, and demographic influences). These variables reflect aggregate risk. They influence the norms, myths, and attitudes that underlie intentions and affect behavior that can differentially influence the probability of transmission or disease progression. For example, the acceptability of anal intercourse, the use of condoms, or prostitution varies depending on context. In addition, the acceptability of health care systems (which directly affects the time before diagnosis and treatment and therefore the duration of infection) is also mediated in part by social and cultural attitudes toward health care and the delivery system. Sociocultural risk factors are also discussed in this book.

Social context also reflects history and the concomitant political, economic, and biotechnological forces. For example, in societies characterized by political change and the reorganization of social structures, the acceptability of prostitution (which in turn affects the prevalence of STD infection) is increased (4). Ultimately, all these factors shape individual and institutional beliefs, values, intentions, and behaviors.

SUMMARY

The complicated process of identifying risk factors is one of the central goals of epidemiological study for several reasons. First, studies that examine individuals with and without disease can reveal factors that determine disease etiology either by identifying an etiological agent or by establishing risk factors that identify steps along the causal pathway to infection, disease, or the development of long-term sequelae. In addition, specifying such risk factors helps to define the mechanics of transmission, the development of disease, and the progression to sequelae, so that epidemic processes can be characterized. Finally, selecting risk factors that are modifiable is critically important for the development of interventions that result in behavior change and reduction either of initial infection and disease or of long-term sequelae.

LITERATURE CITED

1. **Allard, R.** 1990. A family of mathematical models to describe the risk of infection by a sexually transmitted agent. *Epidemiology* **1:**30–33.
2. **Anderson, R.** 1988. The epidemiology of HIV infection: variable incubation plus infectious periods and heterogeneity in sexual activity. *J. R. Stat. Soc.* **151:**66.
3. **Aral, S., and K. Holmes.** 1984. Epidemiology of sexually transmitted diseases, p. 126–140. *In* K. Holmes, P.-A. Mardh, P. Sparling, P. Wiesner, W. Cates, Jr., S. Lemon, and W. Stamm (ed.), *Sexually Transmitted Diseases*. McGraw-Hill Book Co., New York.
4. **Aral, S., and K. Holmes.** 1990. Epidemiology of sexual behavior and sexually transmitted diseases, p. 19–36. *In* K. Holmes, P.-A. Mardh, P. Sparling, P. Wiesner, W. Cates, Jr., S. Lemon, and W. Stamm (ed.), *Sexually Transmitted Diseases*, 2nd ed. McGraw-Hill Book Co., New York.
5. **Breslow, N., and N. Day.** 1986. *Statistical Methods in Cancer Research*, vol. I, p. 82. IARC Scientific Publications, Lyon, France.
6. **Bruzzi, P., S. Green, D. Byar, L. Brinton, and C. Schairer.** 1985. Estimating the population attributable risk for multiple risk factors using case-control data. *Am. J. Epidemiol.* **122:**904–914.
7. **Cates, W.** 1990. Acquired immunodeficiency syndrome, sexually transmitted disease, and epidemiology. Past lessons, present knowledge, and future opportunities. *Am. J. Epidemiol.* **131:**749–758.
8. **Centers for Disease Control.** 1988. Number of sex partners and potential risk of sexual exposure to human immunodeficiency virus. *Morbid. Mortal. Weekly Rep.* **37:**565–568.
9. **Chow, J., L. Yonekura, G. Richwald, S. Greenland, R. Sweet, and J. Schachter.** 1990. The association between chlamydia trachomatis and ectopic pregnancy. *J. Am. Med. Assoc.* **263:**3164–3167.
10. **Daling, J., N. Weiss, G. Hislop, C. Maden, R. Coates, K. Sherman, R. Ashley, M. Beagrie, J. Ryan, and L. Corey.** 1987. Sexual practices, sexually transmitted diseases, and the incidence of anal cancer. *N. Engl. J. Med.* **317:**973–977.
11. **Hansfield, H., R. Rice, M. Roberts, and K. Holmes.** 1989. Localized outbreak of penicillinase-producing Neisseria gonorrhoea: paradigm for introduction and spread of gonorrhea in a community. *J. Am. Med. Assoc.* **261:**2357–2361.
12. **Harris, R., L. Brinton, R. Cowdell, D. Skegg, P. Smith, M. Vessey, and R. Doll.** 1980. Characteristics of women with dysplasia or carcinoma in situ of the cervix uteri. *Br. J. Cancer* **42:**359–364.
13. **Heathcote, H., and J. Yorke.** 1984. Gonorrhea transmission dynamics and control. *Lecture Notes in Biomathematics*, no. 56. Springer-Verlag, New York.
14. **Holmes, K., J. Karon, and J. Kreiss.** 1990. The increasing frequency of heterosexually acquired AIDS in the United States, 1983–88. *Am. J. Public Health* **80:**858–863.
15. **MacDonald, N., G. Wells, D. Fisher, W. Warren, M. King, J.-A. Doherty, and W. Bowie.** 1990. High-risk STD/HIV behavior among college students. *J. Am. Med. Assoc.* **262:**3155–3159.
16. **May, R., and R. Anderson.** 1987. Transmission dynamics of HIV infection. *Nature* (London) **326:**137–142.
17. **Moscicki, A.-B., B. Winkler, C. Irwin, and J. Schachter.** 1989. Differences in biological maturation, sexual behavior, and sexually transmitted disease between adolescents with and without cervical intraepithelial neoplasia. *J. Pediatr.* **115:**487–493.
18. **Padian, N.** 1990. Heterosexual transmission: infectivity and risk. *In* N. J. Alexander, H. L. Gabelnick, and J. M. Spieler (ed.), *Heterosexual Transmission of AIDS*. Wiley-Liss, New York.
19. **Padian, N., P. J. Hitchcock, R. E. Fullilove, V. Kohlstadt, R. Brunham, and the NIAID**

Study Group on Integrated Behavioral Research for Prevention and Control of STDs. 1991. Part I: issues in defining behavioral risk factors and their distribution. Report of the NIAID Study Group on Integrated Behavioral Research for Prevention and Control of Sexually Transmitted Diseases. *Sex. Transm. Dis.* **17:**200–210.

20. **Padian, N., L. Marquis, D. Francis, R. Anderson, G. Ritherford, P. O'Malley, and W. Winkelstein.** 1987. Male-to-female transmission of human immunodeficiency virus. *J. Am. Med. Assoc.* **258:**788–790.
21. **Padian, N., S. Shiboski, and N. Jewell.** 1990. The effect of number of exposures on the risk of heterosexual HIV transmission. *J. Infect. Dis.* **161:**883–888.
22. **Potterat, J., R. Rothenberg, D. Woodhouse, J. Muth, C. Pratts, and J. Fogle.** 1985. Gonorrhea as a social disease. *Sex. Transm. Dis.* **12:**25–32.
23. **Rothenberg, R.** 1983. The geography of gonorrhea. Empirical demonstration of core group transmission. *Am. J. Epidemiol.* **117:**688–694.
24. **Rothenberg, R.** 1990. Analytic approaches to the epidemiology of sexually transmitted diseases, p. 37–42. *In* K. Holmes, P.-A. Mardh, P. Sparling, P. Wiesner, W. Cates, Jr., S. Lemon, and W. Stamm (ed.), *Sexually Transmitted Diseases,* 2nd ed. McGraw-Hill Book Co., New York.
25. **Susser, M.** 1973. *Causal Thinking in the Health Sciences. Concepts and Strategies of Epidemiology.* Oxford University Press, New York.
26. **Washington, A., S. Gove, J. Schachter, and R. Sweet.** 1985. Oral contraceptives, Chlamydia trachomatis infection, and pelvic inflammatory disease. A word of caution about protection. *J. Am. Med. Assoc.* **253:**2246–2250.
27. **Washington, A. E.** 1984. Risk, health promotion, disease intervention and sexually transmitted diseases. *Mobius* **4:**26–32.
28. **Winkelstein, W., D. Lyman, N. Padian, R. Grant, M. Samuel, J. Wiley, R. Anderson, W. Lang, J. Riggs, and J. Levy.** 1986. The San Francisco Men's Health Study. I. Sexual practices and risk of infection by the human immunodeficiency virus. *J. Am. Med. Assoc.* **257:**321–325.
29. **Wolner-Hanssen, P., D. Eschenbach, J. Paavonen, C. Stevens, N. Kiviat, C. Critchlow, T. DeRousen, L. Koutsky, and K. Holmes.** 1990. Association between vaginal douching and acute pelvic inflammatory disease. *J. Am. Med. Assoc.* **263:**1936–1941.

Age, Gender, and Sexual Risk Behaviors for Sexually Transmitted Diseases in the United States

Anke A. Ehrhardt and Judith N. Wasserheit

PRINCIPLES OF SEXUAL BEHAVIOR OVER THE LIFE CYCLE: EFFECTS OF AGE AND GENDER

Sexuality is an integral part of most people's lives. Sexual behavior is common, frequently practiced by many, and varies by gender and age. While one of the central functions of sexual behavior is reproduction, sexuality is hardly limited or tied to pregnancy and offspring. In fact, the acts of sexual behavior for pleasure, intimacy, and bonding far outnumber those conducted for reasons of achieving pregnancy. Thus, sexual behavior is not solely linked to the reproductive years but is part of many people's lives from childhood to death.

Sexual behavior varies from individual to individual, by social context, and within different societies. One of the critical categories of differentiation is gender. Girls, boys, women, and men not only have different bodies, they are also socialized into different gender roles that significantly influence their sexual behavior. Both age and gender influence physical characteristics and social roles that, in turn, affect the expression of sexual behavior patterns.

Most people establish their sexual identity as heterosexual, bisexual, or homosexual during their adolescent years, although it is not unusual for a person to change his or her sexual orientation during life (A. A. Ehrhardt and R. H. Remien, *in* R. E. McAnarney, D. P. Orr, and G. D. Comerci, ed., *Textbook of Adolescent Medicine*, in press).

Sexual behavior is not only linked to reproduction and to expressions of pleasure and love but also may transmit disease. To avoid unwanted pregnancies, most people in industrialized countries make contraceptive methods part of their lives throughout their reproductive years. Prevention and treatment of sexually transmitted diseases (STDs) require a similar degree of attention, education, and integration into many people's sexual behavior.

The goal of this chapter is to outline some of the important principles of sexual behavior throughout the life cycle, particularly in regard to risk behavior for disease. At the same time, we also summarize physiological risk factors for STDs within the context of age and gender. Finally, we present a synthesis of sexual risk

Anke A. Ehrhardt – HIV Center for Clinical and Behavioral Studies, New York State Psychiatric Institute, and Department of Psychiatry, College of Physicians and Surgeons, Columbia University, New York, New York 10032. *Judith N. Wasserheit* – Sexually Transmitted Diseases Branch, Division of Allergy and Infectious Diseases, National Institute of Allergy and Infectious Diseases, Bethesda, Maryland 20892.

behaviors and physiological changes that predispose to STDs and their implications for intervention.

Early and Middle Childhood

Our society puts a great value on separating infants and, subsequently, children on the basis of gender. Names, colors of baby clothes, and toys are gender dimorphic. By age 18 months to 2 years, children have usually learned that they belong to the category of either girls or boys. By the age of 3 or 4 years, children have firmly established a gender identity that is continuously solidified and reinforced throughout childhood and adolescence. Once gender identity is established, it becomes an integral part of a person's personality and usually is not questioned. In the normal course of events, gender assignment at birth is in congruence with prenatal biological development. However, even in children with prenatal genetic or hormonal anomalies, gender identity is strongly dependent on postnatal rearing, demonstrating the strong effects of learning and social reinforcement (22, 65). The expression of one's gender identity is reflected in gender-role behavior or gender-specific behavior, often referred to as masculine or feminine. Sex differences in behavior are more variable than gender identity; they may change with one's age, social contacts, or cultural norms (56).

In a recent article, Maccoby (55) examined the profound effect of gender on girls' and boys' play behavior and encounters with each other during the prepubertal years. Her observations and insights into the effect of gender on the behavior of young children are relevant here, since they may be seen as roots for some of the sociosexual encounters that occur among adolescents and that now come under scrutiny because they may be barriers to modification of sexual risk behavior.

Maccoby (55) examined the significance of gender in the children's social groupings. From preschool years until puberty, children prefer same-sex play groups. Maccoby and Jacklin (57) described a longitudinal study in which they were able to document that among nursery school children of 4.5 years of age, children spent three times as much time with peers of the same sex. By age 6.5 years, the ratio of same-sex to opposite-sex play time had increased to 11 to 1. One of the likely explanations for this striking phenomenon is the difference in play behavior between boys and girls, with boys tending to engage in more rough-and-tumble, body-contact play than girls. This difference in play style has profound effects on many different social contexts. Maccoby (55) reviewed the observation by Charlesworth and Dzur (13) of children who needed to set up a cooperative system to view a movie through a movie viewer with a one-eye eyepiece. There were four children in each group, and only one child could view the movie at a time. Both boys' and girls' groups managed to achieve cooperation. However, the techniques used were different. In both cases, one child emerged as the dominant one. In boys' groups, dominant boys more often used the technique of shouldering other boys out of the way, while dominant girls used verbal persuasion. It is probably important that the physical dominance behavior of boys was not hostile behavior but was, rather, connected with expressed fun and pleasure. The same experiment on mixed groups of two boys and two girls resulted in the boys achieving the dominant role and the girls occupying helping positions. The verbal persuasion that worked for girls with other girls was not effective with boys.

Jacklin and Maccoby (39) also found that girls' attempts to influence boys often were not very effective even at the early age of 33 months. In mixed-sex groups, if one child expressed an undesirable behavior toward another child such as taking a toy away, a girl would respond to a boy's verbal request and stop, while in the opposite interaction, a girl's vocal prohibition would have no effect on the boy's behavior.

Maccoby's review and interpretation of the strong early effect of gender on social behavior may be relevant in the context of verbal interactions between adolescent boys and girls who engage in sexual encounters. Gender roles obviously are important modifiers in how sexual encounters are negotiated and who determines which sexual practices will prevail.

Generally, in adolescence, girls become more feminine than during childhood and boys more masculine. This has been referred to as the "intensification of gender-related role expectations" during early adolescence (37). Tomboys become more feminine, and the stress of being attractive for dating may lead to more anxiety. Indeed, Rosenberg and Simmons (77) showed that adolescent girls express more anxiety and try to avoid negative reactions from others more than boys do. This sex difference was found to increase with older adolescents.

Puberty and adolescence are the transition to adult gender roles. Some of the childhood sex-dimorphic play gives way to adolescent interests, in particular to sexual interests and activities.

The development of sexuality also starts long before puberty. In fact, reactions of the sex organs occur from infancy on; e.g., erection of the penis has been observed from birth (31). While these erections initially seem to be largely associated with other bodily functions, they subsequently become part of the overall exploration of the body and of pleasant sensation, resulting in masturbation during childhood. Both boys and girls masturbate long before puberty and react in many cases with orgasmlike responses. Children also engage in sexuality with each other throughout the first decade, and the psychoanalytic concept of a sexually latent period between the ages of 5 to 6 years and puberty is in contrast to the empirical evidence (80).

While sexual activities in childhood are exploratory and sporadic, in adolescence sexual concerns and behavior become a major part of everyday life and become linked to falling in love, erotic imagery, and involvement with another person (63).

While sexual exploratory play between same-age children is normative, sexual behavior between adults and children is not. Especially if such sexual encounters involve force by an older person, the effect can be traumatic and may have a variety of short-term and long-term effects. Sexual abuse by strangers or family members has recently received much attention in the media in the United States. We lack comprehensive studies on community-based samples that would enable us to make a firm statement regarding the extent of emotional injury and long-term impact on the subsequent psychosexual development of sexually abused children. From clinical studies, it appears that the extent of the trauma varies and that the effects are nonspecific and may influence later achievement or sexual, emotional, or substance abuse behavior (8).

Since children explore their bodies by themselves and with each other from infancy on, sex education should ideally be taught at all levels in an age-appropriate way. Such education or communication with children should go on at home and at school. Children are curious about the anatomy of their bodies and about pregnancy and childbirth and should be taught this information as part of their routine curriculum. In addition, middle childhood may be an ideal time to have children learn about gender differences in verbal expression, negotiation, and emotional needs. This may set the stage for greater understanding between adolescent girls and boys and may pave the way for increased shared responsibility in contraception and disease prevention once sexual intercourse has been initiated.

Adolescence

Adolescence is the transition between childhood and adulthood and extends roughly through the entire second decade. Within the context of prevention of STDs and human immunodeficiency virus (HIV) infection, adolescence is the time when behavior patterns associated with disease transmission become established. It is the period of life when many individuals begin to have sexual relations and may become involved in so-called risk behavior for STDs and HIV infection. Adolescents also frequently begin to experiment with drugs, alcohol, cigarettes, and, in some cases, intravenous drugs.

To design the most appropriate and timely prevention programs, it is important to review some of the fundamental principles of adolescent development.

Early adolescence

Since the 1970s (32), early adolescence has been defined as a distinctive phase during which the most dramatic changes occur in a young person's physiology, physical appearance, cognitive development, and psychosexual and emotional functioning. In fact, early adolescence has been described as possibly the most dramatic transition phase in a person's life history, with striking changes only comparable to infancy (53).

Hamburg (32) argued that early adolescence (approximately 12 to 15 years of age) is a time of great stress and vulnerability. She defined the field when she argued,

> Early adolescence is clearly a critical period of development that involves the negotiation of unique, psychological, and social demands. The adaptive challenge posed by *superimposed* tasks in this era has been underestimated.

Since then, early adolescence has become an accepted, distinct phase of development. Some researchers distinguish two (early versus middle/late adolescence) or three phases of adolescent development: early, 10 to 14 years; middle, 15 to 16 years; late, 17 to 20 years (61). The age ranges may differ, but there is consensus that adolescence may be divided into different phases with different developmental events.

Early adolescence has been singled out as a particularly critical period not only because of the major biological and emotional changes within the individual but also because major changes occur in the environment at the same time. Adults' expectations and reactions to the adolescent become different, and institutional transitions are the norm, such as a shift from elementary school to junior high school.

Early adolescents vary greatly regarding timing of pubertal events, and society's reactions vary in response. Rather than conceptualizing pubertal events as determining behavioral response, many researchers have taken an interactive or reciprocal approach in which biological markers may affect behavior and behavior and societal norms may influence biological changes (21). Endocrine functioning and physical maturity have been shown to be influenced by stress and other psychosocial factors (5, 75), and pubertal events, such as menarche in girls, may have marked effects on a girl's psychosexual and emotional responsiveness (6).

This early phase of transition from childhood to adolescence is seen as a time of plasticity and vulnerability. The major aspects of developmental change that have been delineated for early adolescents are pubertal events, psychosexual development, cognitive changes, and emotional and personality functioning. Early adolescence is differentiated from middle adolescence, the time when some of the major physical changes occur. Middle adolescents are preoccupied with independence issues and with finding their own identity. Late adolescents (17 years and older) typically have attained their adult body habitus, and many of them have experienced love and sexual relations, have a greater sense of their own individuality, and are well on their way to making a transition to adulthood (48).

Early adolescence has critical importance for the prevention of STD and HIV infection, since this is the phase during which many adolescents develop coping strategies.

Physical development plays a key role in early adolescence. In fact, as Hamburg (32) stated, and as has since been documented by many other researchers, psychological development is closely connected to pubertal maturation and body characteristics (5).

In addition to the adolescent's immediate world, the larger societal context shapes particular generations and cohorts of adolescents (70). One wonders whether one of the critical features for the cohort of the late 1980s and 1990s will be HIV, STDs, and drugs.

Pubertal changes

Several excellent reviews have described the somatic and hormonal changes of puberty (46, 63, 93, 94). The physical changes are mediated at four levels of hormonal control. According to current knowledge, the highest level of control takes place in the hypothalamus, influencing the next level, the pituitary gland, which in turn regulates the gonads (ovaries and testes) and the adrenal gland to release the so-called sex hormones that mediate most of the physical changes of puberty.

The specific features of puberty are predictable and uniform enough between individuals to form a standard pattern, although onset and sequence of pubertal events vary greatly between and within the sexes. Therefore, it is customary to report the timing of pubertal events in ranges that usually span several years. The onset of external manifestations of puberty is reported as 8.5 to 13 years for girls and 9.5 to 15 years for boys (46). Breast development in girls is typically the first sign, followed by pubic hair and menarche. For boys, puberty is signaled by testicular growth and scrotal changes, followed by pubic hair and penile growth. The onset of puberty is consistently earlier in girls than in boys, with a time lag of about 2 years (50) based on the beginning of the height spurt. If one compares breast budding with the onset of testicular growth, the sex difference is only 6 months.

It has been shown that the timing as well as the nature of puberty has psychological significance. For instance, some studies have shown that early-maturing boys have a slight advantage in personality development (62). They tend to be more popular, more relaxed, more good-natured, and generally more poised. In contrast, late-maturing boys are less self-confident and more anxious (44, 68, 100). This picture is far less consistent in girls; the differences between early and late maturers seem less marked and vary according to age, with early maturation being sometimes an advantage and sometimes a disadvantage (45).

The reason for the significance of timing in puberty in personality development is not entirely understood, although it makes good sense that the superiority of athletic abilities in boys who undergo early puberty, associated with muscular physique, plays an important part (62, 92). Girls' reactions to early or late puberty are more complex and may be related to self-consciousness resulting from looking different before any of their peers do, moodiness associated with the menstrual cycle, and having to deal with sexuality at an early age.

It is also possible that temporal trends in onset of puberty are a factor in the decreasing age of coital debut and that this, in turn, may facilitate the spread of STDs (see below). Over the last 150 years, onset of puberty (specifically assessed by age of menarche) has continually become earlier. Improvement of environmental conditions, chiefly nutritional, is an important factor and explains some differences between industrialized and developing countries, although typically age of menarche varies within countries among poor, undernourished versus well-off adolescents (95). In addition to nutritional factors, racial differences may contribute to variations of onset of puberty; e.g., menarche now occurs at 12.77 $\pm$ 1.0 years of age in the United States; it occurs about 0.1 year earlier in black children and 0.1 year later in whites (78).

Sexual behavior during adolescence

An acceleration of timing in achieving the various sexual milestones during adolescence has been observed in many Western societies over the last 30 years (81), and the reactions of authorities in different societies have varied. Usually in this country the reactions toward adolescent sexuality are negative, with an expressed hope or implied message that it would be best for adolescents to completely abstain from sexual behavior in order not to experience potentially negative consequences, such as unwanted pregnancies, STDs, and HIV infection. The opposite view, that sexual behavior needs to be learned like any other behavior, is expressed much more seldom. Rutter (81) addresses this issue and points to the fact that sexual competence is not governed by some innate mechanism but needs to be learned. Indeed, Schofield (84) in his general population study in Britain found that one-third of the boys and one-half of the girls did not like their first experience of sexual intercourse. Schofield (85) did a follow-up study on the same group and found that people who first experienced sexual intercourse after age 21 were less likely to enjoy it than those who first experienced it in their teens. Schofield also found that sexual intercourse was most pleasurable within the context of a loving relationship.

Although the right time for adolescents to experience sexual intercourse may be controversial, almost everyone agrees that early adolescence is too young for most youths to engage in sociosexual encounters because these may often be stressful and difficult to cope with.

Adolescent sexual behavior is usually assessed by age of first sexual intercourse and by patterns of sexual practices and number of partners. Findings of recent national surveys (11, 64) provide estimates of average age of initiation of sexual intercourse in the United States. Most adolescents report having engaged in sexual intercourse by age 19, with a higher percentage of males than females at any age and with ethnic differences of earlier intercourse among black compared with white teenagers.

The stereotype of adolescents being nondiscriminate and "highly sexual" is not supported by existing data. Many adolescents have only one partner. Young men tend to have more partners than young women, but even for them the most common pattern for adolescents can be described as "serial monogamy" (88) rather than a pattern of simultaneous affairs with more than one partner. Furthermore, sexual intercourse for adolescents often occurs sporadically rather than on a regular basis. On the other hand, once sexual intercourse has been initiated, sexual activity is continued. Thus, it is uncommon that teens become completely abstinent once they have engaged in sexual intercourse.

While most adolescents initiate sexual intercourse during middle or late adolescence, there is a subgroup of teens who initiate sexual intercourse at a much younger age during early adolescence, a behavior that is often associated with multiple other problems, including substance abuse and leaving school (35). Obviously, this group is at particularly high risk of acquiring disease or having unwanted pregnancies. Further, it is believed that earlier age of onset of intercourse is associated with higher total numbers of lifetime sexual partners. However, we are lacking definitive evidence in this regard. Kinsey et al. (47) documented for adolescent males who started sexual behavior early a lifetime pattern of greater sexual activity than their peers who developed their sexuality at a later age. Sexual activity, however, may have been either within a single long-term relationship or with numerous partners (47). More recent data confirm that adolescents who initiate sexual intercourse earlier have higher numbers of partners than do those who postpone coital debut, but longitudinal information was not available to indicate whether this pattern was sustained beyond the adolescent period to result in higher numbers of lifetime partners (11).

Consistent contraceptive use among American adolescents is low and much less frequent in comparison with teens from other developed countries (43). Moreover, young teens are less likely to use contraception than older adolescents at first sexual intercourse. However, a recent comparison between the 1988 National Survey of Family Growth and 1982 data (25) reveals an encouraging increase of contraceptive use at first sexual intercourse among American teens. For instance, in 1982, 48% of sexually experienced women between 15 and 19 years of age used a contraceptive method at first intercourse, mainly condoms and withdrawal by their male partner. By 1988, the percentage was 65% for this age group, and the increase was almost entirely due to condom use. The increase in condom use was true for both poor and nonpoor teenagers and for black, white, and Hispanic adolescents. The most pronounced increase in condom use occurred among Hispanics, from 13% in 1982 to 42% in 1988.

These positive changes in condom use among teens have important implications for STD and HIV prevention efforts. They strengthen the argument that prevention can work even with a highly vulnerable group such as teens having their first sexual intercourse.

Young Adulthood (the Reproductive Years)

Our knowledge about the sexual behavior of adult American men and women is severely hampered by lack of recent survey data. However, based on available information from small-scale studies, we are able to identify some of the important characteristics of sexual behavior that may be relevant for the purpose of prevention strategies to combat STDs and HIV.

The transition from late adolescence to young adulthood is somewhere around age 19 to 20, when many young people move out of their family homes to go off to college, to take a job, or to get married. The age of first marriage in the United States has increased, and the age of first sexual intercourse has decreased, thus extending the duration of premarital sexual activity and partner change. Most people get married in their twenties but may be single again at a later point in their lives because of divorce (the first-marriage divorce rate in the United States is close to 50%) and widowhood. Thus, based on household survey data in 1988 (25), 50% of women between the ages of 15 and 44 were currently married and 13% were divorced, separated, or widowed, while 36% had never been married. In addition, one-third of all the women reported that they had cohabited at some point in their lives. Approximately two-thirds of all women who had ever had sexual intercourse had two or more sexual partners in their lifetime, with the highest proportion of women between the ages of 20 and 34. Thirty-four percent of women aged 18 to 19 and 50% of men in the same age group had had multiple partners during a 1-year period.

When people live in a coupled relationship (marriage or cohabitation), partner frequency drops and many restrict their sexual activity to the primary partner relationship at least for a while. Overall, partner frequency among Americans drops with age, with 5% of women and 13% of men aged 40 to 44 reporting multiple partners within 1 year. After the first 4 years of marriage, frequency of sexual intercourse drops, even among young people, and this is often attributed by the couples to children in the household, career demands, and making sexual interactions part of the routine (96).

Extramarital sex is practiced by both men and women and may be completely secretive or more or less acknowledged. This type of sexual behavior is often taboo and, according to opinion polls, is not deemed acceptable although it is practiced by many American men and women at work or away from home on trips (54). Therefore, extramarital relations need to receive special attention in education and prevention efforts. Since they are not acknowledged and are often practiced spontaneously and without preparation, they may lead to high-risk behavior for both the partners in casual sexual encounters and their primary relationships.

While we lack data on large sets of women and men on the measures they use to protect themselves against STDs and HIV, we have information on contraceptive use (25). In 1988, approximately 10% (compared with 12% in 1982) of women between 15 and 44 years of age risked an unintended pregnancy, i.e., did not use reversible methods of contraception and were not sterilized. Fifty-five percent of the women relied on a reversible birth control method, e.g., the pill, the intrauterine device, withdrawal, and condoms, while 35% relied on contraceptive sterilization (male and female procedures). Sterilization increases with age and lower socioeconomic status. More poor women rely on being sterilized as their contraceptive method rather than having a partner who has had a vasectomy. Also, compared with more affluent women, poor women more frequently use no contraception at all (15% versus 8%). In 1988, 40% of births were unintended, being either mistimed or unwanted. Thus, contraceptive use in the United States is still far from the desired level. This has important implications for disease prevention. Obviously, many Americans are sexually active without protection against STDs and HIV.

So far, we have discussed sexual behavior within the context of exclusively heterosexual relations. Homosexual men are at higher risk for certain STDs (74) and so far in industrialized countries have been disproportionately affected by HIV. While gay men (at least the predominantly white urban groups) have dramatically changed their high-risk sexual behavior (64), many women and men are not exclusively heterosexual or homosexual (26) and may not use protection outside their primary partnership and outside their predominant sexual orientation (heterosexual or homosexual). For instance, lesbian women who occasionally have sexual intercourse with men may see themselves at low risk because of their sexual identity rather than their sexual practices (A. A. Ehrhardt, unpublished data). Overall, lesbian women have been neglected in public health efforts of prevention against STDs and HIV. This is based on an erroneous assumption that sexual orientation as homosexual or heterosexual is a dichotomy that does not overlap.

Both men and women, and especially women, often report dramatic changes in their sexual identity and may in midlife enter a couple relationship with a person of their own sex after years of heterosexual identity, activity, and marriage. Lesbian women have not been targeted for health care and prevention because they are at lower risk for male-transmitted STDs. However, this is only true if they engage exclusively in homosexual behavior. In addition, lesbian women often appear to be discriminated against because of insensitive and inappropriate management by the medical profession and consequently may avoid seeking routine care.

Special STD and HIV prevention efforts also have to be designed for those who have had the traumatic experience of rape. Many more women than men are raped, but in prison men also frequently are assaulted. We obviously need special programs of education, prevention, and care for both women and men who are forced to engage in behavior that puts them at high risk for acquiring infection.

The Middle Years

Americans are becoming older and are engaging in sexual behavior during their advanced years. Our knowledge of sexual behavior among older Americans is particularly hampered by prejudice and an inordinate focus on youth and young people (54).

Both men and women undergo physiological and sociological changes that may affect their sexual interest, behavior, and performance. Between 45 and 55 years of age, most women undergo menopause, with significant hormonal changes that lead to cessation of menstrual bleeding. Hormonally, women stop cyclical production of estrogen and progesterone and end up with lower levels of sex hormones. Menopause may affect women to varying degrees and may make a woman more or less uncomfortable because of irregular bleeding and hot flashes. The lower levels of estrogen ultimately put women at risk for osteoporosis and account for decreased vaginal lubrication and decreased thickness of the vaginal epithelium.

Sexual interest in older women varies and cannot be fully explained by hormonal changes. Numerous older women lose their male partners, and for many a new partner may not be available or desirable. General physical health is obviously another important factor and may negatively influence sexual behavior. In a classic study of 100 women between the ages of 43 and 53, Neugarten (71) reported that two-thirds of the women described no effect of menopause on sexuality, with the other third being split, one-half attributing a positive effect to the end of pregnancy concerns and the other half judging sexuality as less important. In a small study of women over 50 years old, sexual interest remained high (4).

Some women complain about weaker orgasmic contractions that can be counterbalanced by extended foreplay. Vaginal dryness during sexual intercourse may be improved with a lubricant. Obviously, a vagina that is too dry can be injured by penile penetration and puts the woman at increased risk for transmission of STDs and HIV from an infected partner.

Middle-aged men also experience hormonal changes, especially a decrease in testosterone (19). It may take them longer to achieve erections, or they may experience sporadic impotence that may produce so much anxiety that some men begin to reduce or avoid sexual behavior. Others continue a very active sex life and compensate for any slowing down of their physiological responses. However, condom use may be avoided by some because it may be seen as an additional impediment to erectile performance and thus becomes an important issue for STD and HIV prevention.

Old Age (over 70)

People in their seventies, eighties, and nineties probably vary in their sexuality as much as younger people do. Life circumstances and physical health are of increasing importance in determining whether they engage in sexual behavior with another person. Our knowledge about sexuality in old people is extremely fragmentary (see reference 54 for one of the few reviews on this subject).

One of the isolated studies on this part of the population was conducted by J. Bretschneider and N. McCoy (paper read at the Sixth World Congress of Sexuality, Washington, D.C., 1983), who collected information on 102 women and 100 men between the ages of 80 and 102 years. This was a well-educated group who lived in different retirement facilities in California and were in good physical and mental health. Two-thirds of them had been married, with many more men than women still married at the time of the study. More men than women still masturbated, and 70% of the women and 38% of the men did not have sexual intercourse. More men than women who had sexual intercourse enjoyed it, while there had not been any difference regarding sexual enjoyment between men and women when they were younger. For both men and women there was a high correlation between sexual enjoyment in earlier years and in old age: those who had enjoyed sex when they were younger were more likely to do so in old age.

This study on old age shows what is true throughout the life cycle, i.e., sexual interest and behavior vary greatly in frequency, enjoyment, and sexual practice. Physiological and sociological factors affect both men and women in different ways. One cannot attribute changes in sexual behavior to any one main factor; rather, they have to be seen as the result of an interplay of different effects, partly hormonal and partly life experiential.

The great variability in sexual behavior makes it imperative that we tailor our prevention strategies for STDs and HIV infection to different patterns among men and women and are cognizant of the fact that to be effective we need specific programs that are aimed at the specific risk behaviors we want to change.

STDs FROM A DEVELOPMENTAL PERSPECTIVE

Just as changes in sexual behavior over the life cycle may affect transmission of STDs (including HIV infection) and development of sequelae, the normal sequence of physiological changes in the genital tract and age-related patterns of health behaviors influence these outcomes. In adolescence, these behavioral and biomedical factors act synergistically to dramatically increase the risk of sexually transmitted infections and their complications among sexually active individuals. Subsequently, however, these factors often contribute differentially. In the adult reproductive years, sexual and health behaviors may outweigh biological factors as determinants of disease incidence, while in the elderly, physiological changes with the potential to facilitate transmission of STDs including HIV are usually offset by behavioral patterns that are relatively protective.

Childhood and Adolescence

In the female, susceptibility to STDs and their sequelae is a function of a number of physiological factors, including the type of epithelial lining in the lower genital tract; the resident flora and acidity (pH) of the vagina; the characteristics of the cervical mucus; the patency of the endocervical canal; the phase of the menstrual cycle; and the immunological repertoire of the individual (14). During the cascade of developmental events that stretches from birth through adolescence, there are significant alterations in each of these.

The striking changes that occur in cellular morphology in the vagina and the cervix have a direct effect on the spectrum of STDs found at each stage of development. In the first several weeks of life, because of the residual effect of maternal estrogen, the vagina of the neonate is lined by stratified squamous epithelium similar to that of adults (38, 87). These cells are resistant to chlamydial and gonococcal infection but are susceptible to trichomoniasis and candidiasis. From about 1 month of age until menarche, the squamous epithelium is replaced by thin, atrophic columnar epithelium that supports chlamydial and gonococcal growth. Beginning with the estrogen stimulation associated with puberty, thicker, glycogen-containing stratified squamous epithelium again covers the vaginal vault and columnar epithelium is limited to the cervix.

The interface between these two types of epithelium is called the squamocolumnar junction, and age-related changes in its location may also influence susceptibility to STDs. During adolescence, this junction is often exposed on the surface of the cervix (the ectocervix). With aging, it usually migrates into the endocervical canal. Ectocervical columnar epithelium is referred to as the zone of ectopy, and because of the affinity of gonococci and chlamydiae for columnar cells, its size is believed to correlate with risk of cervical infection (20, 34, 38).

From infancy to adolescence, vaginal ecology shifts from a normal or endogenous flora dominated by enteric organisms to one in which lactobacilli are the most common species (18, 33). Over this same period, probably due to lactic acid production by the lactobacilli, vaginal fluid becomes more acidic, with a fall in pH from about 7.0 during childhood to the 4.0 to 4.5 range after puberty. This shift, together with lactobacillus production of hydrogen peroxide and other antibacterial products, inhibits the growth of some genital tract pathogens in vitro (60, 82). However, the clinical relevance of resident flora in susceptibility to STDs remains unclear. Gonococcal infection rates in women exposed to men with gonorrhea, for example, do not appear to vary with patterns of cervicovaginal flora (15).

Cervical mucus production, the third potential defense against infection, also fluctuates in response to hormonal changes from birth to adolescence. Paralleling the epithelial changes described above, cervical mucus is abundant through the first month of life and then relatively scant until puberty (58). Around puberty, high levels of estrogen stimulate copious mucus secretion, but in contrast to the mucus of older adolescents or adult women, this mucus is easily penetrable by organisms as well as by sperm. After menarche, a monthly cycle of mucus production is established, with maximal secretion and minimal viscosity during the periovulatory phase (midcycle) (97).

These changes in cervical mucus may affect transmission of STDs or development of sequelae in several ways. Perhaps most important, cervical mucus provides a functional barrier both against attachment of pathogens to epithelial surfaces and against ascent of organisms into the uterus and fallopian tubes. The former is probably facilitated by the lubricating effect of the mucus and by binding of organisms to carbohydrate complexes in the matrix (14). Mucus also appears to provide support for other defenses against infection, such as antibacterial enzymes, antibodies, and leukocytes (14, 15, 97).

Patency or opening of the endocervical canal occurs at approximately 9 or 10 years of age (30) and explains the dramatically increased risk of upper tract infection (pelvic inflammatory disease, or PID) observed in peripubertal girls with cervical infection compared with younger children. The penetrability of peripubertal cervical mucus mentioned above and immunological naivete are probably the major biological reasons for the higher incidence of PID in this group than in older adolescents and adult women.

Unfortunately, in the male, little is known about analogous physiological changes that might affect an individual's risk of STDs or their sequelae. For example, while the epithelial lining of the male urethra has been well characterized (16), we could find no data on developmental changes over the life cycle. Similarly, although a few investigators have examined the normal urethral flora in adolescent males (12), little information is available on normal flora at earlier ages or on the role of these organisms in protection against STDs. Finally, there is evidence that seminal and prostatic fluids contain factors with marked antibacterial activity (17, 24, 49, 59) but no understanding of when or how boys begin to exhibit significant levels of these factors in genital secretions. The dearth of data on developmental changes in the anus and rectum also limits discussion of biological risk factors for STDs associated with anal intercourse in homosexual men and heterosexual women.

One factor that does appear to alter risk of acquisition of STDs in males is circumcision. Most studies have not controlled for potentially confounding behavioral variables and therefore cannot be considered definitive. However, both in industrialized countries and in the developing world, lack of circumcision has been linked repeatedly to an increased risk of a broad spectrum of STDs including chancroid, syphilis, herpes, gonorrhea, penile warts, and HIV infection (2, 3). The biological mechanisms for these associations are not yet well understood but may include the tendency of the foreskin to serve as a reservoir for STD pathogens and the susceptibility of the nonkeratinized foreskin to trauma and secondary microbial invasion. The presence of a foreskin may also decrease detection of STDs, thereby increasing the likelihood both of complications and of additional transmission. It is likely that part of the STD risk associated with lack of circumcision can be circumvented by careful genital hygiene and self-examination. Yet the weight of the evidence suggests that the foreskin is also a site of biological vulnerability to STDs and that in communities in which there is a high population prevalence of infection, circumcision may have significant personal and public health benefits.

Health behaviors of children and adolescents often compound the impact of physiological factors on STD morbidity. Most children and many adolescents are unable to recognize or understand the significance of STD symptoms. Frequently, they either have no independent access to health care or are afraid of the consequences of utilizing care that is available. Instead, many self-medicate with inadequate or inappropriate antibiotic regimens obtained from friends. Those who do present for care often do not complete their therapy or comply with follow-up instructions (72).

Finally, sexual abuse of children or young adolescents may be more likely than rape of adult women to result in transmission of STDs (41, 42). This may be because penetration is more likely to be traumatic in children or because abuse is more commonly a repeated event.

Adulthood and the Reproductive Years

In women, during the adult reproductive years, physiological changes that affect risk of STDs are related primarily to the menstrual cycle, to pregnancy, and to contraceptive use. In men, few analogous changes are believed to occur during this period, but the dearth of data on males mentioned above pertains throughout the life cycle.

The menstrual cycle appears to influence risk of upper tract infection in women. Several studies suggest that symptomatic gonococcal or chlamydial PID occurs most frequently during the first week of the cycle (23, 91; L. Westrom, thesis, Studentlitteratur, Lund, Sweden, 1976). The reasons for this are poorly understood but may include the relative penetrability of the cervical mucus plug during menses and the reflux of potentially contaminated blood into the fallopian tubes, a phenomenon that often accompanies menstrual uterine contractions. In gonococcal infection, two other factors may be important. Iron, which is abundant in menstrual blood, may promote gonococcal growth. In addition, the type of gonococcus that causes tubal infection (transparent phenotype) proliferates at the cervix during menstruation (40).

Pregnancy is associated with immunological, anatomical, and microbiological changes that affect risk of STDs and their sequelae (10). Host defenses, for example, are normally suppressed during pregnancy, probably as a maternal adaptation to avoid immunological rejection of the fetus as a foreign body. Suppression increases with duration of pregnancy and appears to be mediated primarily by a decrease in the number and function of lymphocytes (9, 89). This immune suppression often affects the course of genital tract infections. It is thought to be responsible for the accelerated progression or expression of human papillomavirus (76, 83), the augmented frequency and severity of recurrences of genital herpes (herpes simplex virus) (7, 98), and the relatively benign course of syphilis (67) observed during pregnancy.

Gestational anatomical changes may increase susceptibility to cervicitis but tend to protect the upper tract from infection. Cervical infection may be facilitated by hormone-driven increases in the size of the zone of ectopy (86). Simultaneously, decreased penetrability of the cervical mucus plug (97) and obliteration of the uterine cavity by the growing fetus decrease the risk of PID. After week 16 of pregnancy, however, the fetal membranes rest over the internal cervical opening, and infection of these membranes (chorioamnionitis) increases in frequency.

The microbiological changes that occur during pregnancy may have evolved primarily to provide a safe cervicovaginal environment for the infant during delivery but may also protect the woman from acquisition of some STDs. In the lower genital tract, changes such as decreased pH, increased glycogen stores, and increased vascularity facilitate growth of lactobacilli and suppress growth of several other bacterial species, particularly anaerobes. As discussed above, products of lactobacilli inhibit growth of pathogens such as gonococci in vitro (82).

Finally, contraceptives are often important factors in altering risk of STDs during the reproductive years (29). Condoms and diaphragms serve as mechanical barriers to attachment of genital pathogens. Laboratory testing of spermicides indicates that compounds such as nonoxynol-9 can kill most sexually transmitted organisms, including gonococci, chlamydiae, treponemes, trichomonads, herpes simplex virus, and HIV (1, 29). Clinical studies of the efficacy of spermicides in prevention of STDs support these findings with respect to gonorrhea and chlamydia but have been inconclusive with respect to HIV (J. Kreiss, I. Ruminjo, E. Ngugi, P. Roberts, J. Ndinya-Achola, and F. Plummer, Vth International Conference on AIDS, Montreal, Quebec, Canada, abstr. MAO36, 1989). One issue may be that with very frequent use, spermicides may cause local inflammation and genital ulceration, possibly offsetting the decreased number of viable organisms with an increased likelihood of infection per organism.

Intrauterine devices and hormonal contraceptives influence risk of STDs and their sequelae principally via effects on host defenses (29). Users of intrauterine devices run a 1.5- to 2-fold-increased risk of PID compared with women who are not using contraceptives (28). This risk appears to be greatest around the time of insertion (51) and is due to contamination of the uterine cavity with cervicovaginal flora. Intrauterine devices may also impair uterine clearance mechanisms when organisms do breach the cervical barrier. Oral contraceptive pills may increase risk of cervical chlamydial infection by increasing the size of the zone of ectopy (34, 99). Oral contraceptive pills, however, appear to decrease both the frequency and severity of PID (79, 90, 101). Possible mechanisms for these protective effects include reduced penetrability of cervical mucus, reduced uterine contractions during menses, and alteration of immunological responses. The impact of injectable hormonal agents on STDs has not been examined systematically.

The Postmenopausal Years and Senescence

With aging beyond the reproductive years, hormonal changes in women and waning immune defenses in both sexes predispose to increased incidence and severity of genital tract infections. These increases are, however, largely theoretical and generally have not been reflected in studies of older populations. Probably the most important reason for this is that the sexual behaviors discussed above place individuals over 50 years of age at low risk of exposure to STD pathogens. The tendency of health care providers to omit testing for STDs in geriatric patients and the small number of studies of STDs in this age group may also contribute to this impression.

At menopause, a sharp decline in estrogen levels heralds atrophic changes in the vagina, with thinning of the epithelium, reduced lubrication, and narrowing and shortening of the vaginal canal (38, 66). These changes may be less pronounced in postmenopausal women who continue to be sexually active (52), but it is not clear whether level of sexual activity is modulated by discomfort secondary to senescent changes or whether degree of atrophy is modulated by sexual activity. Decreases in vascularity and glycogen content in the lower genital tract have been postulated to result in alterations of cervicovaginal flora in postmenopausal women, but most studies have failed to confirm major shifts (37, 73).

GENDER DIFFERENCES IN STDs

Gender not only influences sexual behaviors but also affects the efficiency of transmission of some STDs, the ease with which infection is detected, and, as discussed by Amaro and Gornemann (this volume), care-seeking behaviors.

Gender Differences in Transmission of STDs

Rigorous studies of transmission of STDs are scarce because they are difficult to perform both logistically and ethically. Available data, which are not definitive, suggest that transmission of STD pathogens that cause a discharge or reside in genital secretions (e.g., gonococci, chlamydiae, trichomonads, HIV) is generally more efficient from male to female than from female to male. Transmission of STD pathogens that cause genital ulcers or lesions (e.g., herpes simplex virus, treponemes, and *Haemophilus ducreyi*, the causative organism of chancroid) appears to be equally efficient between the sexes. In the former case, the more efficient transmission from male to female may be partly due to more extended contact with pathogens after sexual exposure among women with infected partners than among men with infected partners: if the male partner has one of these STDs, infected semen is deposited in the vagina and remains there following intercourse; in contrast, if the female partner is infected, the male's exposure to organisms is largely limited to the duration of coitus. It is also possible that the cervix is more easily infected than the urethra of the male. The absence of differential transmission in the latter case may be due to the facts that genital ulcer pathogens depend on small breaks in the epithelium to establish infection and that microtrauma probably occurs in both partners during vigorous sexual intercourse.

Gender Differences in Detection of STDs

Detection of STDs is frequently more difficult in women than in men. Symptoms, signs, and laboratory test results may all be less reliable in women. For anatomical reasons, for example, both abnormal discharge and painless genital lesions are more likely to go unnoticed in women than in men. Even traditionally painful syndromes like chancroid are frequently associated with milder symptoms in women.

Gender difference in the predictive value of clinical signs and of laboratory tests presents additional problems. While clinical diagnosis in the absence of laboratory testing is often useful in men with STDs and in women with genital lesions, the two most common syndromes in women, vaginitis and cervicitis, cannot be diagnosed reliably on clinical criteria alone. Furthermore, the large number and variety of cells and bacteria that are normally present in the vaginal vault reduce the sensitivity of methods such as Gram staining and fluorescent monoclonal antibody staining of lower tract specimens. Cultures of cervicovaginal secretions are also more likely than cultures of the male urethra to be uninterpretable because of contamination by resident nonpathogenic organisms.

Gender Differences in Health Care-Seeking Behaviors

Although overall, women are more likely than men to seek health care (36, 69), care for STDs appears to be an important exception for several reasons. As mentioned above, women infected with STDs are far more likely than men to be asymptomatic. When symptoms of STDs do occur, these are generally less obviously attributable to STDs in women than in men. Even among infected women who do interpret symptoms as potential cues to action, presentation to a public STD clinic may be so stigma laden that it is not considered a viable option. In many societies around the world, contracting an STD is considered a rite of passage to manhood for an adolescent boy or an insignificant nuisance for an older man but an extremely shameful occurrence for a young girl and her whole family.

Women also have health care alternatives that are not available to men. Many women who can afford to do so consult private gynecologists for symptoms of STDs. Too often in the past, these providers have had limited expertise, interest, and laboratory capability in this area and have failed to provide adequate counseling or partner notification. Another alternative has been use of over-the-counter douches or other intravaginal preparations as home remedies for symptoms of STDs. Unfortunately, their use often masks rather than cures infection, and since no specific diagnosis is made, partners are not notified. Recent studies also suggest that douching is linked to an increased incidence of upper tract infection, either because of incomplete eradication of pathogens or because organisms are forced up into the uterus by the pressure with which the douche is applied (102).

From an intervention standpoint, however, one might anticipate that it would be easier to motivate changes in health care behaviors among women than among men. Since the irreversible and potentially fatal consequences of STDs (e.g., infertility, ectopic pregnancy, cervical cancer, and adverse outcomes of pregnancy, see Chapter 1) disproportionately affect women and their infants, efforts to educate adolescents and young adults about the impact of STDs may elicit a greater change in behavior among women than among men.

IMPLICATIONS FOR INTERVENTIONS

Risk factors for STDs and HIV vary with age and gender. They consist of an increased vulnerability because of physiological characteristics or behavioral patterns. They may be compensatory (low behavioral risk and high physiological risk) or synergistic (high behavioral risk and high physiological risk). Strategies of prevention, intervention, and health care need to be tailored and specific rather than global and general to have the highest probability of impact. They also need to be interdisciplinary rather than designed and executed from a purely behavioral science, infectious disease, or public health perspective.

The following considerations are grouped by developmental phase and are research priorities rather than exhaustive recommendations.

Childhood

While exploratory sexual play behavior may potentially put a child at risk for trauma and infection, these problems are rare and therefore this behavior does not warrant any special attention.

On the other hand, sexual abuse by an adult requires diligent medical attention and preventive care for STDs and HIV, especially for the young girl around menarche when hormonal and genital tract changes put her at heightened risk for cervical infections and PID. In addition, the emotional trauma must be addressed in expert counseling to prevent subsequent behavioral problems.

We suggest that the highest priorities be given to the long-term tasks of (i) preventing risk behaviors that can result in acquiring STDs and HIV and (ii) developing effective health care behaviors. Childhood is an ideal time for establishing protective behavioral patterns that may have a strong modifying effect on risk behavior in later years. Since school children are a captive audience, the basics of risk prevention strategies can become a routine part of the mandatory educational curriculum. Ideally, all these efforts will be reinforced and coordinated both by parents at home and by society at large in messages communicated via magazines, radio, and television.

Since the onset of the AIDS epidemic, there has been a call for an AIDS prevention curriculum for kindergarten through high school, but this effort has been hampered by reluctance to discuss sexual matters with children at a young age. Usually, therefore, such curricula have either been reduced to information about diseases or remained completely undeveloped.

Instead, we propose the development of model programs that modify gender-related behaviors that lead to such sexual scripts as man, the seducer, ignoring the objections of his female partner, or of spontaneous, unplanned sexual encounters as the ultimate ideal of romance and eroticism. During childhood, such a program may consist of playful modifications of typical encounters between girls and boys and reinforcing improved communication and an understanding between the sexes. Subsequently, during adolescence, such "gender bending" should include role playing and training for sexual encounters that do not put the girl and boy at risk for STDs and HIV.

Adolescence

During the second decade of life, those who should receive the highest priority are early adolescents. Unprotected sexual intercourse during early adolescence puts young girls at high risk for STDs and unwanted pregnancy. Physiological vulnerability and emotional immaturity necessitate development of effective prevention programs that lead to delay of sexual intercourse, early and consistent use of barrier methods if intercourse is initiated, and health care behaviors that foster early detection of disease. Early and nonjudgmental sex education that includes the discussion of sexual behavior other than sexual intercourse, such as kissing and touching, is a cornerstone of such prevention efforts. In addition, we need interdisciplinary studies on young adolescent boys, a group that has been neglected in research on developmental factors predisposing to STDs.

The majority of teens during middle and late adolescence will be engaging in sexual intercourse. Therefore, a priority of prevention must be "safer sex," i.e., consistent condom use. In addition, we must integrate sexual behavior with health care behavior for STD and HIV prevention.

Adolescents also need to develop skills to select their partner, to negotiate safer sex, and to share the responsibility of protection against disease and pregnancy. Many of the basic skills are critical in nonsexual interactions and, ideally, will have been developed during childhood and can now be applied to sexual encounters.

Strategies for coordinated and comprehensive delivery of adolescent health care are needed. These should include evaluation of school-based and neighborhood clinics that assess basic health needs, including STD risk assessment, and provide contraceptives, STD care, certain vaccines such as hepatitis B vaccine in high-risk settings, and other general health screening such as hypertension and cholesterol screening.

Young Adulthood

In the United States, young men and women in their twenties have the highest partner frequency, especially before they get married or commit to a primary relationship. It is imperative, therefore, that knowledge about disease protection and contraceptive behavior is established early and reinforced at college, at work-training places, during athletic activities, and during routine health care.

Presently, one of the major obstacles to effective prevention is the sole reliance on condom use. While we need to enhance condom appeal for both men and women, we also need to develop new methods that are under a woman's control. Women with reluctant or resistant partners often do not have the power to enforce condom use.

We also need to test existing female-controlled methods of contraception (diaphragm, pill, etc.) for their efficacy in preventing STDs and HIV infection (89a), and when we obtain these data, we must make them widely available to family planning clinics, STD clinics, and the general public.

Young couples who are planning pregnancy and are not sure whether they have been exposed to STDs or HIV should be routinely counseled to be screened.

Health care providers, both for adolescents and for young adults, must learn to take sexual histories in a sensitive and nonjudgmental way that accepts sexual variety such as heterosexual or homosexual behavior and multiple partners or no partner at all. Subsequent care and referral should be tailored to clients' individual needs.

In considering pregnancy, both the woman and her partner (if available) should be informed about the risk of sexual behaviors for acquisition of STDs and the risk of STDs for adverse outcomes of the pregnancy.

The Middle Years

During the middle years as well as during young adulthood, preventive messages should be specific to the life circumstances of the individual. For instance, a couple that is mutually monogamous except for an occasional extramarital relationship should be encouraged to communicate with each other about this and to be consistent in practicing safer sex outside of the primary relationship.

Divorced and widowed women and men who start relationships with new partners may need to relearn negotiation for safer sex even if contraception is no longer of concern. This is particularly true if the woman or man has chosen sterilization and assumes erroneously that no protection is necessary.

It is essential that health care during this period include routine screening (at least through a careful sexual history and physical examination), education, and counseling.

Old Age

The most important issue for the phase of old age is knowledge and acceptance of the fact that sexual behavior continues and that appropriate screening for STDs and HIV should be a routine part of geriatric health care. In light of widespread denial of sexuality during senescence, it is often particularly difficult for both patient and provider to address sexual behavior, STDs, or HIV infection during this phase of the life cycle. Training programs and continuing medical education programs in geriatrics should actively attempt to correct this deficit.

In conclusion, for optimally productive STD and HIV research and optimally effective STD and HIV health care services, it is imperative to apply an interdisciplinary framework. Greater understanding of the interplay among sexual behavior, health care behavior, and biomedical factors that determine the host-pathogen interaction must be brought to bear if prevention and control of STDs and HIV infection are to become a reality. This goal will depend on the development of a team approach that includes both biomedical and behavioral scientists.

Acknowledgments. A.A.E. acknowledges support by grant no. 5-P50-MH43520 from the National Institute of Mental Health/National Institute of Drug Abuse.

LITERATURE CITED

1. **Alexander, N. J.** 1990. Sexual transmission of HIV: virus entry into male and female genital tract. *Fertil. Steril.* **54:**1–18.
2. **American Academy of Pediatrics.** 1989. Report of the Task Force on circumcision. *Pediatrics* **84:**388–391.
3. **Aral, S. O., and K. K. Holmes.** 1990. Epidemiology of sexual behavior and sexually transmitted diseases, p. 19–36. *In* K. K. Holmes, P.-A. Mardh, P. F. Sparling, P. J. Wiesner, W. Cates, Jr., S. M. Lemon, and W. E. Stamm (ed.), *Sexually Transmitted Diseases*. McGraw-Hill Book Co., New York.
4. **Brecher, E. M., and the editors of *Consumer Reports*.** 1984. *Love, Sex, and Aging*. Little, Brown & Co., Boston.
5. **Brooks-Gunn, J., and A. C. Petersen (ed.).** 1983. *Girls at Puberty: Biological, Psychological and Social Perspectives*. Plenum Press, New York.
6. **Brooks-Gunn, J., and D. N. Ruble.** 1983. The experience of menarche from a developmental perspective, p. 155–178. *In* J. Brooks-Gunn and A. C. Petersen (ed.), *Girls at Puberty: Biological, Psychological and Social Perspectives*. Plenum Press, New York.
7. **Brown, Z. A., L. A. Vontver, J. Benedetti, C. W. Critchlow, D. E. Hickok, C. J. Sells, S. Berry, and L. Corey.** 1985. Genital herpes in pregnancy: risk factors associated with recurrences and asymptomatic shedding. *Am. J. Obstet. Gynecol.* **153:**24–30.
8. **Browne, A., and D. Finkelhor.** 1986. Impact of child sexual abuse: a review of the research. *Psychol. Bull.* **99:**66–77.
9. **Brunham, R. C., K. K. Holmes, and J. E. Embree.** 1990. Sexually transmitted diseases in pregnancy, p. 771–801. *In* K. K. Holmes, P.-A. Mardh, P. F. Sparling, P. J. Wiesner, W. Cates, Jr., S. M. Lemon, and W. E. Stamm (ed.), *Sexually Transmitted Diseases*. McGraw-Hill Book Co., New York.
10. **Brunham, R. C., D. H. Martin, T. W. Hubbard, C.-C. Kuo, C. W. Critchlow, L. D. Cles, and D. A. Eschenbach.** 1983. Depression of the lymphocyte transformation response to microbial antigens and to phytohemagglutinin during pregnancy. *J. Clin. Invest.* **72:**1629–1638.
11. **Centers for Disease Control.** 1991. Premarital sexual experience among adolescent women—United States, 1970–1988. *Morbid. Mortal. Weekly Rep.* **39:**929–932.
12. **Chambers, C. V., M. A. Shafer, H. Adger, M. Ohm-Smith, S. G. Millstein, C. E. Irwin, Jr., J. Schachter, and R. Sweet.** 1987. Microflora of the urethra in adolescent boys: relationships to sexual activity and nongonococcal urethritis. *J. Pediatr.* **110:**314–321.
13. **Charlesworth, W. R., and C. Dzur.** 1987. Gender comparisons of preschoolers' behavior and resource utilization in group problem-solving. *Child Dev.* **58:**191–200.
14. **Cohen, M. S., J. R. Black, R. A. Proctor, and P. F. Sparling.** 1985. Host defenses and the vaginal mucosa. *Scand. J. Nephrol.* **86:**13–22.
15. **Cohen, M. S., R. D. Weber, and P.-A. Mardh.** 1990. Genitourinary mucosal defenses,

p. 117–127. *In* K. K. Holmes, P.-A. Mardh, P. F. Sparling, P. J. Wiesner, W. Cates, Jr., S. M. Lemon, and W. E. Stamm (ed.), *Sexually Transmitted Diseases*. McGraw-Hill Book Co., New York.

16. **Colleen, S. L.** 1982. The human urethral mucosa: an experimental study with emphasis on microbial attachment. *Scand. J. Urol. Nephrol. Suppl.* **68:**4–55.
17. **Colleen, S., P.-A. Mardh, and A. Schytz.** 1975. Magnesium and zinc in seminal fluid of healthy males and patients with non-acute prostatitis with and without gonorrhoea. *Scand. J. Urol. Nephrol.* **9:**192–197.
18. **Cruickshank, R., and A. Shaiman.** 1934. The biology of the vagina in the human subject. II. The bacterial flora and secretion of the vagina at various age-periods and their relation to glycogen in the vaginal epithelium. *J. Obstet. Gynaecol. Br. Emp.* **41:**208–226.
19. **Davidson, H. P., J. J. Chen, L. Crapo, G. D. Gray, W. J. Greenleaf, and J. A. Catania.** 1983. Hormonal changes and sexual functioning in aging men. *J. Clin. Endocrinol. Metab.* **57:**71–77.
20. **Draper, D. L., E. A. Donegan, J. James, R. L. Sweet, and G. F. Brooks.** 1980. Scanning electron microscopy of attachment of *Neisseria gonorrhoeae* colony phenotypes to surfaces of human genital epithelia. *Am. J. Obstet. Gynecol.* **138:**818–826.
21. **Ehrhardt, A. A.** 1984. The psychobiology of gender, p. 81–96. *In* A. S. Rossi (ed.), *Gender and the Life Course*. Aldine Publishing Co., Hawthorne, N.Y.
22. **Ehrhardt, A. A.** 1985. Gender differences: a biosocial perspective. *Psychol. Gender* **32:**37–57.
23. **Eschenbach, D. A., J. P. Harnisch, and K. K. Holmes.** 1977. Pathogenesis of acute pelvic inflammatory disease: role of contraception and other risk factors. *Am. J. Obstet. Gynecol.* **128:**838–850.
24. **Fair, W. R., J. Couch, and N. Wehner.** 1976. Prostatic antibacterial factor. *Urology* **7:**169–177.
25. **Forrest, J., and S. Singh.** 1990. The sexual and reproductive behavior of American women, 1982–1988. *Fam. Plann. Perspect.* **22:**206–214.
26. **Gagnon, J. H., S. Lindenbaum, J. L. Martin, R. M. May, J. Menken, C. F. Turner, and L. S. Zabin.** 1989. Trends in sexual behavior among persons of the same gender, p. 113–136. *In* C. F. Turner, H. G. Miller, and L. E. Moses (ed.), *AIDS, Sexual Behavior, and Intravenous Drug Use*. National Academy Press, Washington, D.C.
27. **Galask, R. P., and B. Larsen.** 1981. Identifying and treating genital tract infections in postmenopausal women. *Geriatrics* **36:**69–79.
28. **Grimes, D. A.** 1987. Intrauterine devices and pelvic inflammatory disease: recent developments. *Contraception* **36:**97–109.
29. **Grimes, D. A., and W. Cates, Jr.** 1990. Family planning and sexually transmitted diseases, p. 1087–1094. *In* K. K. Holmes, P.-A. Mardh, P. F. Sparling, P. J. Wiesner, W. Cates, Jr., S. M. Lemon, and W. E. Stamm (ed.), *Sexually Transmitted Diseases*. McGraw-Hill Book Co., New York.
30. **Gutman, L. T., and C. M. Wilfert.** 1990. Gonococcal diseases in infants and children, p. 803–810. *In* K. K. Holmes, P.-A. Mardh, P. F. Sparling, P. J. Wiesner, W. Cates, Jr., S. M. Lemon, and W. E. Stamm (ed.), *Sexually Transmitted Diseases*. McGraw-Hill Book Co., New York.
31. **Halverson, H. M.** 1940. Genital and sphincter behavior of the male infant. *J. Genet. Psychol.* **56:**95–136.
32. **Hamburg, B. A.** 1974. Early adolescence: a specific and stressful stage of the life cycle, p. 101–124. *In* G. V. Coelho, D. A. Hamburg, and J. E. Adams (ed.), *Coping and Adaptation*. Basic Books, New York.
33. **Hammerschlag, M. R., S. Alpert, I. Rosner, P. Thurston, D. Semine, D. McComb, and W. M. McCormack.** 1978. Microbiology of the vagina in children: normal and potentially pathogenic organisms. *Pediatrics* **62:**57–62.
34. **Harrison, H. R., M. Costin, J. B. Meder, L. M. Bownds, D. A. Sim, M. Lewis, and E. R. Alexander.** 1985. Cervical *Chlamydia trachomatis* infection in university women:

relationship to history, contraception, ectopy, and cervicitis. *Am. J. Obstet. Gynecol.* **153:**244–251.

35. **Hayes, C. D. (ed.).** 1987. *Risking the Future: Adolescent Sexuality, Pregnancy, and Childbearing,* vol. 1. National Academy Press, Washington, D.C.
36. **Hibbard, J. H., and C. R. Pope.** 1983. Gender roles, illness orientation and use of medical services. *Social Sci. Med.* **17:**129–137.
37. **Hill, J. P., and M. E. Lynch.** 1983. The intensification of gender-related role expectations during early adolescence, p. 201–228. *In* J. Brooks-Gunn and A. C. Petersen (ed.), *Girls at Puberty: Biological, Psychological and Social Perspectives.* Plenum Press, New York.
38. **Holmes, K. K.** 1990. Lower genital tract infections in women: cystitis, urethritis, vulvovaginitis, and cervicitis, p. 527–545. *In* K. K. Holmes, P.-A. Mardh, P. F. Sparling, P. J. Wiesner, W. Cates, Jr., S. M. Lemon, and W. E. Stamm (ed.), *Sexually Transmitted Diseases.* McGraw-Hill Book Co., New York.
39. **Jacklin, C. N., and E. E. Maccoby.** 1978. Social behavior at 33 months in same-sex and mixed-sex dyads. *Child Dev.* **49:**557–569.
40. **James, J., and J. Swanson.** 1978. Color opacity colonial variants of *Neisseria gonorrhoeae* and their relationship to the menstrual cycle, p. 338–343. *In* G. F. Brooks, E. C. Gotschlich, K. K. Holmes, W. D. Sawyer, and F. E. Young (ed.), *Immunobiology of Neisseria gonorrhoeae.* American Society for Microbiology, Washington, D.C.
41. **Jenny, C.** 1990. Child sexual abuse and STD, p. 895–900. *In* K. K. Holmes, P.-A. Mardh, P. F. Sparling, P. J. Wiesner, W. Cates, Jr., S. M. Lemon, and W. E. Stamm (ed.), *Sexually Transmitted Diseases.* McGraw-Hill Book Co., New York.
42. **Jenny, C., T. M. Hooton, A. Bowers, M. K. Copass, J. N. Krieger, S. L. Hillier, N. Kiviat, L. Corey, W. E. Stamm, and K. K. Holmes.** 1990. Sexually transmitted diseases in victims of rape. *N. Engl. J. Med.* **322:**713–716.
43. **Jones, E. F., J. D. Forrest, N. Goldman, S. K. Henshaw, R. Lincoln, J. I. Rosoff, C. F. Westoff, and D. Wulf.** 1985. Teenage pregnancy in developed countries: determinants and policy implications. *Fam. Plann. Perspect.* **17:**53–63.
44. **Jones, M. C., and M. Bayley.** 1950. Physical maturing among boys as related to behavior. *J. Educ. Psychol.* **41:**129–148.
45. **Jones, M. C., and P. H. Mussen.** 1958. Self-conceptions, motivations, and interpersonal attitudes of early and late maturing girls. *Child Dev.* **29:**491–501.
46. **Katchadourian, H.** 1977. *The Biology of Adolescence.* W. H. Freeman & Co., San Francisco.
47. **Kinsey, A. C., W. B. Pomeroy, and C. E. Martin.** 1948. *Sexual Behavior in the Human Male.* The W. B. Saunders Co., Philadelphia.
48. **Kreipe, R. E., and J. Strauss.** 1989. Adolescent medical disorders, behavior, and development, p. 98–142. *In* G. R. Adams, R. Montemayor, and T. P. Gullotta (ed.), *The Biology of Adolescent Behavior and Development.* Sage Publications, Newbury Park, Calif.
49. **Krieger, J. N., and M. F. Rein.** 1982. Canine prostatic secretions kill *Trichomonas vaginalis. Infect. Immun.* **37:**77–81.
50. **Kulin, H. E.** 1972. Endocrine changes at puberty, p. 1120–1122. *In* H. B. Barnett and A. H. Einhorn (ed.), *Pediatrics.* Appleton-Century-Crofts, New York.
51. **Lee, N. C., G. L. Rubin, H. W. Ory, and R. T. Burkman.** 1983. Type of intrauterine device and the risk of pelvic inflammatory disease. *Obstet. Gynecol.* **62:**1–6.
52. **Leiblum, S., G. Bachmann, E. Kemmann, D. Bolburn, and L. Swartzman.** 1983. Vaginal atrophy in the postmenopausal woman: the importance of sexual activity and hormones. *J. Am. Med. Assoc.* **249:**2195–2198.
53. **Lerner, R. M.** 1984. *On the Nature of Human Plasticity.* Cambridge University Press, New York.
54. **Luria, Z., S. Friedman, and M. D. Rose.** 1987. *Human Sexuality.* John Wiley & Sons, Inc., New York.
55. **Maccoby, E. E.** 1988. Gender as a social category. *Dev. Psychol.* **24:**755–765.
56. **Maccoby, E. E., and C. M. Jacklin.** 1974. *The Psychology of Sex Differences.* Stanford University Press, Stanford, Calif.
57. **Maccoby, E. E., and C. M. Jacklin.** 1987. Gender segregation in childhood, p. 239–287.

In E. H. Reese (ed.), *Advances in Child Development and Behavior*, vol. 20. Academic Press, Inc., New York.

58. **Madile, B. M.** 1976. The cervical epithelium from fetal age to adolescence. *Obstet. Gynecol.* **47:**536–539.
59. **Mardh, P.-A., S. Colleen, and J. Sylwan.** 1980. Inhibitory effect on the formation of chlamydial inclusions in McCoy cells by seminal fluid and some of its components. *Invest. Urol.* **17:**510–513.
60. **Mardh, P.-A., and L. V. Soltesz.** 1983. In vitro interactions between lactobacilli and other microorganisms occurring in the vaginal flora. *Scand. J. Infect. Dis. Suppl.* **40:**47–51.
61. **McAnarney, E. R.** 1985. Social maturation: a challenge for handicapped and chronically ill adolescents. *J. Adolesc. Health Care* **6:**90–101.
62. **McCandless, B. R.** 1960. Rate of development, body build, and personality. *Psychiatr. Res. Rep.* **13:**42–57.
63. **Meyer-Bahlburg, H. F. L.** 1980. Sexuality in early adolescence, p. 61–82. *In* B. B. Wolman and J. Money (ed.), *Handbook of Human Sexuality*. Prentice-Hall, Inc., Englewood Cliffs, N.J.
64. **Miller, H. G., C. F. Turner, and L. E. Moses (ed.).** 1990. *AIDS: The Second Decade*. National Academy Press, Washington, D.C.
65. **Money, J., and A. A. Ehrhardt.** 1972. *Man and Woman, Boy and Girl: the Differentiation and Dimorphism of Gender Identity from Conception to Maturity*. The Johns Hopkins University Press, Baltimore.
66. **Mooradian, A. D., and V. Greiff.** 1990. Sexuality in older women. *Arch. Intern. Med.* **150:**1033–1038.
67. **Moore, J. E.** 1923. Studies on the influence of pregnancy in syphilis. I. The course of syphilitic infection in pregnant women. *Johns Hopkins Med. Bull.* **34:**89–99.
68. **Mussen, P. H., and M. C. Jones.** 1957. Self-conceptions, motivations, and interpersonal attitudes of late- and early-maturing boys. *Child Dev.* **28:**243–256.
69. **Neighbors, H. W., and C. S. Howard.** 1987. Sex differences in professional help seeking among adult Black Americans. *Am. J. Community Psychol.* **15:**403–417.
70. **Nesselroade, J. R., and P. B. Baltes.** 1974. Adolescent personality development and historical change: 1970–1972. *Monographs of the Society for Research in Child Development*, 39 (1, serial no. 154).
71. **Neugarten, B. L.** 1963. Women's attitudes towards the menopause. *Vita Hum.* **6:**140–153.
72. **O'Reilly, K. R., and S. O. Aral.** 1985. Adolescence and sexual behavior: trends and implications for STD. *J. Adolesc. Health Care* **6:**262–270.
73. **Osborne, N. G., R. C. Wright, and L. Grubin.** 1979. Genital bacteriology: a comparative study of premenopausal women with postmenopausal women. *Am. J. Obstet. Gynecol.* **135:**195–198.
74. **Ostrow, D. G.** 1990. Homosexual behavior and sexually transmitted diseases, p. 61–69. *In* K. K. Holmes, P.-A. Mardh, P. F. Sparling, P. J. Wiesner, W. Cates, Jr., S. M. Lemon, and W. E. Stamm (ed.), *Sexually Transmitted Diseases*. McGraw-Hill Book Co., New York.
75. **Petersen, A. C., and B. Taylor.** 1980. The biological approach to adolescence, p. 117–155. *In* J. Adelson (ed.), *Handbook of Adolescent Psychology*. John Wiley & Sons, Inc., New York.
76. **Rando, R. F., S. Lindheim, L. Hasty, T. V. Sedlacek, M. Woodland, and C. Eder.** 1989. Increased frequency of detection of human papillomavirus deoxyribonucleic acid in exfoliated cervical cells during pregnancy. *Am. J. Obstet. Gynecol.* **161:**50–55.
77. **Rosenberg, F. R., and R. G. Simmons.** 1975. Sex differences in the self-concept during adolescence. *Sex Roles* **1:**147–160.
78. **Rosenfeld, R. L.** 1982. The ovary and female sexual maturation, p. 217–268. *In* S. A. Kaplan (ed.), *Clinical Pediatric and Adolescent Endocrinology*. The W. B. Saunders Co., Philadelphia.
79. **Rubin, G. L., H. W. Ory, and P. M. Layde.** 1982. Oral contraceptives and pelvic inflammatory disease. *Am. J. Obstet. Gynecol.* **144:**630–635.
80. **Rutter, M.** 1971. Normal psychosexual development. *J. Child Psychol. Psychiatry* **11:**259–283.

81. **Rutter, M.** 1980. Psychosexual development, p. 322–339. *In* M. Rutter (ed.), *Scientific Foundations of Developmental Psychiatry*. Heinemann Medical, London.
82. **Saigh, J. H., C. C. Sanders, and W. E. Sanders, Jr.** 1978. Inhibition of *Neisseria gonorrhoeae* by aerobic and facultatively anaerobic components of the endocervical flora: evidence for a protective effect against infection. *Infect. Immun.* **19:**704–710.
83. **Schneider, A., M. Hotz, and L. Gissmann.** 1987. Increased prevalence of human papillomaviruses in the lower genital tract of pregnant women. *Int. J. Cancer* **40:**198–201.
84. **Schofield, M.** 1965. *The Sexual Behaviour of Young People*. Longmans, London.
85. **Schofield, M.** 1973. *The Sexual Behaviour of Young Adults*. Allen Lane, London.
86. **Singer, A.** 1975. The uterine cervix from adolescence to the menopause. *Br. J. Obstet. Gynaecol.* **82:**81–99.
87. **Singleton, A. F.** 1980. Vaginal discharge in children and adolescents. *Clin. Pediatr.* **19:**799–804.
88. **Sorenson, R. C.** 1973. *Adolescent Sexuality in Contemporary America*. World Publishing Co., New York.
89. **Sridama, V., F. Pacini, S. L. Yang, A. Moawad, M. Reilly, and L. J. DeGroot.** 1982. Decreased levels of helper T cells. A possible cause of immunodeficiency in pregnancy. *N. Engl. J. Med.* **307:**352–356.
89a. **Stein, Z. A.** 1990. HIV prevention: the need for methods women can use. *Am. J. Public Health* **80:**460–462.
90. **Svensson, L., and L. Westrom.** 1984. Contraceptives and acute salpingitis. *J. Am. Med. Assoc.* **251:**2553–2555.
91. **Sweet, R. L., M. Blankfort-Doyle, M. O. Robbie, and J. Schachter.** 1986. The occurrence of chlamydial and gonococcal salpingitis during the menstrual cycle. *J. Am. Med. Assoc.* **255:**2062–2064.
92. **Tanner, J. M.** 1962. *Growth at Adolescence*, 2nd ed. Blackwell Scientific Publications Ltd., Oxford.
93. **Tanner, J. M.** 1970. Physical growth, p. 77–155. *In* P. H. Mussen (ed.), *Carmichael's Manual of Child Psychology*, 3rd ed., vol. 1. John Wiley & Sons, Inc., New York.
94. **Tanner, J. M.** 1974. Sequence and tempo in the somatic changes in puberty, p. 448–470. *In* M. M. Grumbach, G. D. Grave, and F. E. Mayer (ed.), *The Control of the Onset of Puberty*. John Wiley & Sons, Inc., New York.
95. **Tanner, J. M., and P. B. Eveleth.** 1975. Variability between populations in growth and development at puberty, p. 256–273. *In* S. R. Berenberg (ed.), *Puberty*. H. E. Stenfert Kroese B.V., Leiden.
96. **Udry, J. R.** 1980. Changes in the frequency of marital intercourse from panel data. *J. Sex. Behav.* **9:**319–325.
97. **Vickery, B. H., and J. P. Bennett.** The cervix and its secretion in mammals. *Physiol. Rev.* **48:**135–154.
98. **Vontver, L. A., D. E. Hickok, Z. A. Brown, L. Reid, and L. Corey.** 1982. Recurrent genital herpes simplex virus infection in pregnancy: infant outcome and frequency as asymptomatic recurrences. *Am. J. Obstet. Gynecol.* **143:**75–84.
99. **Washington, A. E., S. Gove, J. Schachter, and R. L. Sweet.** 1985. Oral contraceptives, *Chlamydia trachomatis* infection and pelvic inflammatory disease. *J. Am. Med. Assoc.* **253:**2246–2250.
100. **Weatherley, D.** 1964. Self-perceived rate of physical maturation and personality in late adolescence. *Child Dev.* **35:**1197–1210.
101. **Wolner-Hanssen, P.** 1986. Oral contraceptive use modifies the manifestations of pelvic inflammatory disease. *Br. J. Obstet. Gynaecol.* **93:**619–624.
102. **Wolner-Hanssen, P., D. A. Eschenbach, J. Paavonen, C. E. Stevens, N. B. Kiviat, C. Critchlow, T. DeRouen, L. Koutsky, and K. K. Holmes.** 1990. Association between vaginal douching and acute pelvic inflammatory disease. *J. Am. Med. Assoc.* **263:**1936–1941.

Sexual Behaviors: Temporal and Cross-Cultural Trends

Manuel Carballo, Oussama Tawil, and King Holmes

The emergence of human immunodeficiency virus (HIV) and AIDS as a global pandemic has highlighted, perhaps more so than any other recent communicable disease, the need for public health strategies to be based on up-to-date knowledge of the behaviors that underlie disease transmission. In HIV and AIDS, sexual transmission of the virus has become the most common, if not the most efficient, mode, and information on patterns of sexual behavior is being increasingly sought. The fact that the transmissibility of HIV is accentuated in individuals with other sexually transmitted infections (see Brunham and Ronald, this volume) has made information on sexual behavior all the more important. In the absence of country- and community-specific information on patterns of sexual behavior, understanding the epidemiology of sexually transmitted diseases (STDs) will remain difficult and make projections about the possible future course of the disease and the populations that might be affected even more tenuous.

Of all human behaviors, sexual behavior is one of the most complex and least well studied. A function of physical, cultural, social, economic, and political as well as personal factors and conditions, human sexuality is in many ways a mirror of society, family, and individual experience. On the one hand, there is the physiological capacity to engage in sexual acts and the biological need to do so. On the other hand, there are external forces and conditions that impose time- and situation-specific choices and opportunities for different modes of sexual expression. Local history, traditions, values, and patterns of social organization all play a role. They help define the types of sexual behavior that are considered functional to society and the limits to which variations will be tolerated. The ages at which sex is considered appropriate, with what types of partners, under what circumstances, and with what quality of fulfillment and meaning are all in some way or another dictated by these forces and conditions.

Perhaps more so than with any other human behavior, then, variations in sexuality can be anticipated to occur across cultures, within cultures, and over time. Education, socioeconomic background, family background, age, gender, and access to health-related information and health care services all influence the ways in which people perceive sexual behavior, what they consider to be acceptable and normative, and what value and priority they allocate to sex. Policies regarding marriage and procreation also play a determining role. These also change over

---

Manuel Carballo and Oussama Tawil – Programme on Substance Abuse, Research and Development Unit, World Health Organization, CH-1211 Geneva 27, Switzerland. ***King Holmes*** – Center for AIDS and STD, Seattle, Washington 98122.

time, on some occasions adapting to demographic needs, while at others responding more to political and religious imperatives.

In the context of the HIV and AIDS pandemic, it has also become more apparent than ever before that most societies are essentially heterogeneous systems made up of many different subgroups and subcultures. Not only are these groups often demographically different, they sometimes also differ in their psychosocial and health experiences, their views of the world, and their political interests and sexual preferences.

Perhaps in part because of this potential for cultural variability, as well as sociopolitical and methodological reasons, the comparative study of human sexual behavior has been relatively neglected. As a result, today there is generally a paucity of information of the type and quality that health planners could effectively use in formulating STD and AIDS prevention strategies. Until recently, for example, there have been few population-based surveys. Instead, currently available information primarily comes from small and often unrepresentative ethnographic studies that are by definition descriptive and noncomparative, studies of physical development in which ancillary questions on sexual behavior have been asked, or fertility-related surveys from which extrapolations to sexuality can be made. While valuable in their own right, they do not always or easily lend themselves to estimations of global trends, and although they contribute to an understanding of the biosocial context in which sexual behavior occurs, it is difficult to generalize from them.

TEMPORAL TRENDS TOWARD EARLIER ONSET OF SEXUAL MATURITY AND SEXUAL INTERCOURSE

Sexual maturity, as measured by physical and endocrine development, is not in itself a sufficient indicator of sexual behavior. Nevertheless, information on changing patterns of menarche and spermarche can serve as a marker of the predisposition or readiness for sexuality. In this regard, there is evidence that the age at menarche has decreased in many parts of the world (70), especially in highly industrialized countries where the secular decline in age at menarche has been attributed to changing patterns of health and nutrition (60) and to better health care in general. Over approximately 100 years, the average age at which girls experience their first menstruation (although not necessarily their first ovulation) has fallen from around 16 to 17 years to 12 to 13 years (60).

Similar declines in the age of menarche have been reported in selected developing countries where marked urban and rural and socioeconomic differences have further suggested that nutrition and overall health status are important correlates of sexual maturation. This earlier onset of menarche (and spermarche in the male, which appears to occur approximately 2 years later than menarche in the female) deserves to be noted as an event and a process that may predispose young people to earlier sexual intercourse. Indeed, the earlier onset of maturity has been linked, although not in terms of any direct association, with reported increases in rates of unwanted pregnancy, induced abortion, premature parenthood, and STDs.

Available data also indicate that the age at first sexual intercourse has decreased in recent decades in developed and developing countries (63, 64; E. R. Allgeier, unpublished report for the International Development and Research Center, Ottawa, Ontario, Canada, 1989). Especially high prevalences of early sexual activity among unmarried teenagers, for example, have been noted in Western Europe and North America (64).

Nationally representative data on young people aged between 11 and 21 years in Canada (29), for example, point to a secular trend toward younger age at first sexual intercourse, and survey data for Scotland (4) suggest that the age at first sexual intercourse has progressively decreased with each 5-year cohort from 1926 to 1930 to 1961 to 1965. Data on sexual activity among college students throughout much of this century corroborate other findings that in developed countries there has been an increase in premarital sex (15). This relationship between age and sexual behavior is further discussed by Ehrhardt and Wasserheit in this volume.

PATTERNS OF SEXUAL BEHAVIOR AND INFLUENCE OF SOCIAL CHANGE

Although information on patterns of sexual behavior among young people in developing countries is not as abundant as that for developed countries, data nevertheless suggest that similar trends have occurred and that age at first sexual intercourse has generally decreased in recent decades (63), even though there are relatively marked differences between countries and regions. For example, higher rates of sexual activity are reported for adolescents in sub-Saharan Africa than in Latin America and parts of Asia. Within Africa, the numbers of women who say they had premarital sex by late adolescence are high. In Gambia, Nigeria, Tanzania, and Uganda, more than two-thirds of the women interviewed in World Fertility Surveys said they had had sexual relations by the age of 19 to 20 years. Similar findings have been reported for female students in Liberia and Sierra Leone (63).

With the exception of Jamaica and Honduras, where the prevalence of sexual activity among female adolescents is comparable to that in countries in Africa, population-based findings for Latin America indicate that between one-third and one-half of the women studied had sexual intercourse by the age of 19 years. In Southeast Asia, a generally lower level of sexual activity was reported among adolescents; in Hong Kong, for example, only 12% of the women studied reported having had sexual intercourse between the ages of 15 and 19 years (63). Data from Indonesia (W. Sittitrai and J. Barry, unpublished report for the International Development and Research Center, Ottawa, Ontario, Canada, 1989), where traditional cultural and religious values are still encouraged, indicate that less than 2% of the females studied reported premarital sex. In Japan and South Korea (25), the percentages of women 21 years old and under who say they have had premarital sexual intercourse are also low, being 4 and 7%, respectively. In other societies in the same region, on the other hand, survey data for Taiwan (11), Hong Kong (59), and the Philippines and Thailand (47) suggest that higher proportions of female students have had sexual intercourse before marriage.

Given the roles ethnicity, religion, exposure to communication, and place of residence play in determining much of human behavior, patterns of human sexuality can also be expected to vary according to these factors. In new and still-evolving urban communities, where the role of religion may be less marked and where new information and ideas are regularly communicated, young men and women may need to formulate their own codes of sexual conduct. In the absence of the support, guidance, and traditional control they would have received from rural family systems, they may be compelled to innovate. Sittitrai and Barry (1989), for example, report that in many parts of Southeast Asia, young urban males are more sexually active than those living in rural areas. Recent World Health Organization collaborative studies on sexual behavior have also found similar differences between urban and rural men; in Rwanda (Programme National de Lutte Contre le SIDA [PNLS], Kigali, Rwanda, 1988), Central African Republic (PNLS, Bangui, Republique Centrafricaine, 1990), Ivory Coast (PNLS, Abidjan, Côte d'Ivoire, 1990), Kenya (National AIDS Control Programme, Nairobi, Kenya, 1990), and Togo (PNLS, Lome, Togo, 1989), for example, urban men reported higher rates of premarital and extramarital activity than did rural respondents. Similar patterns have been reported for parts of Latin America and Europe, where marked rural-urban and sex-selective migrations have also occurred (63, 64).

INCREASING AGE OF MARRIAGE IN THE CONTEXT OF DECLINING AGE OF FIRST COITUS

Age at marriage has traditionally reflected a wide range of factors including land tenure patterns, inheritance customs, the perceived value of procreation, the role of women, and patterns of education, as well as opportunities and aspirations for occupational mobility. Industrial and socioeconomic development has been instrumental in changing much of this. It has attracted people away from agricultural life-styles, has made inheritance and land tenure less important, has opened up opportunities for educational and occupational improvement, and has reduced the influence of childbearing in determining the status of women in the family and community. As a result, one of the relatively constant corollaries of industrialization has been the gradual postponement of age at marriage for both men and women.

Thus, with the exception of the "marriage boom" that characterized many Western European and North American societies in the 1950s and 1960s, developed regions of the world have experienced a steady trend toward postponement of marriage (64). Between 1950 and 1980, fewer than 10% of marriages in these regions involved people in their teens; for example, the percentage of teenage marriages in the United States declined from 17 to 8.8%. Sweden and Denmark currently report the lowest percentages (less than 1%) of teenage marriages in the world (64).

At the same time, countries with relatively strong agricultural economies and large rural populations, such as Greece, Portugal, Spain, and Ireland, have experienced a slight increase in teenage marriages during the period 1950 to 1980 (64). In parts of Eastern Europe, the proportion of adolescents who are married has always been relatively high and continued to be so during the same period (64).

The picture in other parts of the world also varies according to country, but in general there has been a similar trend toward postponement of marriage (63). In much of North Africa, the Middle East, Asia, and the Pacific, the proportion of married teenagers has decreased (12, 55, 56). In industrialized countries of the Far East, such as Japan, South Korea, Hong Kong, and Singapore, the proportions of people marrying in their teenage years are similar to those reported for Western Europe (63). Similarly low rates have been reported in China, where recent social and economic policies have systematically encouraged delaying marriage and childbearing; in parts of the Indian subcontinent and sub-Saharan Africa, on the other hand, teenage marriage is still very common, even though the ideal age at marriage is considered to be between 20 and 24 years (63).

The postponement of age at marriage during a historical period when the age of both menarche and spermarche has decreased has also probably contributed to an increased opportunity for multiple sexual partnerships. The geographical and social mobility of young people and the fact that they move away from families of origin earlier than ever before also must be taken into account. Young people often find themselves in new urban situations where cultural and social definitions of "acceptable" and "appropriate" patterns of sexuality may be poorly structured and where "opportunistic" relationships become more necessary and possible.

In some societies, however, postponement of marriage has occurred concurrently with an increasing social recognition of nonlegal unions. Often termed consensual unions, cohabitation, common law unions, free unions, or simply living together, nonlegal unions appear to have replaced the need for traditional marriage. The proportion of young people reporting such unions has increased markedly within Europe, for example. In the United Kingdom, 27% of women who married in the late 1970s reported that they had lived together with a partner before marriage; the proportion in France was 31%, in Norway 47%, in Denmark 80%, and in Sweden, where the practice has become much more institutionalized, 89% (65).

Information for other regions is less precise, but the situation in much of Latin America suggests that the postponement of age at marriage has also occurred in a context of increasing acceptance of consensual unions. Indeed, in much of the Caribbean and Central America, consensual unions constitute the most common type of relationship among young people and are only later converted into legal marriages (63). To what extent cohabitation or nonlegal unions provide the same degree of economic interdependence as traditional legal marriages is not clear, but the data suggest that in all other respects, cohabitation introduces the same constraints on extra-union sexual behavior as does traditional marriage.

Any consideration of the potential for STDs also needs to take into account the mediating effect of condoms. In the context of the AIDS pandemic, condoms have received increasing attention by public health prevention programs. Patterns of condom use, however, have traditionally been variable between and within countries. Before the AIDS pandemic, there had not been much active promotion of condoms outside of family planning programs, and even within these, other contraceptive methods had become more common because of their greater perceived use-effectiveness and social acceptability. Among adolescents and young adults, both single and married in the developing world, oral and other contraceptive methods are, as a result, more frequently used than condoms (63).

Relatively high prevalences of condom use are reported for countries such as Singapore, Hong Kong, Costa Rica, and Trinidad and Tobago, where 22, 15, 13, and 12%, respectively, of couples reported that they regularly used condoms. Much lower use-prevalence rates are reported for other countries in Asia, the Middle East, Latin America, and most of Africa (26). Particularly in sub-Saharan Africa, where the prevalence of STDs is high and where STDs account for a high proportion of the reported sterility (21, 28), the acceptance of condoms is low and few advances have been made with respect to their promotion (5, 37, 48–53).

A variety of reasons may account for the low rates of condom use in Africa; among them have been concerns about their pricing, their continued availability and distribution, and the fact that many people see them as foreign to the mores and values of many local African cultures. Perhaps in part responding to this, the majority of family planning programs in sub-Saharan Africa have depended more on female methods. It should nevertheless be noted that the success of family planning programs in general has been limited irrespective of the contraceptive method in question (5, 34, 54).

While familiarity with condoms has increased in many regions (26), there is little evidence that use patterns in sub-Saharan Africa are changing. Recent AIDS-related survey data from African countries continue to indicate low use patterns. For example, in Lesotho (National AIDS Control Programme, Maseru, Lesotho, 1989), Uganda (31), and Togo (PNLS, 1989), only 4.6, 3, and 8.2%, respectively, of respondents of both sexes reported ever using a condom. Somewhat higher proportions of respondents reported having used condoms in Zaire (J. T. Bertrand et al., unpublished report, Tulane University, New Orleans, La., 1989), Senegal (PNLS, Dakar, Senegal, 1988), the Congo (PNLS, Brazzaville, Congo, 1989), and the Central African Republic (PNLS, 1990), but even in these countries the health benefits of condoms appear to be ignored. In the Central African Republic (PNLS, 1990), for example, 84% of the respondents in one survey said they had made changes in their sexual behavior, but only 3% mentioned use of condoms as a part of these changes. In Chad, condoms were spontaneously mentioned as a means of contraception by only 6% of respondents and as a means of preventing HIV transmission by a comparably low proportion (PNLS, N'Djamena, Tchad, 1989).

In all these surveys, marked urban-rural differences in awareness and use of condoms have emerged; in general, familiarity with condoms and their use is higher in urban communities than in rural areas. This may reflect differences in education, exposure to information about condoms, and the availability of family services.

PATTERNS OF PROSTITUTION

Within the context of STDs, frequency and type of exposure are critical risk indicators. Men and women who provide sex, be it for money, goods, favors, services, or other forms of compensation (2), and do so regularly are inevitably at greater risk of exposure to STDs than other people (16). Providing sex for financial or other rewards is an integral part of most social systems, and most societies, at one time or another, have institutionalized the practice even if they have not necessarily acknowledged or approved of it.

The size and nature of the population of men and women providing sex for money are difficult to assess. In some parts of the world, socioeconomic development and other occupational opportunities have made prostitution less attractive and possibly more geographically selective. Developing countries, or countries going through economic hardship, may present a different image. A recent report (1) estimated the prostitute population of Bangkok, Thailand, to be on the order of 100,000.

The term prostitution, however, is broad and relatively generic. It covers and at the same time can hide a range of cultural and social variations that are important from a health perspective. To better disaggregate these variations, Plant et al. (46) proposed a distinction according to the extent to which the practice is a principal source of income for the individual concerned and the extent of the commitment made by the person to prostitution as a professional activity. Additional distinctions can be made on the basis of socioeconomic background, stratification within the "profession" (32), place and type of work performed, and clientele (18). Further classifications based on the type of sexual services provided are also probably justified according to the health implications that both providers and clients are exposed to.

A common theme characterizing prostitution globally is economic need. Especially in developing countries, few other alternatives may exist, especially for women, at particular periods in life. As a result, working as prostitutes is sometimes seen as a necessary phase or economic rite of passage, in which women and men move to large cities for a time to support families or save money for marriage (2, 18, 61). In other situations, however, demographic factors also play an important role. Many major urban centers in developing countries are characterized by large concentrations of young single men who have recently migrated from rural traditional communities in search of employment (65). Alone or with few social networks to draw on, they may have few opportunities for sexual relationships other than with prostitutes. Similar conditions have also been observed in large industrial cities of Europe where over the past 20 years there has been a policy of essentially male "guest labor" recruitment from less-developed countries.

Within the practice of providing sex for money, however, clear distinctions between regular and irregular sex work are difficult to make. This is especially the case in situations of economic hardship, in which the need to seek alternative sources of support affects large numbers of people representing different socioeconomic backgrounds. In some African communities, it is difficult to differentiate "femmes libres" or "good-time girls" from those who provide sex for money on a regular basis (36, 68), and place of work may be the only reasonable indicator. Women working in well-defined areas of the city from their own rooms for fixed prices; those who frequent bars and exchange sex for drinks or other gifts; and those who work hotel lounges and serve a more selective and usually foreign clientele probably constitute relatively different groups, types of service provided, and risk exposure.

The data suggest that in addition to economic need, another common characteristic of women practicing prostitution in sub-Saharan African countries is widowhood or separated or divorced status. Studies in Kenya and Nigeria (68) and Ghana (35) report that approximately 44 and 85%, respectively, of the prostitutes interviewed were divorced. It is noteworthy that similar findings have also been reported for prostitutes in Liverpool, England (45).

In some communities, the AIDS pandemic could contribute to a broadening of this phenomenon. This is especially so in poor communities if large numbers of women become widowed or separated from their husbands because they suspect them, or are suspected themselves, of being HIV infected. Where the opportunities for other employment or income are limited, the number of women having to resort to prostitution could increase (7).

In many Western societies, prostitution has become increasingly professionalized even though its criminalization has meant that sex for money is often provided covertly and thus remains difficult to assess in terms of magnitude and distribution.

From the point of view of its implications for STDs, contemporary prostitution also needs to be considered from the point of view of geographical mobility of both providers and clients. Because economic need is often the precipitating force behind decisions to provide sex for money, many of the people involved in sex work do so for limited periods and then return to their communities of origin. The fact that they do so while still sexually active may be an important factor in the spread of STDs from one geographical region and population group to another, and especially from large metropolitan areas to rural communities.

The health implications of prostitution nevertheless vary. For although providing sex for money is a relatively universal practice, the types of sexual services provided differ and do not always or necessarily fit the general model of vaginal intercourse. Information on sub-Saharan Africa suggests that vaginal intercourse is the dominant service provided by prostitutes and that oral sex is rare (44, 67). On the other hand, in some Western societies, oral and other nonvaginal types of sexual interaction appear to be increasingly common. In New York City and New Jersey, for example, oral sex is one of the services most frequently sought by clients of prostitutes (19; L. T. Leonard, M. Freund, and J. J. Platt, *Am. J. Public Health,* Letter, **97**:903, 1989). Similar findings have been reported from Amsterdam (66), London (18), and Guadalajara, Mexico (B. M. Torres-Mendoza, E. Vázquez-Valls, M. N. Ayala-Chavira, and G. Ayala y de Landeros, IVth Int. Conf. AIDS, abstr. 5070, p. 332, 1988), where 70, 63, and 34%, respectively, of the female prostitutes interviewed said that oral sex was requested by clients. In some cities of the United States where "crack" cocaine is used widely among certain groups, there have been suggestions that oral sex is more common than vaginal sex in sex-for-money relationships.

Anal sex appears to be relatively uncommon among female prostitutes, especially in societies in which it is also reportedly uncommon among the general population. Studies undertaken in the Philippines (O. T. Monzon, J. M. Capellan, E. Navarro-Almario, R. Zeta, E. Sotucua, and P. Casuela, 1st International Congress on AIDS in Asia, Manila, 1987) and the United Kingdom (18), for example, indicate a low range of between 2 and 7%. On the other hand, a study of 113 female prostitutes in Brazil, where anal intercourse is not uncommon among heterosexual couples (38), indicated that 27% of those interviewed provided anal sex (L. Castello-Branco, M. I. L. Carvalho, E. A. de Castilho, H. E. Pereira, M. S. Pereira, and B. Galvro-Castro, IVth Int. Conf. AIDS, abstr. 5144, p. 350, 1988).

Frequency of exposure is a determinant of risk of STDs, but data are relatively limited and it is difficult to discern any national or regional patterns or trends in the frequency of sexual intercourse among prostitutes. What data are available suggest that frequency is correlated with socioeconomic background and local economic conditions. In general, the number of sexual contacts is considerably higher than among the nonprostitute female populations in the same countries. Female prostitutes in Sydney reported having up to 250 partners per month (median frequency of 24.5), while for a matched population of nonprostitutes, the frequency was between 1 and 4, with a median of 1.5 (42). Relatively similar findings (20 partners per month) were reported by Carswell (10) in a study of barmaids in Lyantode, Uganda. In a study of prostitutes in a northern Italian city, Pordenone (U. Tirelli, E. Vaccher, A. Carbone, P. De Paoli, G. F. Santini, and S. Monfardini, Letter, *Lancet* **i**:1424, 1985), frequencies of between 40 and 70 contacts per month were found. A study in Mali indicated that "professional" prostitutes had five or six clients per day (unpublished report, AIDSTECH Project, Family Health International, Durham, N.C., 1987), and in the Pumwani district in Nairobi, they had four to six clients per day (55a).

Recent studies among drug users suggest that providing sex for money is relatively common in some population groups. The variability in prevalence from one country and city to another makes any generalization difficult, however. Although the evidence suggests that drug use may lead to prostitution, this is not always clear (45). Goldstein's review (27) indicated that the percentage of female prostitutes who also use drugs ranges from 40 to 85%, depending on location and group, but drug injecting appears to be more common among street sex workers than those working from homes or other establishments. In Amsterdam, a study of STD clinic clients reported that 80% of 117 prostitutes were injecting drugs (66), and relatively high prevalences have been reported for selected groups in Sydney, Australia (41), Bangkok, Thailand (43), and Glasgow, Scotland (26). A New York City study of street prostitutes similarly estimated that approximately 50% of them had injected drugs (19). Meanwhile, a study of drug users in Italy indicated that prostitution was low and more sporadic (62).

Other studies have suggested that when drug abusers do provide sex for money, they may be more willing than other prostitutes to engage in high-risk sex if this is demanded by their clients. When this is the case, the likelihood of condom use being insisted upon by either provider or client may be lower than in other paid sexual relationships (45). This topic is discussed in further detail by Aral et al. (this volume).

SEX TOURISM

Perhaps as a result of modern communication and travel facilities, a recent development in the domain of sex work has been the emergence of sexual tourism. As a source of employment and income, sex tourism has become pronounced in some cities of developing countries, especially in Southeast Asia (Sittitrai and Barry, unpublished report, 1989). Originally associated with military movements in the region, large segments of the sex industry in this region now cater primarily to a visiting foreign tourist clientele. Of 1,770 female prostitutes recruited for HIV screening in three locations in the Philippines, for instance, 41% said they only had sex with foreign clients (Monzon et al., 1st Int. Cong. AIDS Asia, 1987). In some cases, it also appears that sexual tourism attracts clients who not only have a particular preference for foreign prostitutes (33) but who might not frequent prostitutes at all in their own countries.

The facility of contemporary international travel has also made it feasible for sex workers themselves to move in search of employment (18), and the international migration of prostitutes has become an important facet of today's sex industry. Just as with the migration of sex workers within countries, the corollary opportunities for the geographic spread of STDs, including HIV, has become an issue of increasing public health concern. In the Dominican Republic, the results of a 1985 study suggest that the prevalence of HIV infection among prostitutes who had worked abroad was 25 times higher than among those who had not worked outside the country (E. R. Koenig, Letter, *Lancet* **i**:782–783, 1989). A similar picture is reported among sex workers in the Ivory Coast (J. K. Anarfi, Ph.D. thesis, Université d'Abidjan, Abidjan, Ivory Coast, 1990) and Senegal (35).

HOMOSEXUALITY AND BISEXUALITY

In response to the AIDS pandemic, far more attention has begun to be given to questions of same-gender sex, particularly men who have sex with men, and bisexuality among men. Although information on these issues is sparse, it has nevertheless become clear in recent years that both homosexuality and bisexuality are more common than had been popularly believed, even in cultures with strong social and religious taboos. Whitman (69) suggests that the proportion of men practicing sex with other men is likely to be relatively constant across cultures. Early estimates (30) suggested that approximately 10% of men in the United States had been exclusively homosexual for some period in their adult lives and that between adolescence and old age approximately 37% of the total male population had had some overt homosexual experience leading to orgasm. More recent data, however, suggest lower estimates of 20.3% of adult men having experienced sexual contacts with other men leading to orgasm (22). Data from Southeast Asia indicate a range from 1% of adult men in Singapore (National AIDS Control Programme, Singapore, 1989) to 12% of male students in Thailand (Sittitrai and Barry, unpublished report, 1989) having had homosexual sexual relations.

Definition problems may account for some of these variations, as may cultural reluctance to discuss the matter with interviewers. For although homosexuality has recently found greater public expression in larger and more sociopolitically pluralistic societies, it is clear that historically it has been, and remains, a relatively covert behavior. Contemporary research and the possibility for more open discussion of homosexuality and bisexuality have also suggested that these rubrics encompass far wider ranges of relationships and practices than had been previously described (17).

The meaning and significance of these behaviors appear to differ by both culture and socioeconomic background. In some cultures, the choice of sexual partner (male or female) seems to be less important than the sexual roles played by the two partners. Where this is the case, the distinction between the active or passive role (insertive or receptive) becomes more meaningful than the concepts of homosexuality and heterosexuality, the active role often being equated with masculinity and the passive role with femininity (40). Same-gender sex, however, may be age, time, and situation specific rather than typical of an ongoing or continued sexual preference. Imprisonment, military service, and sexually segregated schools, in which heterosexual relationships have to be postponed, may lend themselves to same-gender sexual relationships even if they do not necessarily determine the pattern of sexual life once the individuals leave those situations.

While sexual practices such as oral sex and mutual masturbation are common features of sexual relationships between men, anal sexual intercourse is central to the concept of homosexuality. As for female prostitution, however, the prevalence of anal intercourse between men may reflect and be influenced by its traditional prevalence in the wider heterosexual population (39). Male prostitutes in Brazil (Castello-Branco et al., IVth Int. Conf. AIDS, abstr. 5144, 1988) and the Philippines (B. Modan, R. Goldschmidt, A. Vonsover, T. Gotlieb-Stematsky, M. Zinn, R. Guttman, and E. Guttman, IVth Int. Conf. AIDS, abstr. 4051, p. 272, 1988), for example, reported high frequencies of anal intercourse with clients just as did female prostitutes (see above).

In the context of the AIDS pandemic, these practices may be changing, and a number of studies in the United States and elsewhere indicate that the prevalence of unprotected anal intercourse may have decreased in recent years, especially in epicenters of the disease (1a). In other settings where AIDS has not been as prevalent and where the same channels of informal information and peer group pressure and support have not evolved, however, similar changes may not have occurred (6), and risk of HIV transmission, as well as other STDs, as a result of anal intercourse should not be assumed to have systematically decreased.

From the point of view of HIV infection and its potential spread to a larger heterosexual and pediatric population, bisexuality has also become a major issue of concern. As with the term homosexuality, the notion of bisexuality has been used to cover a variety of experiences and practices. Sexual experimentation in youth, situational same-gender relationships between otherwise heterosexual men, bisexual male prostitutes, their married male clients, and men who do not identify as bisexual as well as those who do have all at some time or another been included within this rubric.

For the purposes of this discussion, bisexual behavior and bisexual identity are differentiated. The former refers to same- and opposite-gender sexual activity over a given period; bisexual identity refers to the way in which an individual sees himself and relates to a group with which he identifies. A series of studies indicate the two are not necessarily consistently related. In the United States, Lever et al. (J. Lever, W. Roger, S. P. Carson, R. Hertz, and D. Kanowe, Vth Int. Conf. AIDS, abstr. TDP18, 1989) reported that only 28% of 7,484 behaviorally bisexual men identified themselves as bisexual. Conversely, Winkelstein et al. (W. Winkelstein, J. A. Wiley, N. Padian, and J. Levy, Letter, *J. Am. Med. Assoc.*, **255**:901, 1986) showed that while 16.3% of 1,035 men said they were bisexual, only 10.4% had had a female partner during the previous 2 years.

While accurate estimates are difficult to derive, the proportion of men in Western countries who engage in bisexual behavior appears to be small. National surveys of sexual behavior in Norway (58) and the United States (T. Wilkie, *The Independent*, London, United Kingdom, 20 February 1990) report that less than 6% of men have sexual contact with both men and women at any time in their lives. Other studies report marked geographical and social variability in bisexual behavior. While Winkelstein et al. (*J. Am. Med. Assoc.*, **255**:901, 1986) reported that 16.3% of their sample of single men in San Francisco saw themselves as bisexual, Forman and Chilver's (24) study of men living in different areas of England and Wales reported that only 1.5% of men had had both homosexual and heterosexual partners at any time in their lives.

Studies of self-identified homosexual men indicate that many of them have had a female partner at some point in their lives and that approximately 10 to 15% report having had one in the previous year (57; P. M. Davies, A. Hunt, M. Macourt, and P. Weatherburn, Final Report, Department of Health, London, United Kingdom, 1990). Clinic-based studies tend to give higher estimates, with 10 to 30% of homosexually active men classified as behaviorally bisexual (13, 20; J. Welch, S. Palmer, and J. E. Banatvala, *Br. Med. J.* **293**:924, 1986).

Cultural factors emerge as important in the definition and prevalence of bisexuality. Carrier (8, 9) suggests that over 30% of single Mexican men aged 15 to 25 have had sexual contact with both male and female partners and that 25% of the homosexual men studied have had heterosexual intercourse in the course of a year. Garcia et al. (M. L. Garcia, J. A. Izazola, J. L. Valdespino, C. Magis, G. Ornelas, P. Uribe, and J. Sepulveda, Vth Int. Conf. AIDS, abstr. WGP25, p. 1014, 1989) found that of 1,676 homosexually active men attending an HIV testing center in Mexico City, 56% said they had had sexual relations with both men and women; 19% (n = 325) reported sexual contact with male and female partners in the previous 6 months, a rate twice that (9%) reported in a roughly equivalent sample in London (20).

As for homosexual men, the effect of the AIDS pandemic and information campaigns about high-risk sexual behavior may have been to modify patterns of behavior, albeit at a slower pace. In Melbourne, Australia, in 1989, a wide range of sexual practices was still being reported by bisexual men; they also appeared to have lower levels of knowledge about safe sex than homosexual men (W. Palmer,

Vth Int. Conf. AIDS, abstr. MEP43, p. 840, 1989). Data among black homosexual and bisexual men in San Francisco also indicated a continuing high prevalence of unsafe sex among the latter (J. L. Peterson, R. Fullilove, J. Catania, and T. Coates, Vth Int. Conf. AIDS, abstr. WDP27, p. 747, 1989).

Other studies in the United Kingdom (23) and Australia (14), on the other hand, have reported less marked differences in patterns of homosexual behavior between behaviorally bisexual men and exclusively homosexual men. The frequency of active (insertive) anal intercourse was similar in both groups, and unprotected intercourse was more common with regular partners than others. Among non-self-identified bisexual (or homosexual) men, however, the prevalence of high-risk sexual behavior may be still high. Bennett et al. (3) reported that 63% of the 54 bisexual men in their study had had insertive and 65% had had receptive anal intercourse with a casual male partner. In about 53 and 37% of these men, respectively, sexual intercourse was unprotected.

As with homosexual men and prostitutes, self-perception and identification appear to be critical to any process of behavior change. Those who do not so identify often remain outside the networks of information and peer group support that seem to have been instrumental in bringing about or making behavior change possible. In general, however, it is probably true that bisexual male networks are less common than among homosexual men and that self-identification as bisexual may be culturally and socially more difficult.

CONCLUSION

Evidence from different countries and regions around the world suggests that fairly marked changes have taken place in patterns of sexual behavior over the past 50 years. In part, this may have been influenced by the fact that the age at sexual maturation in girls and boys has decreased. Prompted by improved health and nutrition, changes in the onset of menarche and spermarche have taken place in both developed and developing countries. Many of these physical changes have taken place in evolving social environments that give rise to new needs and opportunities for sexual expression.

Throughout much of the world, patterns of family organization, including concepts of ideal size, have also changed. Large, extended family systems have given way to smaller, nuclear families. With them have gone many of the traditional ways of preparing and socially controlling young people in their reproductive and sexual life. In the meantime, modern communication has made the sexual values and mores of industrial society universally known. Increasingly associated with the concept of modernism, these values have become increasingly normative, especially for young people, irrespective of social, cultural, or economic environment.

Many of these changes have occurred in an era of rapid urbanization and industrialization that has precipitated new social and economic relationships. Opportunities for alternative employment have inspired major rural-urban population movements in which migration has become an age- and usually sex-selective process. In some major urban centers, the result has been the emergence of demographically skewed urban populations with new social and sexual needs.

With the movement away from agricultural life, the economic value of children has become less important. In part as a result of this, as well as the new opportunities presented for educational and occupational mobility, ideal family size has decreased, while the ideal age at marriage has increased. Meanwhile, there have been profound developments in modern contraceptive technology; the notion, if not the fact, of sex without fear of conception has become more of a reality than ever before.

In an era of AIDS and the need for innovative prevention strategies, it has become clear that society is becoming socially and culturally more pluralistic. There have been profound changes in the politics of sexual relations, especially, but not only, in industrialized countries. Behaviors and practices previously considered antisocial and condemned to be covert are finding new public expression and legitimacy. At one and the same time they are giving rise to new public health problems and yet also new possibilities for the prevention of the sexual transmission of disease.

Yet despite these changes and the growing realization that sexual behavior is an important key to understanding this current public health dilemma, the systematic study of sexual behavior remains the exception rather than the rule. The study of STDs continues to be constrained even though STDs are now a global problem affecting the reproductive health and the well-being of children as well as adults. Attitudes and values more appropriate to a utopian world free of communicable diseases than to modern society continue to make the study of human sexuality and STDs politically and socially difficult. Before the AIDS pandemic, few countries had seen fit to undertake the type of large population-based survey that might have thrown more light on the nature and magnitude of behaviors that place people at risk of STDs and AIDS.

These sociopolitical constraints have combined with real methodological problems. For if the study and tracking of STD transmission have proved technically difficult, the conceptual and methodological concerns implicit in the study of human sexuality have been even more so. Of all human behavior, sexuality has remained the most private and least open to any straightforward description and analysis. Often linked to quasi-mystical concepts of reproduction and to gender politics and status, sexuality has remained one of the unspoken, albeit fundamental, aspects of human society. Often caught up in a mix of religion, dogma, superstition, and ignorance, it has tended to escape scientific scrutiny and be peripheral to much of contemporary biosocial science. As a result, much of the information currently available is drawn from research that was not explicitly set up to study sexuality. It often lacks the depth, precision, and cross-cultural character that are required in the fight against STDs in general and AIDS in particular.

And yet, reliable methods and techniques relevant to the study of sexual behavior have become more available. Health research in general has increasingly benefited from the combination of qualitative and quantitative social science research approaches. Drawing upon anthropological and ethnographic experiences as well as more social-psychological and epidemiological survey methods, it is now possible to focus on critical issues from different perspectives and levels of analysis. Today it is more feasible than at any time in the past to map and describe human behavior of all types. It is well within the domain of science today to assess the nature and force of the factors and conditions that determine the social presentation of biological needs.

To continue to negate the importance of research on sexual behavior and its impact on health would be to deny an opportunity of understanding (among other things) the nature of STD transmission and AIDS. It would greatly reduce the possibility of developing new and innovative approaches to their prevention, treatment, and control.

Future public health research agendas should seek to give more priority to the study of the relationships among social environment, human sexuality, the distribution of STDs, the nature of health care-seeking behavior, and the willingness to modify individual practices. Much more also needs to be known about how different individuals at different times in their lives and in various social circumstances perceive the notion of risk and are willing to participate in acts that increase or decrease their exposure to that risk. For although sexuality is universal and primal, its significance for different people remains ill-defined.

Whether a vaccine for HIV and AIDS will emerge and become widely available in the coming years remains to be seen. Given the limited success in the past with what are otherwise proven, safe, and effective treatments for other STDs, as well as with the promotion and use of condoms as a prophylactic measure, the answer to prevention will depend on a better comprehension of the factors that determine exposure to disease and health care-seeking behavior. Only through such a research approach will it become possible to design and provide the type and quality of prevention and treatment services that are socially acceptable and medically effective.

LITERATURE CITED

1. **Anonymous.** 1987. Thailand's double fear. *New Sci.* **1562:**29.

1a. **Becker, M. H., and J. G. Joseph.** 1988. AIDS and behavioral change to reduce risk: a review. *Am. J. Public Health* **78:**394–410.

2. **Bennett, F. J.** 1962. The social determinants of gonorrhoea in an East African town. *East Afr. Med. J.* **39:**332–342.

3. **Bennett, G., S. Chapman, and F. Bray.** 1989. Sexual practices and "beats": AIDS-related sexual practices in a sample of homosexual and bisexual men in the western state of Sydney. *Med. J. Aust.* **151:**307–314.

4. **Bone, M.** 1986. Trends in single women's sexual behaviour in Scotland. *Popul. Trends* **43:**7–14.

5. **Caldwell, J., and P. Caldwell.** 1988. Is the Asian family planning program model suited to Africa? *Stud. Fam. Plann.* **19:**19–28.

6. **Carballo, M.** 1990. Psychosocial aspects of AIDS: policy implications. *AIDS* **4**(Suppl.)**:** 529–533.

7. **Carballo, M., and M. Carael.** 1988. Impact of AIDS on social organization, p. 81–93. *In* A. F. Fleming, M. Carballo, D. W. FitzSimons, M. R. Bailey, and J. Mann (ed.), *The Global Impact of AIDS.* Alan R. Liss, London.

8. **Carrier, J. M.** 1989. Sexual behavior and spread of AIDS in Mexico. *Med. Anthropol.* **10**:129–142.
9. **Carrier, J. M.** 1985. Mexican male bisexuality. *J. Homosex.* **11**:75–85.
10. **Carswell, J. W.** 1987. HIV infection in healthy persons in Uganda. *AIDS* **1**:223–227.
11. **Cernada, G. P., M. C. Chang, H. S. Lin, T. H. Sun, and C. C. Cernada.** 1986. Implications for adolescent sex education in Taiwan. *Stud. Fam. Plann.* **17**:181–187.
12. **Coale, A. J.** 1983. Recent trends in fertility in less developed countries. *Science* **221**:828–832.
13. **Collaborative Study by the Consultants in Genitourinary Medicine and the Public Health Laboratory Service.** 1989. HIV infection in patients attending clinics for sexually transmitted diseases in England and Wales. *Br. Med. J.* **298**:415–418.
14. **Connell, R., J. Crawford, G. Dowsett, S. Kippax, V. Sinnott, P. Rodden, D. Baxter, P. Berg, and L. Watson.** 1989. Unsafe anal sexual practice among homosexual and bisexual men. *Social Aspects of the Prevention of AIDS Study, Report no. 6.* Macquarrie University, New South Wales, Australia.
15. **Darling, C. A., D. J. Kallen, and J. E. Van Dusen.** 1984. Sex in transition: 1900–1980. *J. Youth Adolesc.* **3**:385–399.
16. **Darrow, W. W.** 1984. Prostitution and sexually transmitted diseases, p. 109–115. *In* K. K. Holmes, P.-A. Mardh, P. F. Sparling, and P. J. Wiesner (ed.), *Sexually Transmitted Diseases.* McGraw-Hill Book Co., New York.
17. **Davis, D. L., and R. G. Whitten.** 1987. The cross-cultural study of human sexuality. *Annu. Rev. Anthropol.* **16**:69–98.
18. **Day, S.** 1988. Prostitute women and AIDS: anthropology. *AIDS* **2**:421–428.
19. **Des Jarlais, D. C., and S. R. Friedman.** 1987. HIV infection among intravenous drug users: epidemiology and risk reduction. *AIDS* **1**:67–76.
20. **Evans, B. A., K. A. McLean, S. G. Dawson, S. A. Teece, R. A. Bond, K. D. MacRae, and R. W. Thorp.** 1989. Trends in sexual behaviour and risk factors for HIV infection among homosexual men, 1984–7. *Br. Med. J.* **298**:215–218.
21. **Farley, T. M., and E. M. Belsey.** 1988. The prevalence and aetiology of infertility. African Population Conference, Dakar, 1988. *Int. Union Sci. Study Popul.* **2**:15–30.
22. **Fay, R. E., C. F. Turner, A. D. Klassen, and J. H. Gagnon.** 1989. Prevalence and patterns of same-gender sexual contact among men. *Science* **243**:338–348.
23. **Fitzpatrick, R., G. Hart, M. Boulton, J. McLean, and J. Dawson.** 1989. Heterosexual sexual behaviour in a sample of homosexually active men. *Genitourin. Med.* **65**:259–262.
24. **Forman, D., and C. Chilvers.** 1989. Sexual behaviour of young and middle aged men in England and Wales. *Br. Med. J.* **298**:1137–1142.
25. **Friedman, H. L.** 1985. The health of adolescents and youth: a global overview. *World Health Stat. Q.* **38**:256–266.
26. **Goldberg, H. I., N. C. Lee, M. W. Oberle, and H. B. Peterson.** 1989. Knowledge about condoms and their use in less developed countries during a period of rising AIDS prevalence. *Bull. W.H.O.* **67**:85–91.
27. **Goldstein, P. J.** 1979. Prostitution and drugs. Lexington Books, Lexington, Mass.
28. **Guest, I.** 1978. Special report: infertility in Africa. *People* **5**:23–34.
29. **King, A. J., R. P. Beazley, W. K. Warren, C. A. Hankins, A. S. Robertson, and J. L. Radford.** 1988. *Canada Youth & AIDS Study.* Queen's University, Kingston, Ontario, Canada.
30. **Kinsey, A. C., W. B. Pomeroy, and C. E. Martin.** 1948. *Sexual Behavior in the Human Male.* The W. B. Saunders Co., Philadelphia.
31. **Konde-Lule, J. K., S. F. Berkley, and R. Downing.** 1989. Knowledge, attitudes, and practices concerning AIDS in Ugandans. *AIDS* **3**:513–518.
32. **La Fontaine, J.** 1974. The free woman of Kinshasa: prostitution in the city of Zaire, p. 89–113. *In* J. Davis (ed.), *Choice and Change: Essays in Honour of Lucy Mair. LSE Monographs in Social Anthropology,* no. 50. Athlone Press, London.
33. **Mansson, S. A.** 1980. *The Man in Sexual Commerce.* Lund University, Lund, Sweden.

34. **Maudlin, W. P., and S. J. Segal.** 1988. Prevalence of contraceptive use: trends and issues. *Stud. Fam. Plann.* **19:**335–353.
35. **Neequaye, J. E., A. R. Neequaye, S. Wein, and M. Polts.** 1986. Sexual habits and social factors in local Ghanaian prostitutes which could affect the spread of human immunodeficiency virus (HIV). *Ghana Med. J.* **23:**12–15.
36. **Nzilambi, N., K. H. Dalock, D. N. Forthal, H. Francis, R. W. Ryder, I. Malebe, J. Getchell, M. Laga, P. Piot, and J. B. McCormick.** 1988. The prevalence of infection with human immunodeficiency virus over a 10 year period in rural Zaire. *N. Engl. J. Med.* **318:**276–279.
37. **Ondo State, Nigeria.** 1989. *Demographic and Health Survey, 1986.* Institute for Resource Development/Westinghouse, Columbia, Md.
38. **Parker, R. G.** 1989. Youth, identity, and homosexuality: the changing shape of sexual life in contemporary Brazil. *J. Homosex.* **17:**269–289.
39. **Parker, R. G.** 1985. Masculinity, femininity and homosexuality: on the anthropological interpretation of sexual meaning in Brazil. *J. Homosex.* **11:**155–163.
40. **Parker, R. G., and M. Carballo.** 1991. Qualitative research on homosexual and bisexual behavior relevant to HIV/AIDS. *J. Sex Res.* **27:**497–525.
41. **Perkins, R., and G. Bennett.** 1985. *Being a Prostitute.* George Allen and Unwin, Sydney, Australia.
42. **Philpot, C. R., C. Harcourt, J. Edwards, and A. Grealis.** 1988. Human immunodeficiency virus and female prostitutes, Sydney 1985. *Genitourin. Med.* **64:**193–197.
43. **Phongpaichit, F.** 1982. *From Peasant Girls to Bangkok Masseuses: Women, Work and Development 2.* International Labour Organization, Geneva.
44. **Piot, P., F. A. Plummer, M. A. Rey, E. N. Ngugi, C. Rouzioux, J. O. Ndinya-Achola, G. Veracauteren, L. J. D'Costa, M. Laga, H. Nsanze, L. Fransen, D. Haase, G. van der Groen, R. C. Brunham, A. R. Ronald, and F. Brun-Vézinet.** 1987. Retrospective seroepidemiology of AIDS virus infection in Nairobi population. *J. Infect. Dis.* **155:**1108–1112.
45. **Plant, M. L. (ed.).** 1990. *AIDS, Drugs and Prostitution.* Tavistock/Routledge, London.
46. **Plant, M. L., M. A. Plant, D. F. Peck, and J. Setters.** 1989. The sex industry, alcohol and illicit drugs: implications for the spread of HIV infection. *Br. J. Addict.* **84:**53–59.
47. **Population Center Foundation.** 1985. Young adult fertility in the Philippines. *YAFS Report Series,* no. 1. The Foundation, Manila, The Philippines.
48. **Republic of Liberia.** 1988. *Liberia Demographic and Health Survey, 1986.* Institute for Resource Development/Westinghouse, Columbia, Md.
49. **Republic of Uganda.** 1989. *Uganda Demographic and Health Survey, 1988/1989.* Institute for Resource Development/Macro Systems, Inc., Columbia, Md.
50. **République du Burundi.** 1988. *Enquête Démographique et de Santé au Burundi, 1987.* Institute for Resource Development/Westinghouse, Columbia, Md.
51. **République du Mali.** 1989. *Enquête Démographique de Santé au Mali, 1987.* Institute for Resource Development/Westinghouse, Columbia, Md.
52. **République du Sénégal.** 1988. *Enquête Démographique et de Santé au Sénégal, 1986.* Institute for Resource Development/Westinghouse, Columbia, Md.
53. **République du Togo.** 1989. *Enquête Démographique et de Santé au Togo, 1988.* Institute for Resource Development/Macro Systems, Inc., Columbia, Md.
54. **Ross, T. A., M. Rich, J. P. Molzan, and M. Pensak.** 1988. *Family Planning and Child Survival: 100 Developing Countries.* Columbia University, New York.
55. **Senderowitz, J., and J. M. Paxman.** 1985. Adolescent fertility: worldwide concerns. *Popul. Bull.* **40:**1–51.

55a. **Simonsen, J. N., F. A. Plummer, E. N. Ngugi, C. Black, J. K. Kriess, M. N. Gakinya, P. Waiyaki, L. J. D'Costa, J. O. Ndinya-Achola, P. Piot, and A. Ronald.** 1990. *AIDS* **4:**139–144.

56. **Smith, P. C.** 1980. Asia marriage patterns in transition. *J. Fam. Hist.* **2:**58–92.
57. **Soskolne, C., R. Coates, and A. Sears.** 1986. Characteristics of a male homosexual/bisexual study population in Toronto, Canada. *Can. J. Public Health* **77:**12–16.

58. **Sundet, J., I. Kvalem, P. Magnus, and L. Bakketeig.** 1988. Prevalence of risk-prone sexual behaviour in the general population of Norway, p. 53–60. *In* A. F. Fleming, M. Carballo, D. W. FitzSimons, M. R. Bailey, and J. Mann (ed.), *The Global Impact of AIDS*. Alan R. Liss, London.
59. **Tang, G. W.** 1982. Abortion in single girls in Hong Kong. *J. Adolesc. Health Care* **2:**213–216.
60. **Tanner, J. M.** 1982. *Growth of Adolescents*. Blackwell Scientific Publications, Oxford.
61. **Thorbek, S.** 1987. *Voices from the City: Women of Bangkok*. Zed Books, London.
62. **Titti, F., G. Rezza, P. Verani, S. Butto, L. Sernicola, M. Rapicetta, B. Sarrecchia, C. Oliva, and G. B. Rossi.** 1988. HIV, HTLV-1, and HBV infections in a cohort of Italian intravenous drug abusers: analysis of risk factors. *J. Acquired Immune Defic. Syndr.* **1:**405–411.
63. **United Nations.** 1989. *Adolescent Reproductive Behaviour: Evidence from Developing Countries*, vol. II. *Population Studies* no. 109/Add. 1. United Nations, New York.
64. **United Nations.** 1988. *Adolescent Reproductive Behaviour: Evidence from Developed Countries*, vol. I. *Population Studies* no. 109. United Nations, New York.
65. **United Nations.** 1988. *World Population Trends and Policies: 1987 Monitoring Report*. Population Studies no. 103. United Nations, New York.
66. **Van den Hoek, J. A., H. J. van Haastrecht, B. Scheeringa-Troost, J. Goudsmit, and R. A. Coutinho.** 1989. HIV infection and STD in drug addicted prostitutes in Amsterdam: potential for heterosexual HIV transmission. *Genitourin. Med.* **65:**146–150.
67. **Van de Perre, P., M. Carael, M. Robert-Guroff, P. Freyens, R. C. Gallo, N. Clumeck, E. Nzabihimana, P. De Mol, J.-P. Butzler, and J.-B. Kanyamupira.** 1985. Female prostitutes: a risk group for infection with human T-cell lymphotropic virus type III. *Lancet* **ii:**524–526.
68. **Verhagen, A. R., and W. Gemert.** 1972. Social and epidemiological determinants of gonorrhea in an East African country. *Br. J. Vener. Dis.* **48:**277–286.
69. **Whitman, F. L.** 1983. Culturally invariable properties of male homosexuality: tentative conclusions from cross-cultural research. *Arch. Sex. Behav.* **12:**207–226.
70. **World Health Organization.** 1983. *Adolescent Reproductive Health: an Approach to Planning Health Service Research*. WHO offset publication no. 77. World Health Organization, Geneva.

Health Care Utilization for Sexually Transmitted Diseases: Influence of Patient and Provider Characteristics

Hortensia Amaro and Isolde Gornemann

The assessment of factors that influence utilization of services for the prevention and treatment of sexually transmitted diseases (STDs), including human immunodeficiency virus (HIV) infection and AIDS, is a major area of scientific and practical relevance for the prevention and control of STDs. Education and behavior change among persons not infected with an STD are frequently necessary to reduce the risk of infection and for the prevention of STDs. Among infected persons, screening and treatment directly influence the duration of infectiousness and therefore the transmission as well as the sequelae of STDs (54). Discrepancies between estimates of the prevalence of STDs and the rates of use of STD clinics reflect the reality that many individuals in need of service never reach treatment, reach treatment at later stages of disease, self-medicate, or are not able to access services. Despite the central importance of health care seeking in the control of STDs, relatively little theoretical or empirical attention has been given to this topic (15).

The purpose of this chapter is to examine research regarding factors that impede or facilitate entry into treatment for STDs. First, a classification of risk factors that serve as forces toward or away from seeking help is presented. Second, the research literature dealing with selected factors in the classification framework is reviewed.

FACTORS AFFECTING UTILIZATION OF STD PREVENTION AND TREATMENT SERVICES

An understanding of what factors predispose individuals to seek or not to seek treatment is critical for the effective control of STDs, because to control the spread of STDs, those affected must seek and obtain effective treatment and those at high risk of infection must seek preventive health care (14). However, individuals who need medical care and those at high risk will not always seek or accept medical care; the consumer's knowledge, attitudes, and behavioral patterns play a key role in STD transmission and in seeking health care services (14). Despite this, the investigation of psychosocial and behavioral factors that influence health care seeking and treatment continuation for STDs has lagged behind other areas of research (e.g., drug treatments, epidemiology of risk behaviors).

Hortensia Amaro and Isolde Gornemann – Social and Behavioral Sciences Department, Boston University School of Public Health, Boston, Massachusetts 02118.

Some experts (14, 77) have suggested that equally important to understanding patient characteristics is the need to understand the characteristics and activities of health care professionals and the role of psychosocial and environmental factors (e.g., social atmosphere and interpersonal communication and relationship between provider and client), which can determine health care-seeking behavior among individuals in need of services. Yet, research on determinants of provider behaviors and on the impact of provider behaviors on patient health care-seeking and compliance behaviors regarding treatment of STDs is virtually nonexistent.

The absence of comprehensive efforts to investigate factors that affect utilization of services for prevention and treatment of STDs stands as a glaring problem in STD research. Despite existing theoretical models for understanding health care utilization, most research on STDs has focused narrowly on investigation of high-risk behaviors and factors that determine individual behavior change. Past research has suffered from several limitations. First, the omission of individuals who do not enter treatment from study samples has not allowed investigation of the factors that facilitate or inhibit treatment entry. Second, study samples have often been limited to unrepresentative samples of clients from one or a small number of clinics, limiting the generalizability of findings. Third, most relevant research on STDs has not investigated the relationship of provider and service characteristics to health care seeking. Fourth, research questions have often been limited to issues of compliance. For example, distinctions in health care seeking among symptomatic and asymptomatic patients have not been investigated and health care-seeking behaviors outside return for test of cure have not been studied.

To guide discussion in this chapter, we provide a classification scheme that describes factors affecting utilization of services for the prevention and treatment of STDs (Fig. 1). The scheme encompasses components of prior models such as the model of Anderson and Newman (1) of social and individual determinants of medical care utilization, the health belief model (4, 5), the theory of reasoned action (22, 23), and other relevant factors not considered by these models (3). The scheme proposed here can be employed to investigate relationships between independent variables and utilization of services as well as interrelationships among groups of variables. We examine selected variables as they are hypothesized to affect utilization of services for STDs.

The potential antecedents of seeking treatment for STDs are specified in Tables 1 and 2. This classification scheme identifies factors expected to affect client utilization of health care services for prevention or treatment of STDs (Table 1). Also considered are factors that influence health care providers, which in turn shape the quality and quantity of services offered and which can facilitate or inhibit client utilization of services (Table 2). Many of these factors have been related to health care behaviors; however, there is a dearth of information regarding how these factors influence health care seeking for STDs.

To seek help for the treatment or prevention of an STD, a person must first perceive the existence of an STD or the risk of acquiring an STD and be willing to address the problem through contact with the treatment system. Characteristics of the potential client, such as knowledge and beliefs regarding health, STDs,

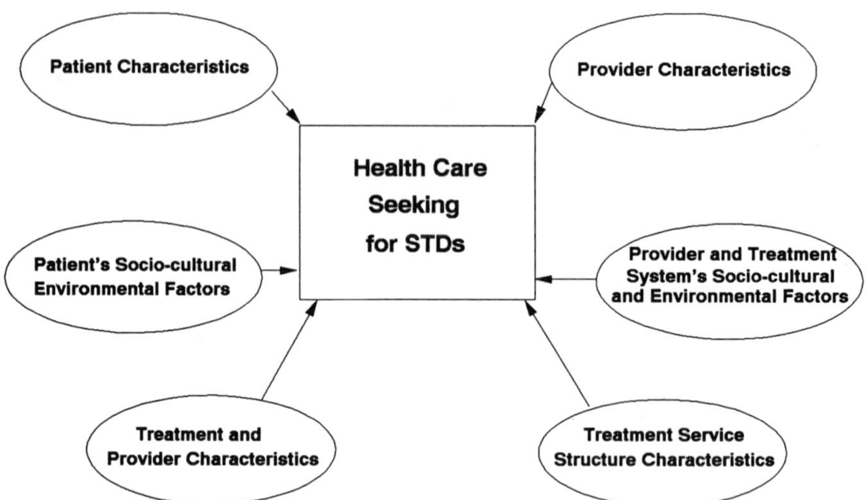

Figure 1. Factors influencing health care utilization for STDs.

symptom recognition, availability of services, and the efficacy of treatment, can influence an individual's judgment regarding whether a health problem exists and whether treatment will be helpful. Other factors, such as the individual's previous experiences with the health care system, balance of personal priorities, partner referral, perceived efficacy of prevention and treatment efforts, and mental health status, also influence seeking of medical care.

In addition, the individual must have other personal resources necessary to secure the services and overcome potential barriers to treatment (e.g., economic resources, language skills). These characteristics can affect an individual's willingness to initiate treatment-relevant actions and success in accessing services. Once the client is in contact with treatment systems, he or she must be willing to remain in treatment and adhere to the prescribed prevention or medical regimens if the medical condition warrants sustained treatment. Social enabling factors (e.g., social support, social norms, child care), the characteristics of treatment services, and the characteristics of the providers (e.g., knowledge, communication style, language, diagnostic and treatment ability) also can affect the client's willingness and success in accessing and effectively utilizing services.

CLASSIFICATION OF RISK MARKERS AND RISK FACTORS

Patient characteristics that affect the person's ability to secure and motivation to use services are listed in Table 1. The first set of patient characteristics are sociodemographic risk markers (e.g., education, income, employment status,

Table 1. Factors that influence patient utilization of health care for STDs

- I. Patient characteristics
  - A. Sociodemographic risk markers
    1. Education
    2. Income
    3. Employment status
    4. Ethnicity/race
    5. Sex
    6. Age
    7. Religion
    8. Marital status
    9. Sexual orientation
  - B. Knowledge and skills
    1. Knowledge about reproductive health
    2. Knowledge about transmission and symptoms of STDs
    3. Knowledge of available treatment and services for treatment of STDs
    4. Ability to recognize symptoms of STDs
    5. Skills and experience in assessing the health care delivery system, especially for treatment of STDs, and satisfaction with services and service providers
  - C. Beliefs, attitudes, and values
    1. Perceived severity of STDs and their consequences
    2. Perceived susceptibility to STDs
    3. Perceived personal efficacy in prevention and treatment efforts
    4. Evaluation of probable efficacy of treatment
    5. Perceived possible cost of seeking or continuing treatment in relation to financial considerations, stigma, relationship with partner, and health
    6. Perceived possible cost of not seeking or continuing treatment in relation to financial considerations, stigma, relationship with partner, and health
    7. Beliefs and values regarding personal responsibility for public health efforts to prevent transmission to others
    8. General beliefs and attitudes concerning scientific or medical approaches; STDs, their causes and treatment; health services and health care providers; and general health
    9. Attitudes and values regarding sexuality
  - D. Psychological and psychosocial factors
    1. Mental health including self-esteem, depression, anxiety, alienation, and addiction
    2. Sex role traditionalism
- II. Sociocultural and socioenvironmental factors
  - A. Norms in the culture, community, among significant others and sexual partner(s) regarding sexuality, illness, STDs, and health care services
  - B. Nature and importance of role of informal networks and significant others (including partner[s]) in facilitating or inhibiting health care utilization and seeking and continuing treatment for STDs
  - C. Situational factors such as child care responsibilities, access to transportation, and availability of time
- III. Treatment and provider characteristics
  - A. Access to treatment (cost, availability, type of service, linguistic access)
  - B. Availability of support services (child care, transportation)
  - C. Characteristics of the physical space where services are provided, such as atmosphere and comfort
  - D. Procedural encounters needed for engaging in services, including length of wait for appointments and scheduling full patient quotas
  - E. Type and quality of outreach procedures and referral sources
  - F. Role of community in development and delivery of services to improve quality and appropriateness
  - G. Characteristics of staff

Table 2. Factors that influence behaviors of STD service providers

- I. Provider characteristics
  - A. Sociodemographic characteristics
    1. Sex
    2. Religion
    3. Age
    4. Ethnicity/race
    5. Marital status
    6. Education
    7. Income
    8. Employment
    9. Sexual orientation
  - B. Knowledge and skills
    1. Knowledge regarding client population
    2. Knowledge and expertise in establishing rapport communicating with client, including speaking the client's primary language, and ability to personalize health recommendations
    3. Knowledge and expertise in diagnosis and treatment of STDs
  - C. Beliefs, attitudes, and values
    1. Beliefs, attitudes, and values regarding sexuality
    2. Beliefs, attitudes, and values regarding the client population
    3. Beliefs, attitudes, and values regarding the role of providers in discussing sexuality, prevention, assessment of STD risk, diagnosis, and treatment
  - D. Psychological and psychosocial factors
    1. Sex role traditionalism
    2. Personality characteristics
    3. Job stress
- II. Sociocultural and socioenvironmental factors
  - A. Institutional norms and policies regarding STD services
  - B. Competing provider role demands and work load
  - C. Cost and benefit to provider
- III. Treatment service structure characteristics
  - A. Support provided for STD prevention services
  - B. Support services for diagnosis (length of time required to perform test and to obtain results)
  - C. Support services for treatment (length of time to provide treatment)
  - D. Cost and benefit of providing STD services to the system

ethnicity/race, sex, age, religion, marital status, and sexual orientation). The second type of factors includes knowledge and skills. This includes knowledge regarding health, reproductive health, transmission and symptoms of STDs, and available treatment and services for STDs. Skills pertaining to a person's ability to perform the tasks necessary to access prevention or treatment services are included here. Such skills will be influenced by personal history related to previous STDs and treatment experiences and include the ability to recognize symptoms and the ability to access STD services. The third grouping of patient characteristics includes beliefs, attitudes, and values regarding health, STDs, and treatment. Beliefs specific to STDs include perceived severity, perceived susceptibility, perceived personal efficacy in prevention and treatment efforts, perceived efficacy of treatment, perceived efficacy in accessing treatment, perceived costs and benefits of seeking or not seeking treatment, and beliefs and values regarding personal responsibility to prevent transmission to others. Other beliefs and attitudes concerning scientific or medical approaches, STDs and their causes and treatment, health services and health care providers, and attitudes and values regarding sexuality are also considered. The last group of patient characteristics is composed of psychological and psychosocial factors that can affect utilization of services. These include mental health and personality characteristics such as self-esteem, depression, anxiety, alienation, addiction, and sex role traditionalism.

Some of the characteristics discussed above are not changeable (e.g., age, sex, ethnicity), while others can be changed through individual (e.g., marital status), policy (e.g., socioeconomic status), or educational (e.g., knowledge, attitudes, beliefs) efforts.

The second major group of factors considered are the social and environmental factors that impinge on the potential client, such as norms regarding sexuality, illness, STDs, and health care services in the culture and community and among the individual's social network; the nature and extent of social support networks and their role in facilitating and/or inhibiting seeking treatment for STDs; and situational factors such as child care responsibilities, access to time, and transportation.

The third factor affecting help seeking for prevention or treatment of STDs concerns the treatment and provider characteristics. Both characteristics of the treatment service structure and characteristics of the provider can affect entry into treatment. Factors in the treatment service structure include (i) access to treatment as determined by cost, geographical distribution, and multilingual staff; (ii) availability of support services such as child care and transportation; (iii) characteristics of the physical space; (iv) procedural encounters, waiting time, atmosphere of clinic, privacy; (v) type and quality of outreach procedures and referral sources; (vi) degree of target community involvement in development and implementation of services; and (vii) sociodemographic and professional background of the staff.

Table 2 presents service provider characteristics that influence delivery of services and that in turn can influence client utilization of health care services for STDs. The provider's sociodemographic characteristics (e.g., sex, ethnicity/race, religion, sexual orientation) are the first group of factors considered as potential determinants of provider behaviors. Second, provider knowledge and skills are also considered. These include the provider's knowledge and expertise regarding the client population, ability to establish rapport and communicate with the client, ability to speak the client's primary language, and ability to tailor the prevention message or regimen to the client. There is a growing appreciation of the need for systematic training of service providers in techniques of assessment of risk of STDs and HIV infection; thus, medical expertise in prevention, diagnosis, and treatment of STDs and symptom management also needs to be considered. Third, providers' beliefs, attitudes, and values can influence their behaviors. For example, beliefs, attitudes, and values regarding sexuality, the client population, and the role of providers in discussing sexuality, prevention, assessment of STD risk, diagnosis, and treatment should be considered.

Provider behaviors are also shaped by social factors such as (i) institutional norms and policies regarding STD services, (ii) competing demands on providers based on their roles and work load, and (iii) professional costs and benefits of providing STD services for the provider.

Finally, characteristics of the treatment service structure that determine the day-to-day mechanics of service delivery may facilitate or inhibit diagnostic and treatment procedures. Such characteristics include support services available for prevention, diagnosis, and treatment and the cost and benefit of providing STD services to the system.

In addition to the patient and provider characteristics and factors discussed above, specific events that serve as cues to action and promote health care-seeking behavior for treatment or prevention of an STD include changes that occur within the patient, in the social environment, or in the treatment setting. Changes in the individual's personal or social context that might promote increased motivation or support for seeking prevention or treatment services are (i) changes in patient characteristics, such as becoming pregnant; (ii) changes in beliefs, such as increased perception of symptom severity resulting from increased pain; and (iii) changes in social factors, such as a new sexual partner who observes symptoms in the client and urges the client to seek treatment for STDs. Changes in the availability of services, changes in service delivery, and changes in how services and/or staff are perceived by potential clients may also serve to change a client's inclination to seek services.

PREDISPOSING FACTORS INFLUENCING PATIENT UTILIZATION OF STD PREVENTION AND TREATMENT SERVICES

Sociodemographic Factors

Socioeconomic factors may present barriers to utilization of STD services for many individuals at high risk. Rates of STDs in ethnic minority populations, who are also more likely to be poor, are two to three times higher than rates in non-Hispanic whites (12, 21, 54, 77). In many countries, including the United States, the incidence of STDs is highest among individuals of lower socioeconomic status (14). Lower financial resources limit access to private health care and may even constrain individuals from seeking treatment in public community clinics.

It is unclear to what extent race and socioeconomic differences in the incidence of STDs can be explained by differences in health care utilization. Sexually active young male adults, who are the group at most risk for STDs, are also the sector of the population with the least contact with the health care system.

The inner city black or Hispanic poor individual is confronted with a multitude of competing and often immediate life concerns, which when combined with lack of appropriate services may result in underutilization of services for treatment of STDs. It is likely that socioeconomic factors play a less central role in health care seeking for medical treatment of STDs in countries where access and quality of medical services are not dictated by the client's ability to pay. A study of patients in STD clinics in Amsterdam, where treatment is provided regardless of ability to pay, found that those with lower educational levels were more likely to seek treatment at an earlier stage of disease than those of higher educational background (70).

In the United States, it has been reported that ethnic minorities and the poor are less likely to engage in recommended health behaviors (15). However, Darrow and Pauli (15) point out that when health care services are made readily available, such as when the Salk poliomyelitis vaccine was made available free of charge to communities in the rural south, health care seeking among ethnic minority and poor communities can even exceed that of white communities. Supporting this example is the finding that among men attending an STD clinic, blacks sought treatment sooner than whites did after becoming symptomatic with gonorrhea or nongonococcal urethritis (39). Unfortunately, the study was limited to a clinic population, and the effects of socioeconomic status and/or ethnicity on health care-seeking behaviors for STD among those not in treatment were not assessed. It is important to recognize that even when financial barriers are removed, other barriers (e.g., language, distrust, complex and inconvenient clinic procedures) hamper utilization of health care services. Among blacks and Hispanics in the United States, suspicion and mistrust of the mainstream white establishment, including public health experts, is evident in the AIDS epidemic (13). According to Bulhan (10), suspicion and mistrust among persons of color is based on the history of oppression through the misuse of science and medicine. In addition to the direct effects of race, ethnicity, and education on health care seeking for STDs, they may also exacerbate indirect effects through other factors that affect utilization of services. For example, in the United States, Hispanics and those with less education have less knowledge and more misconceptions about HIV transmission (16, 17, 29; H. Amaro, L. Strunin, R. Hingson, and L. Mofenson, Abstr. Annu. Meet. Am. Public Health Assoc., abstr. 1148, p. 87, 1988). The lesser knowledge about HIV among Hispanics has been attributed to lack of Spanish language educational materials and lack of prevention efforts targeted at this group.

Gender is associated with seeking of health care services, and it may also influence health care seeking for the prevention and treatment of STDs. While women in general are more likely to report illness symptoms and use health services (52), symptoms of STDs among women (e.g., chlamydia) are more subtle or asymptomatic and more difficult to diagnose than among men. For this reason, women are less likely to identify symptoms and more likely to perceive them as less severe, resulting in the reduced likelihood that they will seek treatment and/or continue treatment. Thus, in the case of STDs, it is unclear whether women are more likely than men to seek and/or continue treatment.

Younger age, another risk factor for STDs, is considered a negative predisposing factor for health care seeking. Individuals younger than 25 years of age account for the majority of cases of STDs (12, 54, 77). Developmental characteristics of individuals in this age range, especially adolescents, may make them less likely to perceive themselves at risk of infection. O'Reilly and Aral (53) argue that cognitive development and fears related to parental notification are barriers to seeking health care among adolescents at risk for STDs. Adolescents who have not developed from cognition that focuses on the present and is associated with the belief that one is omnipotent to cognition that allows one to think realistically about the future will find it difficult to consider the potentially adverse outcomes of risky behaviors. Because they believe they are omnipotent, adolescents with STDs often delay seeking treatment (53). In addition, adolescents' lack of direct and close experience with STDs is likely to render them vulnerable to optimistic biases or the underestimation of personal risk (78). Without awareness of their own risk, adolescents are relatively unlikely to seek health care for STDs. Another age-specific factor, required parental notification for medical treatment for minors, has important ramifications for health care seeking among adolescents with STDs (53). Although parental notification has not been required for STD treatment in the United States, fear of parental notification might contribute to delays in seeking health care among adolescents. Adolescent beliefs regarding parental notification practices for STD treatment and the relation of these beliefs to health care-seeking behaviors need empirical study.

Knowledge and Skills Related to STDs, Services, and Health

There is some evidence that knowledge about STDs is associated with increased health care-seeking behaviors such as improved compliance with follow-up appointments and taking medications (26, 51, 67, 81; R. Blonna, *Dis. Abstr. Int.* **48**:308, 1987). Little to no research exists on the relationship between knowledge and skills relevant to STDs, services, and health and health care seeking among those at risk who are not currently receiving treatment.

Educational interventions that seek to increase knowledge about STDs have shown increased health care-seeking behaviors in clinic samples. One of these studies (66) employed a videotape to increase knowledge in male patients with gonorrhea and found that the treatment group increased their knowledge and were more likely to return for the test of cure than controls. However, this study also noted that knowledge alone could not account for health care-seeking behaviors. Another study employing a videotaped educational intervention found that STD patients in the experimental group showed increased knowledge, positive attitudes toward condom use, and redemption of coupons for condoms (68). A clinic-based study of men with gonococcal urethritis found that the experimental group, which received an educational intervention, demonstrated significantly improved compliance with follow-up appointments and medication regimens (Blonna, *Dis. Abstr. Int.* **48**:308, 1987). One major limitation of these studies is that they have not attempted to ascertain the independent effect of knowledge versus that of other factors (e.g., beliefs, motivation) on improved health behaviors, making it difficult to ascertain which aspect of the educational interventions was most critical in improving health care-seeking behaviors. Also, measures of knowledge that reflect short-term improvement may not be relevant to subsequent behavior. These studies also do not address the impact of knowledge on health care seeking among nonclinic samples.

Results from other studies have been equivocal and suggest that there is no relationship between level of knowledge and some health care-seeking behaviors such as participation in HIV testing among some populations (44) or use of reliable contraceptive methods among adolescents seeking STD services (74). Further research is needed to more fully investigate critical questions related to the role of knowledge regarding STDs, medical services, and general health in promoting seeking of health care among populations at risk. We also need to better understand how patients' previous experiences and skills in accessing the health care delivery system, especially treatment of STDs, affect future use of such services.

Beliefs and Values about STDs, Sexuality, Treatment, and Health

Beliefs about STDs and their treatment, including beliefs related to the severity of STDs, personal susceptibility to an STD, perception regarding personal efficacy in prevention and treatment, the efficaciousness of treatment, and the costs and benefits of seeking treatment or of not seeking treatment, have been hypothesized to be associated with health care seeking. The importance of many of these variables in explaining individual differences in the adoption of health-related behaviors has been best described by the health belief model (5). However, empirical support for the health belief model has been equivocal and at times contradicts the model (34, 38, 42). It is possible that these discrepancies in findings are explained by limited-precision measurements of the variables and by the need to augment the health belief model with variables that consider social and cultural factors that may act as barriers or as facilitators of health-related behaviors (15, 43, 64). The health belief model is thought to represent a limited rational model that does not consider essential factors such as perceived social norms, perceived self-efficacy, and motivation (3, 23).

A few studies have documented the relationship between beliefs regarding STDs and health-related behaviors. A study of college students found that health care seeking as reflected in frequency of checkups for asymptomatic STDs was associated with perceptions regarding susceptibility and barriers to care (64). Similarly, a study (44) of methadone patients reported that, compared with those who chose not to have an HIV antibody test, individuals seeking antibody testing were more likely to be worried about contracting HIV and to hold positive beliefs regarding the test's usefulness. Those who chose to be tested were also more likely to be planning to have children and may have been motivated by the desire to make an informed decision regarding pregnancy.

Health care-seeking behaviors may also be influenced by other beliefs and values regarding the general value of Western scientific and medical approaches to treatment, personal responsibility to prevent transmission, sexuality, and sex roles. The importance of these beliefs in predicting health care-seeking behaviors has received little attention in research on STDs.

A study (60) of homosexual men in Sweden, Australia, Finland, and Ireland reported that masculine sex role orientation was associated with more STD infections. Sex role conservatism was associated with more infections in Finland

and lower rates in Australia, indicating the context-specific meaning of these factors. Among women, a traditional sex role orientation that emphasizes female passivity in sexuality is hypothesized to be a barrier to condom use and to seeking prevention or treatment services for STDs.

Psychological Characteristics

An individual's mental state may also modify health care-seeking behaviors. Feelings of powerlessness, depression, or anxiety and active addiction may serve as barriers to taking action and seeking treatment. The proposed model suggests that mental health and a positive sense of self contribute positively to seeking preventive and treatment services. Some populations (e.g., lower-income individuals, women) most affected by STDs also suffer from high rates of depression. In these groups, psychiatric symptoms may pose additional barriers to health care seeking.

Numerous studies indicate that patients in clinics for STDs have high percentages of psychiatric symptoms for depression and anxiety (11, 24, 30, 31, 44, 47, 59). The high rate of psychiatric symptoms has been explained by some as the direct result of the emotional impact of an STD diagnosis (20, 25). Others have argued that maladjusted individuals are at greater risk for STDs (27). However, case-control studies indicate that once background characteristics are controlled, STD patients do not differ from uninfected individuals in most psychological characteristics (15). Existing studies do not compare rates of psychiatric symptoms between individuals with STDs who seek services and those who do not seek treatment. Therefore, it is not possible to ascertain the impact of psychiatric problems on health care-seeking behaviors. There is a need for research that investigates the extent and nature of the relationship between psychiatric symptoms and seeking of health care services for STDs. Research that focuses on the underlying mechanisms and processes of this relationship would have the most applied value.

Sociocultural and Socioenvironmental Factors

Community norms regarding sexuality, illness, STDs, and utilization of health care services and the nature and importance of informal networks and social support relationships are hypothesized to have effects on health care seeking for the prevention or treatment of STDs. Such norms may facilitate or inhibit health care-seeking behaviors.

Prejudicial norms that stigmatize STDs promote fear of revealing one's STD status and avoidance of related health care services (35, 75). Some STDs are more stigmatized than others and may result in increased inhibition or fear of seeking services or of notifying a sexual partner. Stigmatization of persons with STDs including AIDS and associated discrimination in the United States have been well documented (7, 9, 28, 36). Similar stigmatization, which includes a lack of compassion for persons with AIDS, has been documented in other countries as well (35). Such stigmatization is detrimental to medical care-seeking behaviors because it not only provokes fear among those infected but also results in coercive policies

(35) that negatively affect access to health care (e.g., loss of a job or loss of health insurance).

At the root of the stigmatization of STDs including AIDS are misconceptions regarding transmission as well as long-standing prejudicial attitudes regarding the populations affected by these diseases (e.g., homosexual men, injection drug users, and persons of color) (35). While it is clear that stigmatization has a detrimental effect on those affected by HIV, empirical research is needed to understand the full impact of prejudicial social norms on medical care seeking among individuals at risk or infected with STDs. Social norms that stigmatize STDs, including AIDS, are probably the most powerful existing barrier to seeking health care.

The importance of social networks in promoting health care behaviors is evidenced in the manner in which the homosexual community in the United States responded to the AIDS epidemic. The sweeping changes in sexual behaviors among U.S. homosexual men in the first 10 years of the epidemic (46, 48) were facilitated by the strong community activism and behavioral norms promoting safer sex that developed in the homosexual community as a response to the epidemic. Conversely, social networks can also adopt norms that promote high-risk behaviors and lack of attention to prevention and health care-seeking behaviors (71). This social context hypothesis has been proposed as one explanation for the association between drug use and high-risk behaviors among some subgroups of homosexual men (71).

Other social enabling factors, such as family responsibilities regarding children and lack of transportation, are common barriers, especially for poor women, in accessing services for treatment of HIV (S. Allison-Cooke and J. S. Griffin, Abstr. Annu. Meet. Am. Public Health Assoc., abstr. 3205, p. 287, 1990; A. Carr, research report, Visiting Nurse Association, Chicago, 1990).

Treatment and Provider Characteristics

Many sources cite the importance of location of the clinic, speed with which care can be obtained, and cost of services as factors that affect access to health care services (54, 77). Some studies have attempted to assess the types of STD counseling and medical interventions that are most effective in promoting patient compliance. However, we identified no studies that investigated the characteristics of services associated with health care-seeking behaviors for prevention or treatment of STDs. Research questions related to how services for STDs can be best structured to promote utilization and health care-seeking behaviors among the targeted populations need to be investigated systematically in future research.

FACTORS INFLUENCING PROVIDER BEHAVIORS

While many clinicians and researchers agree that health care providers play a critical role in the treatment of STDs, the paucity of research on the provider- and service-related factors that promote or defer health care seeking indicates that empirical investigations have ignored the critical role of providers. Instead, most relevant research has focused solely on patient characteristics. The rich body of theoretical and empirical work stemming from psychology on provider behavior and health care seeking has not been applied to the study of health care seeking for STDs.

Adherence to medical regimens, for example, is determined not only by characteristics of the patient but also by the communication style of the physician and the patient-provider match (18, 19). Provider attitudes, values, and beliefs regarding STDs and the class and racial background of patients can affect provider behaviors, which may contribute to patient satisfaction, compliance, and aspects of other health care behaviors (18, 19, 49, 55, 65, 80). The powerful stigma associated with STDs, especially HIV infection and AIDS, is an important factor to consider in provider behaviors toward patients. Similarly, prejudicial attitudes and discriminatory practices toward the poor and members of racial, ethnic, and sexual preference groups render these populations especially vulnerable to the negative consequences of provider attitudes and practices. Unfortunately, as members of society, health care providers are not immune to the prejudicial attitudes and discriminatory behaviors shown toward persons affected with or at risk for STDs. There is a clear tendency to ascribe negative attributes such as socially unacceptable behaviors and decreased moral worth to such patients (33). Such attitudes and their subtle or glaring manifestations can directly impair the building of rapport, trust, and effective communication between provider and patient. In addition, aspects of the work environment (e.g., financial and staff resources, work load) and situational factors impinge on the provider's ability, inclination, or attitudes toward performing recommended prevention or treatment procedures and protocols.

Existing studies provide some indications of the potential impact of provider characteristics on patients' utilization of services; however, several limitations must be considered. First, while data exist on providers' knowledge and attitudes regarding STDs in general, attention to this area has been most pronounced only in the last few years as a response to the AIDS epidemic (35). These studies have investigated provider knowledge, attitudes, and beliefs regarding HIV and AIDS and attitudes toward providing services to these patients. We have much more to learn about provider knowledge and attitudes regarding other STDs. Second, studies have not generally investigated the influence of provider knowledge and attitudes on provider behaviors that may affect the likelihood of treatment utilization among patients. Third, most studies have used limited or poorly specified measures to assess dimensions of provider knowledge or attitudes. Finally, inadequate sample size, selective samples, inappropriate statistical analysis, and lack of comparison groups limit the generalizability and validity of these studies.

The first group of individual characteristics that may determine provider behavior consists of sociodemographic characteristics as well as knowledge, attitudes, and beliefs regarding STDs and the client population; knowledge as well as skills in performing sexual risk assessment interventions; knowledge and expertise in communicating with clients and personalizing health recommendations; and beliefs and values regarding sexuality and the role of providers in discussing sexuality and behavioral risk reduction.

Knowledge about the disease is essential to providing quality health care. It seems reasonable to expect that prepared and confident providers communicate most effectively with patients and contribute to patient knowledge about short- and long-term consequences of STDs, the need for altering high-risk behavior, and the need to seek professional help promptly. Yet, few studies have addressed the current status of knowledge about STDs among providers (56, 57, 62, 63). The majority of studies, focused specifically on HIV and AIDS, reveal that lack of knowledge and misconceptions are not uncommon among some groups of providers (56, 58). Lack of knowledge and misconceptions regarding transmission are associated with behaviors such as refusal to perform certain routine medical tasks for fear of contagion (6, 40, 72, 76, 79, 82). Lawrence and Lawrence (40) found that more knowledgeable staff were more confident that HIV cannot be transmitted through casual contact; nevertheless, even knowledgeable staff were not always comfortable touching and giving care to patients with AIDS, suggesting that knowledge is not the only predictor of provider behavior toward patients with HIV or AIDS. Bailey and colleagues (2) found that increased knowledge was related to increased willingness to provide care and to less harsh and judgmental attitudes toward patients with HIV or AIDS. These studies used self-reported measures of willingness to work with persons with HIV or AIDS rather than actual observed behavioral measures of contact with patients and thereby do not speak to the relationship between knowledge and actual behavior.

Provider knowledge and attitudes toward the patient population also may affect provider behaviors and hinder or enhance patient health care utilization. Studies that have examined factors in this area have focused on fear of homosexuality and fear of contagion. These fears are thought to be the source of anxiety and stress for people who provide health care to AIDS patients. Overall, there is no question that fear of homosexuality, or homophobia, has the strongest relationship to fear of AIDS (37, 50, 56, 57). Homophobia appears strong in all the groups studied, including physicians, nurses, medical students, nursing students, and non-health professionals, compared with other groups. Social workers express more accepting attitudes toward homosexuality as an alternative sexual orientation, and in general they are more empathic toward persons with HIV or AIDS (2). Despite these more favorable attitudes among social workers, social work services for patients with AIDS have been found to be deficient (45), and it is not clear how much of this problem is due to fear of AIDS.

While fear of death does not seem to be associated with providers' attitudes toward patients with AIDS or HIV (41), fear of contagion is an important predictor of attitudes (8, 32, 72, 76). The directionality of the relationship between fear and knowledge is unclear. Some studies (41, 45) report that providers who had more experience with AIDS patients were less fearful. However, Pomerance and Shields (57) found that health care workers who had a high level of contact with AIDS patients, and who presumably had more knowledge, were more comfortable dealing with them but also experienced more stress and higher perceived risk of transmission. In part, fear of contagion among providers who care for patients with AIDS may reflect their greater contact with bodily fluids and actual or feared risk of infection. Misconceptions about transmission represent one of the factors consistently associated with fear and negative attitudes among providers (32, 76). There is a lack of research on other factors that predict fear of contagion. One study (76) reported that ethnic minority health care professionals were more fearful of contagion than white health care professionals. However, a second study (57) employing more precise data analyses found that when other factors were controlled, ethnicity was not associated with fear of contagion. Other studies suggest that sex and professional background are associated with homophobia. Males show higher levels of homophobia than females (50), and medical students are more likely than nursing students to have homophobic attitudes and feelings (62).

Health care providers tend to blame AIDS patients more and ascribe more responsibility to them for their disease than they do with other patients (13, 50). Wallack (76) reports that feelings of anger and blame toward homosexual men for causing an epidemic that now threatens the heterosexual population were reported by approximately one-half of the health care professionals surveyed. Eighteen percent of the physicians and 33% of the nurses agreed that homosexual men with AIDS have only themselves to blame. Kelly et al. (37) found that patients with AIDS were significantly more likely than patients with leukemia to be regarded as responsible for their illness, deserving of what happened to them, and deserving to die. In another study (33), respondents rated patients with AIDS lowest of any group in competence and moral worth, in comparison with patients who had diabetes or heart attacks. Attitudes toward patients fluctuate depending on the disease of the patient, their sexual preference, the patient's sociodemographic characteristics as related to the provider's characteristics, the provider's perceived risk, and the provider's own sexual and moral attitudes. The more deviant the patient is perceived to be, the more the provider tends to impute negative thoughts and feelings and be more judgmental, less emphatic, and less willing to care. Providers' attitudes and fear may elicit stress that interferes with quality job performance. The coping behaviors associated with extreme fear of contagion are avoidance, exaggerated barrier precautions, and verbalization of fear. These behaviors have been clearly identified in providers throughout the literature addressing the AIDS crisis and its impact on health care.

Unfortunately, few studies have investigated attitudes and beliefs among providers and the consequences of provider attitudes on quality of health care and patient health care seeking. The role of the providers' skills in communication and their influence on patient health behaviors have been investigated through studies that test the effectiveness of various educational methods on patient behaviors. Solomon and her colleagues (66–68) found that educational strategies are essential to increasing knowledge and compliance in treatment. They also pointed out that educational methods must be emotionally significant and culturally relevant to the population being served. Washington (77) states that "practitioners are in a position to influence patients' illness, medical compliance and public health care behaviors by providing effective education. For example, compliance with medical care instructions is dependent on the clarity, explicitness and rigor with which clinicians deliver messages."

Green (26) pointed out that communication methods directed at the patient or the general public are most often effective in achieving changes in predisposing factors such as knowledge, attitudes, beliefs, and values. Although the Federal Quality Assurance Guidelines for STD clinics clearly determine that patient education should be routinely included in every patient visit and reinforced by every provider the patient sees, the quality and frequency of this practice vary greatly across health care settings. An observational study by Roter and colleagues (61) found that at least 25% of STD clinic patients did not receive any information about treatment and 28% did not receive any information regarding prevention. Preventive information was much less likely to be given by physicians (14.8%) than by nurses (54.1%) or by counselors (48.3%). Only slightly more than one-half of the patients observed in this study could be considered fully informed. While the findings of this observational study are not generalizable to all STD clinics, it should remind us of the need to examine not only patient behavior but also provider behavior and clinic practices as we investigate predictors of patient health care seeking and compliance.

There is a clear lack of information regarding health care providers' perceived severity of STDs and their consequences; perceived susceptibility of patients to STD; evaluation of effectiveness, cost, and convenience of diagnosis and treatment; and perceived risks of contagion. These are all important issues that could affect provider-patient interaction, effectiveness of communication, and the patient's perception of risk and willingness to take action. These factors influence the amount of time and effort a provider puts into making an accurate diagnosis; inquiring about sexual behavior and practices, the patient's sexual contacts, and the patient's willingness to inform the sexual partner; communicating short- and long-term consequences of the disease and the need to rigorously follow treatment regimens; and explaining the importance of partner referral. These efforts on the part of the provider are likely to be influenced by the amount of personal responsibility he or she feels for public health efforts to prevent transmission to others and the perceived implications and consequences either to the provider (e.g., liability) or to the patient of not making appropriate diagnosis or providing effective treatment and counseling. Among the costs to providers, one study showed that physicians who considered that treating AIDS patients in a private office resulted in risk of contaminating examining equipment, losing other patients, and increasing legal liability and other financial risk were less likely to care for AIDS patients (69). Although providers' perceived cost of treating HIV infection may not be comparable to their perception of the cost of treating other STDs, the implications for further research and future intervention in providers' education in this area are too important to dismiss.

Psychological and Psychosocial Factors

Psychological and psychosocial factors such as values regarding sex role traditionalism and sexuality, personality characteristics, and job stress can influence provider behaviors. It is not yet known how job-related stress, perhaps resulting from fear of contagion, long working hours, understaffed clinics, perceived lack of appropriate training and competence, liability, and overcrowded clinics, affects providers' performance and capability to give an accurate diagnosis, competent treatment, and patient education in STD clinics. In the general primary health care setting, it is not known how these factors affect the provider's willingness and ability to undertake a sexual risk assessment when this is indicated.

Social Enabling Factors and Treatment Service Structure

The last factors considered to influence provider behaviors relate to environmental or situational factors, including characteristics of the clinic setting that impinge on the provider. The lack of research on the role of environmental, situational, and treatment structure characteristics in influencing providers of STD services underlines the narrow emphasis in the existing analysis and understanding of factors that affect health care seeking among consumers. There has been a clear bias to study the patient and to ignore the social, contextual, and administrative aspects of delivery of STD services. There is a critical need for research that investigates the individual factors as well as the social, contextual, and structural factors that make up the treatment setting.

CONCLUSION

To increase the effectiveness of STD prevention and control, it will be necessary to improve our understanding of how patient and service characteristics affect health care seeking. This would enable providers to restructure services and prevention strategies to improve health care seeking. It is our hope that STD researchers will increasingly attend to the investigation of behavioral and service factors that influence health care seeking and that the framework and discussion provided in this chapter will serve as a stimulus for the development of research questions in this area.

Acknowledgments. We express our appreciation to King Holmes, Lee Strunin, Dan Merrigan, John Rich, Eugene Washington, and Rami Marx for insightful suggestions and review of an earlier draft of the manuscript and to Felicia Hendrix for preparation of the manuscript.

LITERATURE CITED

1. **Anderson, R., and J. P. Newman.** 1973. Societal and individual determinants of medical care utilization in the U.S. *Milbank Q.* **51:**95–124.
2. **Bailey, L. G., B. C. Johnson, P. L. Starkey, and C. E. Kellogg.** 1989. Health care workers' knowledge and attitudes concerning AIDS. *J. Miss. State Med. Assoc.* **30:**355–359.
3. **Bandura, A.** 1989. Perceived self-efficacy in the exercise of control over AIDS infection, p. 128–141. *In* V. M. Mays, G. W. Albee, and S. F. Schneider (ed.), *Primary Prevention of AIDS: Psychological Approaches*, vol. 13. Sage Publications, Newbury Park, Calif.
4. **Becker, M. H.** 1974. The health belief model and sick role behavior. *Health Educ. Monogr.* **2:**409–419.

5. **Becker, M. H., and L. A. Mainman.** 1983. Models of health related behavior, p. 539–568. *In* D. Mechanic (ed.), *Handbook of Health Care and the Health Profession*. Free Press, New York.
6. **Bell Meisenhelder, J., and C. L. La Charite.** 1989. Fear of contagion: a stress response to acquired immunodeficiency syndrome. *Adv. Nurs. Sci.* **11:**29–38.
7. **Blendon, R. J., and K. Donelan.** 1988. Discrimination against people with AIDS: the public's perspective. *N. Engl. J. Med.* **319:**1022–1026.
8. **Blumenfield, M., S. P. Jordano, J. Milazzo, S. Seropian, and G. P. Wormser.** 1987. Survey of attitudes of nurses working with AIDS patients. *Gen. Hosp. Psychiatry* **9:**58–63.
9. **Brandt, A. M.** 1985. *No Magic Bullet: Social History of Venereal Diseases in the United States since 1980*. Oxford University Press, New York.
10. **Bulhan, H. A.** 1985. Colonial research and medicine, p. 81–99. *In* H. A. Bulhan (ed.), *Franz Fanon and the Psychology of Oppression*. Plenum Press, New York.
11. **Catalan, J., M. Bradley, J. Gallwey, and K. Hawton.** 1981. Sexual dysfunction and psychiatry morbidity in patients attending a clinic for sexually transmitted diseases. *Br. J. Psychiatry* **138:**292–296.
12. **Centers for Disease Control.** 1988. Cases of specified notifiable diseases. United States. *Morbid. Mortal. Weekly Rep.* **37:**709–711.
13. **Dalton, H. L.** 1989. AIDS in blackface. *Daedalus* **118:**205–227.
14. **Darrow, W. W.** 1976. Social and behavioral aspects of the sexually transmitted diseases, p. 134–153. *In* S. Gordon (ed.), *Sexuality Today and Tomorrow*, vol. 12. Duxbury Press, North Scituate, Mass.
15. **Darrow, W. W., and M. L. Pauli.** 1984. Health behavior and sexually transmitted diseases, p. 65–73. *In* K. K. Holmes, P.-A. Mardh, P. F. Sparling, and P. J. Wiesner (ed.), *Sexually Transmitted Diseases*. McGraw-Hill Book Co., New York.
16. **Dawson, D. A., and A. M. Hardy.** 1990. AIDS knowledge and attitudes among Hispanic Americans. Provisional data from the 1988 National Health Interview Survey. *Nat. Ctr. Health Statist. Adv. Data* **166:**1–22.
17. **DiClemente, R., C. Boyer, and E. Morales.** 1988. Minorities and AIDS: knowledge, attitudes, and misconceptions among blacks and Latino adolescents. *Am. J. Public Health* **78:**55–57.
18. **DiMateo, R. M.** 1985. Physician-patient communication. Promoting a positive health care setting, p. 328–365. *In* J. C. Rosen and L. J. Solomon (ed.), *Prevention in Health Psychology*. University Press of New England, Hanover, N.H.
19. **DiMateo, R. M., and D. D. DeNicola.** 1982. *Achieving Patient Compliance: the Psychology of the Medical Practitioner's Role*. Pergamon Press, Inc., Elmsford, N.Y.
20. **Drob, S., and H. S. Bernard.** 1986. Time-limited group treatment of genital herpes patients. *Int. J. Group Psychother.* **36:**133–144.
21. **Fichtner, R. R., S. O. Aral, J. H. Blount, A. A. Zaida, G. H. Reynolds, and W. W. Darrow.** 1983. Syphilis in the United States: 1967–1979. *Sex. Transm. Dis.* **10:**77–80.
22. **Fishbein, M., and I. Ajzen.** 1975. Belief, attitude, intention and behavior: an introduction to theory and research, p. 128–131. *In* V. M. Mays, G. W. Albee, and S. F. Schneider (ed.), *Primary Prevention of AIDS: Psychological Approaches*, vol. 13. Sage Publications, Newbury Park, Calif.
23. **Fishbein, M., and S. E. Middlestadt.** 1989. Using the theory of reasoned action as a framework for understanding and changing AIDS-related behaviors, p. 93–110. *In* V. M. Mays, G. W. Albee, and S. F. Schneider (ed.), *Primary Prevention of AIDS: Psychological Approaches*, vol. 13. Sage Publications, Newbury Park, Calif.
24. **Fitzpatrick, R., G. Ikkos, and D. Frost.** 1985. The recognition of psychological disturbances in a sexually transmitted diseases clinic. *Int. J. Soc. Psychiatry* **31:**306–312.
25. **Goldmeier, D., and A. Johnson.** 1982. Does psychiatric illness affect the recurrence rate of genital herpes? *Br. J. Vener. Dis.* **58:**40–43.
26. **Green, L. W.** 1979. Educational strategies to improve compliance with therapeutic and preventive regimens: the recent evidence, p. 157–173. *In* R. B. Haynes, D. Sackett, and W. Taylor (ed.), *Compliance in Health Care*. The John Hopkins University Press, Baltimore.

27. **Hart, C.** 1977. *Sexual Malady and Disease: an Introduction to Modern Venereology*. Nelson Hall, Chicago.
28. **Herek, G. M., and E. K. Glunt.** 1988. An epidemic of stigma: public reactions to AIDS. *Am. Psychol.* **43:**886–891.
29. **Hingson, R., L. Strunin, L. Craven, T. Mangione, B. Berlin, H. Amaro, and G. Lamb.** 1989. Statewide survey of AIDS knowledge and behavior changes among Massachusetts adults. *Prev. Med.* **18:**806–816.
30. **Houck, E. L., and P. R. Abramson.** 1986. Masturbatory guilt and the psychological consequences of sexually transmitted diseases among women. *J. Res. Pers.* **20:**267–275.
31. **Ikkos, G., R. Fitzpatrick, D. Frost, and S. Nazear.** 1987. Psychological disturbance and illness behavior in a clinic for sexually transmitted diseases. *Br. J. Med. Psychol.* **60:**121–126.
32. **Imperato, P. J., J. G. Feldman, K. Nayeri, and J. A. DeHovitz.** 1988. Medical students' attitudes toward caring for patients with AIDS in a high incidence area. *N.Y. State J. Med.* **88:**223–227.
33. **Katz, I., R. G. Hass, N. Parisi, J. Ashtone, and D. McEvaddy.** 1987. Lay people's and health care personnel's perceptions of cancer, AIDS, cardiac, and diabetic patients. *Psychol. Rep.* **60:**615–629.
34. **Kegeles, S.** 1963. Why people seek dental care: a behavioral model of health and illness behavior. *J. Health Hum. Behav.* **4:**166–173.
35. **Kegeles, S. M., T. J. Coates, A. T. Christopher, and J. K. Lazarus.** 1989. Perception of AIDS: the continuing saga of AIDS-related stigma. *AIDS* **3**(Suppl. 1)**:**S253–S258.
36. **Kegeles, S. M., T. J. Coates, B. Lo, and J. A. Catania.** 1989. Mandatory reporting of HIV testing would deter men from being tested. *J. Am. Med. Assoc.* **261:**1275–1276.
37. **Kelly, J. A., J. S. St. Lawrence, S. Smith, H. V. Hood, and D. J. Cook.** 1987. Medical students' attitudes towards AIDS and homosexual patients. *J. Med. Educ.* **62:**549–556.
38. **Kirscht, J. P., and J. G. Joseph.** 1989. The health belief model: some implications for behavior change with reference to homosexual males, p. 111–127. *In* V. M. Mays, G. W. Albee, and S. F. Schneider (ed.), *Primary Prevention of AIDS: Psychological Approaches*, vol. 13. Sage Publications, Newbury Park, Calif.
39. **Kramer, M. A., S. V. Aral, and J. W. Curran.** 1980. Self-reported behavior patterns of patients attending a sexually transmitted disease clinic. *Am. J. Public Health* **70:**997–1000.
40. **Lawrence, S. A., and R. M. Lawrence.** 1989. Knowledge and attitudes about acquired immunodeficiency syndrome in nursing and nonnursing groups. *J. Prof. Nurs.* **5:**92–101.
41. **Lester, L. L., and B. J. Beard.** 1988. Nursing students' attitudes toward AIDS. *J. Nurs. Educ.* **27:**399–404.
42. **Leventhal, H., R. Zimmerman, and M. Gutmann.** 1984. Compliance: a self regulation perspective, p. 369–436. *In* D. Century (ed.), *Handbook of Behavioral Medicine*. Guilford Press, New York.
43. **Leviton, L. C.** 1989. Theoretical foundations of AIDS-prevention programs, p. 42–90. *In* R. O. Valdiserri (ed.), *Preventing AIDS*. Rutgers University Press, New Brunswick, N.J.
44. **Magura, S., J. Grossman, D. S. Lipton, K. R. Amann, J. Koyu, and K. Gehan.** 1989. Correlates of participation in AIDS education and HIV antibody testing by methadone patients. *Public Health Rep.* **104:**231–240.
45. **Mantell, J. E., L. C. Shulman, M. F. Belmont, and H. B. Spirak.** 1989. Social workers respond to the AIDS epidemic in an acute care hospital. *Health Soc. Work.* **14:**41–51.
46. **Martin, J. L.** 1987. The impact of AIDS on gay male sexual behavior patterns in New York City. *Am. J. Public Health* **77:**578–581.
47. **Mayou, R.** 1975. Psychological morbidity in a clinic for STD. *Br. J. Vener. Dis.* **51:**57–60.
48. **McKusick, L., W. Horstman, and T. J. Coates.** 1985. AIDS sexual behavior reported by gay men in San Francisco. *Am. J. Public Health* **75:**493–496.
49. **Mejta, C. L., E. Denton, M. E. Krems, and R. A. Hiatt.** 1988. Acquired immunodeficiency syndrome (AIDS): a survey of substance abuse clinic directors' and counselors' perceived knowledge, attitudes and reactions. *J. Drug Issues* **18:**403–419.

50. **Merrill, J. M., L. Laux, and J. J. Thornby.** 1989. AIDS and student attitudes. *South. Med. J.* **82:**426–432.
51. **Moran, J. S., R. J. Harlan, T. A. Peterman, and K. M. Stone.** 1990. Increase in condom sales following AIDS education and publicity, United States. *Am. J. Public Health* **80:**607–608.
52. **Nathanson, C.** 1977. Sex, illness, and medical care: a review of data, theory, and methods. *Soc. Sci. Med.* **11:**13–25.
53. **O'Reilly, K. R., and S. O. Aral.** 1985. Adolescence and sexual behavior. *J. Adolesc. Health Care* **6:**262–270.
54. **Padian, N., P. J. Hitchcock, R. E. Fullilove, V. Kohlstadt, R. Brunham, and the NIAID Study Group on Integrated Behavioral Research for Prevention and Control of Sexually Transmitted Diseases.** 1990. Part I: Issues in defining behavioral risk factors and their distribution. *Report of the NIAID Study Group on Integrated Behavioral Research for Prevention and Control of Sexually Transmitted Diseases. Sex. Transm. Dis.* **17:**200–210.
55. **Plaja, A. O., L. M. Cohen, and J. Samora.** 1968. Communications between physicians and patients in outpatient clinics, social and cultural factors. *Milbank Q.* **46:**161–214.
56. **Pleck, J. H., L. O'Donnell, C. O'Donnell, and A. M. Levine.** 1988. AIDS-phobia, contact with AIDS, and AIDS related job stress in hospital workers. *J. Homosex.* **15:**41–54.
57. **Pomerance, L. M., and J. J. Shields.** 1989. Factors associated with hospital workers' reactions to the treatment of persons with AIDS. *AIDS Educ. Prev.* **1:**184–193.
58. **Richardson, J., L. T. Lochner, and K. McGuigan.** 1987. Physician attitudes and experience regarding the care of patients with acquired immunodeficiency syndrome (AIDS) and related disorders (ARC). *Med. Care* **25:**675–685.
59. **Ross, M. W.** 1987. Illness behavior among patients attending a sexually transmitted diseases clinic. *Sex. Transm. Dis.* **14:**174–179.
60. **Ross, M. W.** 1984. Sociological and psychological predictors of STD infection in homosexual men: a study of four countries. *Br. J. Vener. Dis.* **60:**110–113.
61. **Roter, D. L., N. Knowles, M. Somerfield, and J. Baldwin.** 1990. Routine communication in sexually transmitted disease clinics: an observational study. *Am. J. Public Health* **80:**605–606.
62. **Royse, D., and B. Birge.** 1987. Homophobia and attitudes toward AIDS patients among medical, nursing and paramedical students. *Psychol. Rep.* **61:**876–880.
63. **Sherr, L.** 1987. The impact of AIDS in obstetrics on obstetric staff. *J. Rep. Infant Psychol.* **5:**87–96.
64. **Simon, K. J., and A. Das.** 1984. An application of the health belief model toward educational diagnosis for VD education. *Health Educ. Q.* **11:**403–418.
65. **Singh, D. S., D. D. Royse, and T. V. Tran.** 1987–1988. Social work practitioner's attitudes towards AIDS victims. *J. Appl. Soc. Sci.* **12:**108–123.
66. **Solomon, M. Z., and W. DeJong.** 1988. The impact of a clinic-based educational videotape on knowledge and treatment behavior of men with gonorrhea. *Sex. Transm. Dis.* **15:**127–132.
67. **Solomon, M. Z., and W. DeJong.** 1989. Preventing AIDS and other STDs through condom promotion: a patient education intervention. *Am. J. Public Health* **79:**453–458.
68. **Solomon, M. Z., W. DeJong, and T. A. Jodrie.** 1988. Improving drug regimen adherence among patients with sexually transmitted diseases. *J. Compliance Health Care* **3:**41–56.
69. **Somogyi, A. A., J. A. Watson-Abady, and F. S. Mandel.** 1990. Attitudes toward the care of patients with acquired immunodeficiency syndrome: a survey of community internists. *Arch. Intern. Med.* **150:**50–53.
70. **Stadlander, M., and G. Kok.** 1989. Prevention of sexually transmitted diseases: relapse behavior of visitors to the venereal diseases clinics in Amsterdam. *Health Educ. Res.* **4:**267–271.
71. **Stall, R., L. McKusick, J. Wiley, T. J. Coates, and D. G. Ostrow.** 1986. Alcohol and drug use during sexual activity and compliance with safe sex guidelines for AIDS. The AIDS Behavioral Research Project. *Health Educ. Q.* **13:**359–371.

72. **Strunin, L., A. Culbert, and S. Crane.** 1989. First year medical students' attitudes and knowledge about AIDS. *AIDS Care* **1:**105–110.
73. **Syme, S. L., and L. F. Berkman.** 1976. Social class, susceptibility and sickness. *Am. J. Epidemiol.* **104:**1–8.
74. **Tobin, J. M., and R. B. Roy.** 1985. Are we failing our teenagers? Value of a family planning service for teenagers within the sexually transmitted disease clinic. *Br. Med. J.* **290:**376–378.
75. **Turner, C. F., H. G. Miller, and L. E. Moses (ed.).** 1989. *AIDS: Sexual Behavior and Intravenous Drug Use*. National Academy Press, Washington, D.C.
76. **Wallack, J. J.** 1989. AIDS anxiety among health care professionals. *Hosp. Community Psychiatry* **40:**507–510.
77. **Washington, E.** 1989. Risk, health promotion, disease intervention and sexually transmitted diseases. *Mobius* **4:**26–32.
78. **Weinstein, N. D.** 1989. Perception of personal susceptibility to harm, p. 142–167. *In* V. M. Mays, G. W. Albee, and S. F. Schneider (ed.), *Primary Prevention of AIDS: Psychological Approaches*, vol. 13. Sage Publications, Newbury Park, Calif.
79. **Wertz, D. C., J. R. Sorenson, L. Liebling, L. Lester, and T. C. Heeren.** 1988. Caring for persons with AIDS: knowledge and attitudes of 1,047 health care workers attending AIDS Action Committee educational programs. *J. Primary Prev.* **8:**109–124.
80. **Wright, M., and M. Rodway.** 1989. Sexually transmitted diseases: psychological parameters and implications for social work practice. *J. Soc. Work. Hum. Sex.* **6:**21–35.
81. **Yarber, W. L.** 1988. Evaluation of the health behavior approach to school STD education. *J. Sex. Educ. Ther.* **14:**33–38.
82. **Young, E. W., P. B. Koch, and D. B. Preston.** 1989. AIDS and homosexuality: a longitudinal study of knowledge and attitudes change among rural nurses. *Public Health Nurs.* **6:**189–196.

Demographic and Societal Factors Influencing Risk Behaviors

Sevgi O. Aral, Robert E. Fullilove, Roel A. Coutinho, and J. A. R. Van Den Hoek

Risk behaviors for sexually transmitted diseases (STDs) and AIDS, including sexual behaviors, health behaviors, and drug use, are influenced in complex ways by societal, demographic, behavioral (including other risk behaviors), and personality factors. The usual patterns of effect often encompass reciprocal rather than unidirectional influence and bivariate relationships that are conditional on the values of additional variables.

Demographic characteristics often determine the particular social environments individuals live in. For example, a 20-year-old married poor Hispanic woman is rarely in the same social environment as a 35-year-old white Anglo-Saxon Protestant suburban housewife. Conversely, societal factors define the social meaning of demographic characteristics. For example, being a 20-year-old Hispanic woman in New York City is different from being a 20-year-old Hispanic woman in Medellin, Colombia.

Most if not all demographic and societal effects on behavior are time dependent. To simplify data for analysis, we often collapse some of the dimensions relevant to our analysis. Time is frequently thus collapsed, leading to descriptions of instantaneous cross sections of social and epidemiological phenomena. Such instantaneous analyses mask the dynamic nature of social factors and, perhaps more importantly, make it difficult to define and describe the effects of change itself on behavior.

Two types of change are particularly relevant to STD and AIDS risk behaviors: societal evolution, encompassing large-scale processes such as demographic transition, industrial revolution, urbanization, and westernization; and individual psychosocial development or maturation. Sexual behaviors are particularly prone to the influence of developmental factors. For example, adolescence is typically marked by having multiple sex partners and often leads to settling down with a single partner.

The epidemiological importance and intervention implications of risk behaviors shaped by developmental factors may differ from those of other risk behaviors. The multiple-partner activity of adolescence is a life stage rather than a life-style. In contrast, for some groups in the population, having multiple partners may be a way

Sevgi O. Aral – Behavioral and Prevention Research Branch, Division of STD/HIV Prevention, MS E02, Centers for Disease Control, Atlanta, Georgia 30333. ***Robert E. Fullilove*** – College of Physicians and Surgeons, Columbia University, New York, New York 10032. ***Roel A. Coutinho and J. A. R. Van Den Hoek*** – Municipal Health Service, 1000 HE Amsterdam, The Netherlands.

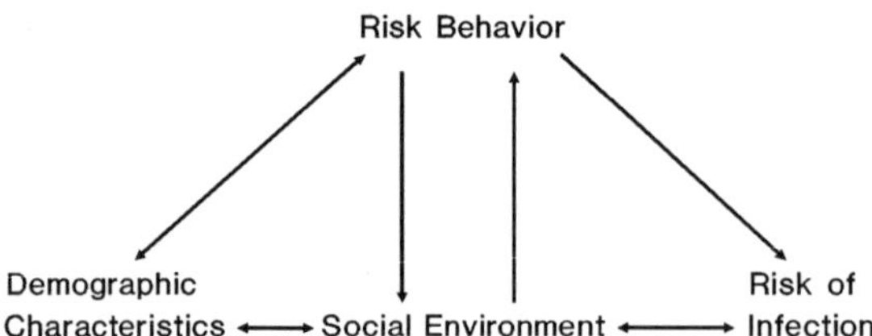

Figure 1. Effect of demographic characteristics on risk behavior.

of life. For example, in the 1970s in most Western countries, having large numbers of sex partners was a life-style for homosexual men. Having multiple sex partners as a life-style may differ in its importance for disease transmission from having multiple sex partners as a developmental stage in adolescence. On the other hand, there may be a strong correlation between the two.

Behavioral interventions aimed at changing sexual life-styles are also different from those aimed at changing behaviors directed by developmental life stages. Moreover, research designs that are appropriate for evaluating change in sexual life-styles may be inappropriate for evaluating change in developmental sexual behaviors. In evaluating life-style changes, we would look especially for long-term change to rule out possible emergence of relapse and to focus on maintained change. In measuring sexual behavior during adolescence, short-term change may be more appropriate, since it would be less affected than long-term change by maturation as an alternative explanation for any change observed.

In this chapter, we discuss the effects of demographic and societal factors, the effects of other behaviors such as drug use and prostitution, and the effects of secular, societal, and individual change on STD and AIDS risk behaviors. We conclude with a discussion of implications of such effects for epidemiological analysis and for interventions and intervention research.

EFFECTS OF DEMOGRAPHIC FACTORS

Demographic characteristics of individuals, including, age, gender, race, marital status, socioeconomic status (SES), and education, affect STD and AIDS risk behaviors (33). To some extent, risk behaviors also influence demographic characteristics. For example, drug use may lead to downward social mobility, thereby affecting SES, or sexual behavior may lead to marriage or divorce. Demographic characteristics influence sexual behavior in indirect ways as well through their effect on the individual's social environment (Fig. 1). (The interaction between indirect and direct risk factors for STDs, based on the proximity of the risk factor to transmission of infection or development of disease, is discussed by Padian et al. in this volume.)

Age and gender are important predictors of the number of sexual partners. According to data from the 1988 to 1989 general social survey (11) of all American men and women aged 18 to 44, 13% of women and 25% of men who had sexual intercourse during the previous 12 months reported two or more sexual partners during that time period. Persons aged 18 and 19 most often reported multiple partners; 34% of women and 50% of men of this age had two or more sex partners over the 12 months. Among 40 to 44 year olds, 5% of women and 13% of men reported two or more sex partners over the past year (11). In 1988, among reproductive-age American women, the proportions reporting two or more partners in the past 3 months were 6% among 20 to 21 year olds, 4% among 25 to 29 year olds, and 2% among 30 to 34 year olds (20). Similarly, in 1987, among women receiving family planning services in Pennsylvania, age was inversely related to number of partners; the proportion of women reporting three or more partners over the past year was 21% among those younger than 15 years, 15% among 15 to 19 year olds, 11% among 20 to 29 year olds, and 10% among women who were 30 years old or older (7). In the same year, 4.6% of 18- to 29-year-old never-married men and 2.9% of 30- to 44-year-old never-married men reported 10 or more sex partners over the preceding 12 months (11).

Age and gender also predict choice of sex partner. In 1988, 6% of men and 1.2% of women aged 18 and older in a random sample of the American population had sex with at least one "casual date or pick-up" within the preceding 12 months. In 1987, among women attending family planning clinics in Pennsylvania, proportions reporting sex with a partner at high risk for human immunodeficiency virus (HIV) infection increased with age. Four percent of those younger than 15 years old and 6% of those 30 years old and older reported sex with an injecting drug user (IDU); 0.5% of those younger than 15 years and 2% of those 30 years old and older reported sex with a bisexual man (7).

Marked gender differentials exist both in the general population and among STD clinic attendees in the recruitment of sex partners (4). Compared with men, women tend to meet their potential partners through less casual associations and know them better and for longer periods before becoming sexually involved with them (4a, 43). A nondiscriminating approach to sex partner recruitment increases the probability of sexual contact with members of high-risk core groups (see chapters by Anderson and by Brunham and Ronald, this volume, for a discussion of core groups) and thus of exposure to sexually transmitted infections.

Race is associated with the incidence of STD, and it has traditionally been assumed that race is a marker for both sexual and health care-seeking behavior (A. E. Washington, S. O. Aral, D. A. Grimes, and K. K. Holmes, *J. Am. Med. Assoc.*, in press). The incidence of STDs among black, Hispanic, and native American citizens of the United States is higher than among whites and appears to be increasing (38, 52). In 1988, for example, blacks constituted 11.5% of the U.S. population but 75.8% of all reported cases of primary and secondary syphilis in the United States, and 78.2% of all reported gonorrhea cases (38). In a study using data from the 1978 National Health and Nutrition Examination Survey, black race emerged as a strong risk marker for syphilis seroreactivity in the U.S. population, independent of other sociodemographic risk markers. This finding was consistent with findings from other studies (26). The incidence of AIDS follows similar trends: blacks and Hispanics are disproportionately represented among persons with AIDS and with HIV infection.

This pattern of disproportionate representation suggests three possible explanations: (i) there are risk behaviors that are peculiar to these minority populations that place them at risk for infection with sexually transmitted pathogens, including HIV; (ii) there is a biological predisposition to acquiring these diseases upon exposure among racial and ethnic groups with increased incidence; and (iii) differential access to or use of health care accounts for the differential incidence of sexually transmitted infections in these groups.

Each of the above explanations can be viewed in the context of the transmission model developed by May and Anderson (34) (see chapters by Anderson and by Brunham and Ronald, this volume). According to this model, $R_0 = \beta c D$; the reproductive rate of infection (R_0) of a particular pathogen depends on the efficiency of transmission (β), the average rate and variability of new sexual partner selection (c), and the duration of infectiousness (D). Hypothetically, parameters β, c, and D may all be higher among racial and ethnic groups that have a high incidence of STD. For example, efficiency of transmission could be higher because of lack of circumcision, higher prevalence of vaginal douching (which might alter the normal, protective flora) and early onset of sexual activity among young women (when the prevalence of ectopy is highest), higher prevalence of other STDs, practice of sexual intercourse in the presence of acute infection, or genetic or biological predisposition that results in higher susceptibility among uninfected persons. The average rate and variability of new partner selection might be higher among blacks, Hispanics, and native Americans than among whites. Finally, duration of infectiousness might be longer among groups with high STD incidence because of relatively poor access to diagnostic and therapeutic services, poor health education, and poor health care-seeking behavior.

Because of the higher overall prevalence of infection among blacks, Hispanics, and native Americans, the risk of any particular individual member of these groups, even those with few sex partners and good health care behaviors, is increased because they tend to have sex within their racial groups. This may be especially true for women (46, 55). For example, compared with white women, black women do not report riskier sexual behavior (2, 3, 4a, 7), but they have higher STD rates.

Factors associated with SES also influence risk behaviors for STDs and AIDS. Such diverse conditions as cancer, diabetes, and cardiovascular diseases as well as accidental injuries and homicides have been shown to be significantly associated with race and SES (35, 50, 53). Are race and SES simply different manifestations of the same phenomenon? The evidence is somewhat equivocal, but it is generally accepted that race, SES, and excess morbidity and mortality are strongly interrelated (6).

While we are able to describe the association between race, social class, and the prevalence and incidence of disease, we are not completely able to explain it. One recent interpretation is that race differences in morbidity are reflections of social class differences and income inequalities (40). However, available data are inconclusive regarding the particular nature of the interrelationships among race and SES, on the one hand, and sexual behavior and STD morbidity on the other. When the effects of all other variables, including SES, are controlled through multivariate analyses, race remains an important predictor of STD morbidity (26) but not of high-risk sexual behavior (7).

A number of investigators (6) have argued that perhaps the best explanation of the interrelationships of race, SES, and disease lies not only with the characteristics of a given disease but also with an understanding of the interrelationships between behavior, social class, and race. Much of the research on AIDS, however, seeks to develop disease-specific explanations for the overrepresentation of blacks and Hispanics among those infected. As a result, efforts to assess the relationship between various measures of sexual behavior and HIV risk behaviors often use race and class as explanatory variables (22). While these variables may be excellent predictors of these behaviors, race and social class are of little utility in the creation of interventions or prevention programs. Even though such characteristics may give general guidance in targeting interventions, they are not subject to manipulation. If we are to limit the spread of STDs including HIV infection, we must progress beyond descriptive research. A critical next step is the identification of variables that will prove useful in the development of prevention and treatment programs.

Finally, marital status is a consistent predictor of many dimensions of sexual behavior. Divorced and separated individuals and never-married individuals apparently engage in riskier sexual behaviors than married individuals (3; S. Seidman, W. D. Mosher, and S. O. Aral, submitted for publication).

EFFECTS OF SOCIETAL FACTORS

Societal factors may influence risk behaviors in several ways. First, society provides the *context* in which behaviors are shaped and conducted; society to a great extent determines the particular social environment an individual lives in. The opportunity structure, the available role models, the reinforcement contingencies that further shape behaviors, the social norms perceived, the beliefs, attitudes, and values, and the self-perception of an individual are for the most part influenced by his or her social environment and in turn affect his or her behavior (55).

Second, the *relational placement* in society greatly affects how the environment, the individual, and the behavioral options are experienced by the individual. For example, the director of an organization stratified into five distinct layers of responsibility and authority experiences life in the organization quite differently than does an employee of the lowest rank. Similarly, individuals who belong in the highest income brackets perceive the same society and the behavioral options it provides quite differently than do those who live in poverty.

Another aspect of relational placement in society involves dyadic social relations. In this context, individuals and groups who are dependent on other individuals and groups for the satisfaction of their needs experience their behavioral options as more limited compared with those who are not dependent. Individuals and groups who have the power to make decisions, to change conditions, experience their environment as more positive and their own behavioral options as less limited compared with those who do not have power. For

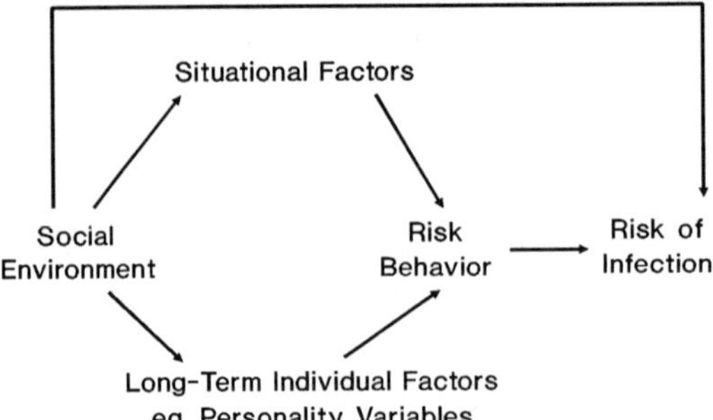

Figure 2. Risk behavior is conjointly affected by situational factors and personality factors.

example, the dominant member of a couple may feel more freedom than the dominated member to introduce change into shared repertoires of activity.

Third, societal factors have short- and long-term effects on behavior. Current social environment defines the situational factors that influence opportunity structures, behavioral options, and perceptions of social norms. The social environment of early childhood may influence more stable characteristics of an individual such as personality (see Jaccard and Wilson, this volume). Situational factors, personality factors, and interactions between them conjointly affect risk behaviors (Fig. 2).

One example of a situational factor that affects the sexual opportunity structure of individuals and, as a result, influences sexual behavior is the population sex ratio. In situations characterized by marked scarcity of one gender, members of the scarce gender tend to have greater numbers of heterosexual partners. The black population of the United States, with a scarcity of men, urban populations of many underdeveloped countries, and migrant labor groups with a scarcity of women all constitute populations with an unbalanced sex ratio. Moreover, given the widespread norm of sexual unions taking place between younger women and relatively older men, the wide-based population pyramids in countries with growing populations contribute a built-in scarcity of older men as potential sex partners.

Social environmental factors also are associated with magnitude of risk directly. They help define the prevalence of infectious pathogens in the environment (e.g., in the sex partner pool) and therefore the probability of being exposed to a sexually transmitted infection during a single act of sexual intercourse (Fig. 2).

THE INTERPLAY OF DEMOGRAPHICS AND SOCIAL ENVIRONMENT: THE RISK ECOLOGY OF STDs

The rather complex interplay among demographic characteristics of the individual, the social environment, situational and personality factors affecting risk behaviors, and the direct effects of social environment on the magnitude of risk of acquiring a sexually transmitted infection are all reflected in the risk ecology of STD, described below.

A landmark study examining the prevalence of gonorrhea in Colorado (41) provides an example of risk ecology and offers important insights into the dynamics that facilitate the spread of many STDs within a given community. Although, as in the general population, gonorrhea was disproportionately concentrated in this city among young nonwhites in lower socioeconomic classes, the disease pattern also demonstrated geographical clustering within core census tracts. Specifically, 51% of the cases were concentrated in four tracts.

These findings mirror results of other studies in which STDs and/or HIV were concentrated in particular neighborhoods and among groups whose members exhibit strong social connections. In a household probability survey of HIV seroprevalence in Belle Glade, Fla., 85 (91%) of 93 AIDS patients resided in the southwest-central part of town (8). For one-third of those infected, contact by needle sharing, sexual intercourse, or maternal-infant transmission was documented (10). Similarly, in Broward County, Fla., the annual number of cases of early syphilis increased from 328 in 1980 to over 1,150 in 1986. Over 70% of early syphilis patients reported in 1985 lived in 11 census tracts that together contained less than 15% of the 1,162,031 residents of Broward County. The median income in these census tracts was less than $15,000 per year (10). Finally, in a case-control study of congenital syphilis among patients at Miami's Jackson Memorial Medical Center, mothers of babies with congenital syphilis were predominantly black Americans (70%) from poor neighborhoods. The vast majority of cases clustered in the central portion of Dade County, where the majority of indigent patients lived (44).

These studies and others indicate that there is a strong ecological component to an individual's risk for exposure to sexually transmitted infections. Being a resident of certain neighborhoods and having social and family ties within these settings (39, 51) may help explain an individual's risk of STD independently of that individual's own specific risk behaviors. Social networks and support systems are strongly associated with neighborhoods and are composed of individuals with similar cultural, ethnic, and social characteristics (18, 19, 25, 27). At the individual level, race, SES, and census tract may all help determine probability of exposure to infectious agents. At this time, data are not available to determine whether or not neighborhood has an effect on STD risk independent of age, race, SES, and marital status.

Data suggest that the research agenda for examining the correlates of sexual behavior and STD risk must pay greater attention to ecological issues than has heretofore been the case. Race, culture, and social class are necessary but not sufficient conditions for examining the variance in STD rates and sexual behaviors. Rather, these variables reflect a complex of forces that influence where members of different groups live as well as how they live together, work together, socialize together, and choose sexual partners.

EFFECTS OF OTHER RISK BEHAVIORS

Drug Use and Prostitution

As we enter the 1990s, there is evidence that the sexual ecology of urban neighborhoods in which STDs are particularly prevalent is changing. For example, the introduction of crack cocaine into many inner city communities has dramatically altered the nature of sexual relationships among many residents. Crack use has been associated with a number of high-risk behaviors that would promote the spread of STDs and HIV. For example, in a 1988 study of black adolescent crack cocaine users conducted in Oakland and San Francisco, Calif. (21), 41% of all respondents reported a history of one or more STDs. Moreover, one respondent in four reported having been engaged as a recipient or as a provider in an exchange of sex for drugs or money.

Crack use is also significantly associated with the incidence of congenital syphilis (9, 44) and primary and secondary syphilis among prostitutes (45). Since 1986, syphilis cases have increased among heterosexuals in several metropolitan areas of the United States (13). Cocaine-addicted female prostitutes apparently played an important role in this rise (15). In a case-control study of risk factors for syphilis in Philadelphia, cocaine use and exchange of drugs or money for sex were found to be risk factors for syphilis, both for men and for women (45). Among men, the strongest association was found with intravenous cocaine use, but nonintravenous cocaine use also appeared to be a risk factor for syphilis. Cocaine users reported more sexual partners and more frequent sex with prostitutes. However, cocaine use remained a risk factor after adjustment for these behaviors.

In a cross-sectional study of drug use among adolescent mothers, drug users were found to be significantly more likely than nonusers to be black, to have a history of abortion and of venereal disease, to report more "negative life events" (e.g., to have been physically threatened or abused), and to have a sexual partner who was a drug user (1). Interestingly, drug-using mothers were more likely to report that they received social support from friends. Since partners of drug-using adolescents were more likely to be drug users themselves, their support may provide a context for continued drug and alcohol use. Friends of adolescent mothers who use drugs may also facilitate drug use (1). In San Francisco, 90% of crack users reported that they had friends who used drugs and 60% reported that they had relatives who used drugs (21). A variety of risk behaviors (not simply those related to STDs) are mediated through contact with friends, relatives, and lovers (R. F. Schilling, N. El-Bassel, and S. P. Schinke, *Public Health Rep.*, in press). To provide successful interventions that will have an impact on the individual and on the individual's social network, a greater understanding of how these networks are created and maintained will be necessary. Since these networks are also typically confined within distinct geographical settings (i.e., the neighborhood), it may also be important to enumerate these networks and determine how their members are interconnected.

The risks imposed by crack use are not simply those that result from the bartering of sexual favors for drugs or money. In the study conducted by Fullilove and colleagues (21, 23, 24), 51% of all crack users surveyed reported that they combined crack use with sexual activity. This pattern of chemical foreplay, that is, of using drugs or alcohol during sexual relations (5), is particularly problematic since the use of psychoactive substances may inhibit the use of safe-sex practices.

How widespread is chemical foreplay? In a probability sample of single adults aged 20 to 44 years in San Francisco (23), 23% of all respondents (n = 1,781) reported using one or more drugs with at least one sexual partner during intercourse in the previous 12 months. This behavior was associated with positive HIV antibody status and with the number of sexual partners reported in the previous 12 months.

Until recently, there has been little interest in the role that IDUs play in the transmission of STDs. This has changed because of the critical position the intravenous-drug-using population occupies in the AIDS epidemic. IDUs, like bisexual men, have been found to form a bridge to the general population through heterosexual transmission of HIV. Of the 2,464 adult AIDS cases reported in the United States from September 1989 through August 1990 and attributed to reported heterosexual contact, 1,374 (56%) were heterosexual partners of IDUs (14). In Europe, data about the risk group of the sexual partners of cases with heterosexually acquired AIDS are generally lacking, but in Italy, where over 50% of the reported cases have occurred among IDUs, a rapid increase in cases attributed to heterosexual transmission was noted in 1989, and it is presumed that the majority of these cases were partners of IDUs (56, 57).

In a large epidemiological study of HIV infection among IDUs in Amsterdam, The Netherlands, the sexual behavior of this population was assessed (54). From September 1988 through March 1989, 243 IDUs were questioned about the frequency of practicing different sexual techniques and condom use. The IDUs were recruited through methadone treatment facilities and through a special STD clinic for drug-addicted prostitutes. Three groups of partners were distinguished: private-steady, private-nonsteady, and commercial partners (30). The study population consisted of 130 male and 113 female IDUs. Their mean ages were, respectively, 31.1 (standard deviation, 5.5) years and 28.6 (standard deviation, 4.9) years, and the majority used heroin and/or cocaine. Exclusive heterosexual preference since 1980 in private relations was reported by 75% of the men and none of the women. Of the 113 female IDUs, 74 (65%) had a steady heterosexual partner, and 31 of these 74 male partners never injected drugs themselves, nor did they have homosexual contacts. Of the 130 male IDUs, 46 (35%) reported a steady partner, and 16 of these partners did not inject drugs.

These findings indicate that IDUs constitute an important bridge to non-drug-using heterosexual populations for the transmission of STDs and AIDS. Prostitution (ever) was reported by 95 (84%) of the women and 21 (16%) of the men. Vaginal contact was the most popular technique in all sexual relationships. Only 20% of the women and 31% of the men used condoms frequently with their nonpaying partners. The use of condoms was much more common during contacts of prostitutes with commercial clients: 86% of the female prostitutes reported frequent condom use while having vaginal contact with clients and 63% reported frequent condom use during orogenital contact. Anal intercourse was practiced rarely.

Donoghoe et al. (17) measured the sexual behavior of 142 IDUs (122 men and 20 women) attending a syringe exchange program in England and Scotland between April 1987 and March 1988. Of this group, 77% had one or more sexual partners in the 3 months prior to the interview and approximately one-half of these partners did not inject themselves. The majority of the sexual partners were private partners; only 5 of 142 reported having been given money or drugs for sex. Condom use was reported by 29% of the sexual contacts, which is comparable with the data from Amsterdam.

Additional studies on the sexual behavior of IDUs have been reported from London (29), San Francisco (32), and Italy (47). In London, one-fourth of the 53 female drug users questioned had exchanged sex for money within the past year. Of 116 IDUs, 102 were sexually active in the previous year and 46 of these had partners who did not use drugs. While condom use with commercial partners was common, only a small minority reported the use of condoms with private partners. The studies in San Francisco and in Italy also found that condom use was infrequent among IDUs. Heterosexual anal intercourse in the preceding 5 years was reported by 56 (38%) of 149 male IDUs in San Francisco, a much higher frequency than was found in Amsterdam (16).

The available data indicate that IDUs are a heterosexually active group. Many have private partners who do not inject drugs and are not otherwise themselves at risk for AIDS, apart from having sexual contact with an IDU. Only a small proportion of IDUs use condoms regularly with their nonpaying partners. Prostitution is one of the ways in which IDUs and especially female IDUs can earn the money they need to buy drugs. Prostitution among IDU women was very frequent in Amsterdam but considerably less frequent in England and Scotland. Some of these differences reflect variations in sampling. Data about the frequency of prostitution among IDUs in other areas are not available. Based on data from Amsterdam and London, it appears that condom use with commercial partners is accepted but certainly not universal.

Thus, although drug-using prostitutes report frequent condom use with commercial partners, sexually transmitted infections still occur in this group. From December 1985 to November 1987, a retrospective study among 117 drug-using prostitutes in Amsterdam found that 73 (62%) reported having had more than 2,000 clients each in the preceding 5 years (54). These prostitutes were enrolled via a special STD clinic for drug-using prostitutes. Ninety percent of 117 female prostitutes reported that condoms were used during vaginal contact at least half the time. Of the 117 prostitutes, 104 attended the clinic during the preceding 6-month period, and during 281 consultations, STDs were diagnosed in 84 of the 104 women. Gonorrhea, *Chlamydia trachomatis* infections, and trichomoniasis were most often diagnosed, but ulcerations resulting from syphilis, genital herpes, or an unknown cause were also frequent. Drug-addicted prostitutes play an important role in the transmission of STDs to their clients, and as 30% of the prostitutes were also found to be infected with HIV, their potential role in transmitting HIV cannot be ignored.

Drug users not engaged in prostitution may play an important role in the transmission of STDs, because such individuals also seem to be at increased risk for STDs. For example, in the Amsterdam study mentioned earlier, 11% of the female drug users who never engaged in prostitution and 6% of men without such a history reported to have had syphilis at least once. A history of gonorrhea was reported by 33 and 29%, respectively. It is important to note that a sizable proportion of drug users have heterosexual partners who do not use drugs themselves. The increased risk among nonprostituting drug users may be associated with a difference in sexual behavior under the influence of drugs. Alternative explanations are that drug users have limited access to health care and/or that they are less health conscious and seek care with more delay than others. Partner notification may be less effective among drug users as well.

Early Age of Sexual Debut

Another behavior that apparently influences STD and AIDS risk behaviors is age of sexual debut. The initiation of sexual intercourse early in life is associated with an increased risk of STD not only because of an increased risk of infection per contact for the young woman owing to the high prevalence of cervical ectopy but also because of an increased number of subsequent sex partners (12). In 1988, American adolescents who had sexual intercourse earlier in life reported greater numbers of sex partners. Among 15 to 24 year olds who initiated sexual intercourse before age 18, 75% reported having had two or more partners and 45% reported having had four or more partners; among those who became sexually active after age 19, only 20% reported having had more than one partner and 1% reported four or more partners (20). Among women aged 15 to 24 years who had been sexually active for the same length of time ($<$ 24 months), 45% of 15 to 17 year olds reported having had two or more partners, compared with 40% of 18 to 19 year olds and 26% of those $\geq$ 20 years of age. The association between early age of sexual intercourse and greater numbers of both recent and lifetime sex partners represents a behavioral link to higher levels of STDs.

Homosexual Behavior among Men

Among men, having sexual intercourse with other men has been associated with higher levels of sexual activity in studies conducted before the AIDS epidemic (49). Men who have sex with men reported higher frequencies of sexual intercourse, greater numbers of current and lifetime sex partners, and more sexual contact with strangers.

From the 1960s through the early 1980s, in the United States, the bathhouse provided a clear picture of the complex, ecologically patterned interactions among demographic and environmental factors and risk behaviors. These factors mutually influenced each other and determined STD and AIDS risk behaviors as well as risk per sexual contact for exposure to sexually transmitted infections. The bathhouse environment where men had sex with men provided opportunities for anonymous sexual intercourse with large numbers of partners (who themselves had anonymous sexual contact with many partners and thus were likely to be infected with sexually transmitted pathogens, including HIV), often under the influence of drugs or alcohol (36), included role models who engaged in this behavior and reinforced these high-risk behaviors.

During the AIDS era, a marked decline in rates of unprotected risky sexual practices was associated with a very rapid decline in rates of gonorrhea, syphilis, and HIV infection among homosexual men and with a near disappearance of those forms of practices attributed to unprotected receptive anal intercourse (37). However, a recent resurgence of HIV infection and of gonorrhea and syphilis as well has been seen in some U.S. cities. This resurgence seems to disproportionately affect younger homosexual men.

SOCIETAL AND INDIVIDUAL CHANGES AS FACTORS INFLUENCING RISK BEHAVIORS

As discussed in the introduction, all cross-sectional presentations of human behavior are shaped simultaneously by several factors, including processes of change taking place in the society surrounding the individual and the developmental processes of change that the individual happens to be undergoing at the time. Unique circumstances such as social or geographical mobility involve additional change processes. Moreover, effects of societal change and individual change interact as they influence individual behavior. For example, being an adolescent in the United States in the post-Depression era was a distinctly different experience from being an adolescent in the United States during the pre-AIDS 1970s.

The place in societal evolution of the society an individual is surrounded by lends meaning to the developmental stage an individual is in. Similarly, the stage of the AIDS epidemic in the group an individual belongs to may influence the individual's stage of readiness (42) to change risk behaviors. For example, as we enter 1991, most homosexual men in the United States are at a more advanced stage of readiness to adopt less risky behaviors in comparison with minority heterosexual men. The former have been confronted with the personal risk the AIDS epidemic presents for a longer time and thus have had a greater likelihood of coming to grips with the personal implications of this epidemic. On the other hand, as noted above, young homosexual men, who have not been confronted with the entire course of the epidemic and who are undergoing the adolescent phase of development, may be less ready to adopt safer behaviors. The particular point in time, in both the history of a society and the biography of an individual, is critical in determining which behaviors the individual engages in.

IMPLICATIONS FOR INTERVENTIONS AND INTERVENTION RESEARCH

Our discussion of the demographic and societal factors influencing risk behaviors points to several important generalizations. First, demographic and societal determinants of behavior mutually influence each other: demographic characteristics influence the social environments that individuals live in, while societal factors define the social meaning of demographic characteristics. Second, both demographic and societal environmental factors influencing risk behaviors are reflected in space, constituting a particular ecological pattern. Third, the demographic and environmental factors create social and sexual networks of human relationships that are also reflected in space, in a particular ecological pattern, and that influence individuals' risk behaviors in important ways.

These generalizations should be considered in drawing conclusions from epidemiological and intervention studies. They point to "ecological fallacy" and "individual reductionism" as two patterns to be avoided in STD-related epidemiological thinking. The ecological fallacy refers to the error of attributing aggregate-level associations between variables to individuals. For example, the conclusion that poor individuals have a higher risk of unwanted pregnancy could be wrong if it is based solely on the observation that low-income census tracts are characterized by high rates of unwanted pregnancy.

Individual reductionism refers to the error of reducing aggregate-level effects to the level of individuals composing the aggregate, thereby assuming that aggregate-level effects do not exist. For example, living in a poor neighborhood independently affects an individual's behavior whether or not the individual is poor, and attributing all such effects to the poverty level of the individual would be erroneous. Other properties of ecological aggregates that should not be reduced to the individual level include, for example, unbalanced population sex ratio, high prevalence of a particular STD, crowded, low-income housing, relatively limited access to health care, and others.

These generalizations should also be considered in developing interventions and evaluating their efficacy. Interventions that succeed in one social network may not necessarily work in another (31). The prevalence of STDs is associated with social and cultural networks. High-risk networks differ along a significant number of dimensions, not the least of which are the ways in which individuals negotiate whether or not to engage in sexual activity and what the nature of that activity is likely to be (22). However, population-based studies of social and sexual networks have not yet provided comprehensive information on sexual behavior.

Our limited understanding of what are potentially acceptable and effective interventions in different social environments argues for a trial-and-error strategy of small-scale behavioral intervention studies covering a wide range of behavioral interventions, demographic subgroups, and social environments. It is nonetheless essential that these trials involve randomization, control groups, and objective outcome measures. On the other hand, some community-based interventions will require large-scale community intervention trials to evaluate their effectiveness (see Green and Washington, this volume). In the light of the important role behaviors and demographic and environmental factors play in the transmission of sexually transmitted infections, including HIV, the need for well-designed large- and small-scale behavioral intervention research is obvious.

Acknowledgments. We thank King Holmes, Mary Lewis, and Stuart Seidman for their help in the preparation of this chapter.

LITERATURE CITED

1. **Amaro, H., B. Zuckerman, and H. Cabral.** 1989. Drug use among adolescent mothers: profile of risk. *Pediatrics* **84:**144–151.
2. **Aral, S. O.** 1990. The changing epidemiology of sexually transmitted diseases. *Curr. Opinion Infect. Dis.* **3:**20–23.

3. **Aral, S. O., and W. Cates.** 1989. The multiple dimensions of sexual behavior as a risk factor for sexually transmitted diseases: sexually experienced are not necessarily sexually active. *Sex. Transm. Dis.* **16:**173–177.
4. **Aral, S. O., and K. K. Holmes.** 1990. Epidemiology of sexual behavior and sexually transmitted diseases, p. 19–36. *In* K. K. Holmes, P.-A. Mardh, P. F. Sparling, P. J. Wiesner, W. Cates, Jr., S. M. Lemon, and W. E. Stamm (ed.), *Sexually Transmitted Diseases*, 2nd ed. McGraw-Hill Book Co., New York.
4a. **Aral, S. O., V. Soskolne, R. M. Joesoef, and K. R. O'Reilly.** 1991. Sex partner selection as risk factor for STD: clustering of risky modes. *Sex. Transm. Dis.* **18:**10–17.
5. **Belcastro, P. A., and T. Nicholson.** 1982. Chemical foreplay among black and white students. *J. Drug Educ.* **12:**373–383.
6. **Berkman, L. F.** 1980. Physical health and the social environment: a social epidemiologic perspective, p. 51–75. *In* L. Eisenberg and A. Kleinman (ed.), *The Relevance of Social Science for Medicine*. Reidel Publishing Co., New York.
7. **Bowen, G. S., S. O. Aral, L. S. Magder, D. S. Reed, K. Dratman, and S. Wasser.** 1990. Risk behaviors for human immunodeficiency virus infection in clients of Pennsylvania family planning clinics. *Fam. Plann. Perspect.* **22:**62–64.
8. **Castro, K. G., S. Lieb, H. W. Jafe, J. P. Narkunas, C. H. Calisher, T. J. Bush, and J. J. Witte.** 1988. Transmission of human immunodeficiency virus in Belle Glade, Florida: lessons for other communities in the United States. *Science* **239:**193–197.
9. **Centers for Disease Control.** 1988. Congenital syphilis—New York City, 1986–1988. *Morbid. Mortal. Weekly Rep.* **38:**825–829.
10. **Centers for Disease Control.** 1987. Early syphilis—Broward County, Florida, *Morbid. Mortal. Weekly Rep.* **36:**221–223.
11. **Centers for Disease Control.** 1988. Number of sex partners and potential risk of sexual exposure to human immunodeficiency virus. *Morbid. Mortal. Weekly Rep.* **7:**565–568.
12. **Centers for Disease Control.** 1991. Premarital sexual experience among adolescent women, United States, 1970–1988. *Morbid. Mortal. Weekly Rep.* **39:**929–932.
13. **Centers for Disease Control.** 1988. Continuing increase in infectious syphilis—United States, 1985–1988. *Morbid. Mortal. Weekly Rep.* **37:**486–489.
14. **Centers for Disease Control.** 1990. HIV/AIDS surveillance. U.S. AIDS cases reported through August 1990, p. 1–18. Centers for Disease Control, Atlanta, Ga.
15. **Centers for Disease Control.** 1988. Relationship of syphilis to drug use and prostitution—Connecticut and Philadelphia, Pennsylvania. *Morbid. Mortal. Weekly Rep.* **37:**755–764.
16. **Coutinho, R. A., E. J. Schoonhoven, J. A. R. Van Den Hoek, and J. A. Emsbroek.** 1987. Influence of special surveillance programmes and AIDS on declining incidence of syphilis in Amsterdam. *Genitourin. Med.* **63:**210–213.
17. **Donoghoe, M. C., G. V. Stimson, and K. A. Dolan.** 1989. Sexual behavior of injecting drug users and associated risks of HIV infection for non-injecting sexual partners. *AIDS Care* **1:**51–58.
18. **Ellis, G.** 1983. Youth in the electronic environment. *Youth Soc.* **15:**3–12.
19. **Folb, E. A.** 1980. *Runnin' Down Some Lines: the Language and Culture of Black Teenagers*. Harvard University Press, Cambridge, Mass.
20. **Forrest, J. D., and S. Singh.** 1990. The sexual and reproductive behavior of American women, 1982–1988. *Fam. Plann. Perspect.* **22:**206–214.
21. **Fullilove, M. T., and R. E. Fullilove.** 1989. Intersecting epidemics: black teen crack use and sexually transmitted disease. *J. Am. Med. Assoc.* **44:**146–153.
22. **Fullilove, M. T., R. E. Fullilove, K. Haynes, and S. Gross.** 1990. Black women and AIDS prevention: a view towards understanding the gender rules. *J. Sex Res.* **27:**47–64.
23. **Fullilove, M. T., M. Weinstein, R. E. Fullilove, R. Goodjoin, B. Bowser, and S. Gross.** 1990. Race/gender issues in the sexual transmission of AIDS, p. 25–62. *In* P. Volberding and M. J. Jacobson (ed.), *AIDS Clinical Review: 1990*. Marcel Dekker, Inc., San Francisco.
24. **Fullilove, R. E., M. T. Fullilove, B. P. Bowser, and S. A. Gross.** 1990. Risk of sexually transmitted disease among black adolescent crack users in Oakland and San Francisco, Calif. *J. Am. Med. Assoc.* **263:**851–855.

25. **Greenbaum, S. D., and P. E. Greenbaum.** 1985. The ecology of social networks in four urban neighborhoods. *Soc. Networks* **27:**47–76.
26. **Hahn, R. A., L. S. Magder, S. O. Aral, R. E. Johnson, and S. A. Larsen.** 1989. Race and the prevalence of syphilis infection in the US population. A national seroepidemiologic study. *Am. J. Public Health* **79:**467–470.
27. **Hammer, M.** 1983. "Core" and "extended" social networks in relation to health and illness. *Soc. Sci. Med.* **17:**405–411.
28. **Harrison, R., M. Costin, J. B. Meder, L. M. Bownds, D. A. Sim, M. Lewis, and E. R. Alexander.** 1985. Cervical *Chlamydia trachomatis* infection in university women: relationship to history, contraception, ectopy, and cervicitis. *Am. J. Obstet. Gynecol.* **153:**244.
29. **Hart, G. J., C. Sonnex, A. Petherick, A. M. Johnson, C. Feinmann, and M. W. Adler.** 1989. Risk behaviors for HIV infection among injecting drug users attending a drug dependency clinic. *Br. Med. J.* **298:**1081–1083.
30. **Hooykaas, C., J. Van Der Pligt, G. J. J. Van Doornum, M. M. D. Van Der Linden, and R. A. Coutinho.** 1989. Heterosexuals at risk for HIV: difference between private and commercial partners in sexual behavior and condom use. *AIDS* **3:**525–532.
31. **Jaffe, H. W., D. T. Rice, R. Voight, J. Fowler, and R. K. St. John.** 1979. Selective mass treatment in a venereal disease control program. *Am. J. Public Health* **69:**1181–1182.
32. **Lewis, D. K., J. K. Watters, and P. Case.** 1990. The prevalence of high risk sexual behavior in male intravenous drug users with steady female partners. *Am. J. Public Health* **80:**465–466.
33. **Liberatos, P., B. G. Link, and J. L. Kelsey.** 1988. The measurement of social class in epidemiology. *Epidemiol. Rev.* **10:**87.
34. **May, R. M., and R. M. Anderson.** 1988. Transmission dynamics of HIV infection. *Nature* (London) **326:**137.
35. **McCord, C., and H. P. Freeman.** 1990. Excess mortality in Harlem. *N. Engl. J. Med.* **322:**1606–1610.
36. **McCusker, J., J. Westenhouse, A. M. Stoddard, J. G. Zapka, M. W. Zorn, and K. H. Nayer.** 1990. Use of drugs and alcohol by homosexually active men in relation to sexual practices. *J. Acquired Immune Defic. Syndr.* **3:**729–736.
37. **McKusick, L., T. J. Coates, S. F. Morin, L. Pollack, and C. Hoff.** 1990. Longitudinal predictors of reductions in unprotected anal intercourse among gay men in San Francisco. *Am. J. Public Health* **80:**978–983.
38. **Moran, J. S., S. O. Aral, W. C. Jenkins, T. A. Peterman, and E. R. Alexander.** 1989. The impact of sexually transmitted diseases on minority population. A national seroepidemiologic study. *Public Health Rep.* **104:**560–565.
39. **National Urban League.** 1990. *State of Black America, 1990.* National Urban League, New York.
40. **Navarro, V.** 1990. Race or class versus race and class: mortality differentials in the United States. *Lancet* **336:**1238–1240.
41. **Potterat, J. J., R. B. Rothenberg, D. T. Woodhouse, J. B. Muth, C. I. Pratts, and J. S. Fogle.** 1985. Gonorrhea as a social disease. *Sex. Transm. Dis.* **12:**25–32.
42. **Prochaska, J. O., and C. C. DiClemente.** 1983. Stages and processes of self-change in smoking: towards an integrative model of change. *J. Consult. Clin. Psychol.* **51:**390–395.
43. **Research and Forecasts, Inc.** 1987. *The Abbot Report: STDs and Sexual Moves in the 1980's.* Research and Forecasts, Inc., New York.
44. **Ricci, J. M., R. M. Fojaco, and M. J. O'Sullivan.** 1989. Congenital syphilis: the University of Miami/Jackson Memorial experience, 1986–1988. *Obstet. Gynecol.* **74:**687–693.
45. **Rolfs, R. T., M. Goldberg, and R. G. Sharrar.** 1990. Risk factors for syphilis: cocaine use and prostitution. *Am. J. Public Health* **80:**853–857.
46. **Rose, G.** 1985. Sick individuals in sick populations. *Int. J. Epidemiol.* **14:**32–38.
47. **Sasse, H., S. Salmaso, S. Conti, and the First Drug User Multicenter Study Group.** 1989. Risk behaviors for HIV-1 infection in Italian drug users: report from a multicenter study. *J. Acquired Immune Defic. Syndr.* **2:**486–496.

48. **Schuster, C. R.** 1988. Intravenous drug use and AIDS prevention. *Public Health Rep.* **103:**261–266.
49. **Schwartz, P., and M. R. Gilmore.** 1990. Sociological perspectives on human sexuality, p. 45–53. *In* K. K. Holmes, P.-A. Mardh, P. F. Sparling, P. J. Wiesner, W. Cates, Jr., S. M. Lemon, and W. E. Stamm (ed.), *Sexually Transmitted Diseases*, 2nd ed. McGraw-Hill Book Co., New York.
50. **Syme, S. L., and L. F. Berkaman.** 1978. Social class, susceptibility, and sickness, p. 398–405. *In* H. D. Schwartz and C. S. Kart (ed.), *Dominant Issues in Medical Sociology*. Addison-Wesley, New York.
51. **Thomas, M. E., and M. Hughes.** 1986. The continuing significance of race: a study of race, class, and quality of life in America, 1972–1985. *Am. Soc. Rev.* **51:**830–841.
52. **Toomey, K. E., M. P. Rafferty, and W. E. Stamm.** 1987. Unrecognized high prevalence of *Chlamydia trachomatis* cervical infection in an isolated Alaskan Eskimo population. *J. Am. Med. Assoc.* **258:**53–56.
53. **U.S. Department of Health and Human Services.** 1986. *Report of the Secretary's Task Force on Black and Minority Health*. U.S. Department of Health and Human Services, Washington, D.C.
54. **Van Den Hoek, J. A. R., H. J. A. Van Haastrecht, B. Scheeringa-Troost, J. Goudsmit, and R. A. Coutinho.** 1989. HIV infection and STD in drug addicted prostitutes in Amsterdam: potential for heterosexual HIV transmission. *Genitourin. Med.* **65:**146–150.
55. **Wallace, R.** 1988. A synergism of plagues: "planned shrinkage," contagious housing destruction, and AIDS in the Bronx. *J. Environ. Res.* **47:**1.
56. **World Health Organization.** 1990. *AIDS in Europe. Quarterly Report 25, Situation by 31 March 1990*. WHO/EC Collaborating Center on AIDS, Paris.
57. **World Health Organization.** 1986. *AIDS Surveillance in Europe by 30th September, 1986. Quarterly Report no. 11*. WHO/EC Collaborating Center on AIDS, Paris.

Personality Factors Influencing Risk Behaviors

James Jaccard and Tracey Wilson

Numerous studies have explored the relationship between personality variables and risk behaviors related to sexually transmitted diseases (STDs). In this chapter, we consider ways in which personality variables can be used for the prediction and understanding of risk behavior and how such variables can be incorporated into intervention efforts designed to reduce STDs. The application of personality variables has several limitations. First, personality variables generally exhibit low correlations with outcomes. In fact, Mischel (38) has coined the phrase *personality coefficient* to refer to correlations of 0.25, reflecting the fact that personality variables rarely account for more than 5% of the variance in outcomes. Second, personality variables, because they are traditionally conceptualized as stable, enduring dispositions, are difficult to change. Most health interventions must be short, one-shot efforts owing to limited time, resources, and other practical constraints. This generally is not conducive to changing major dispositions of individuals. Thus, it makes little sense to focus on variables that cannot be modified easily. Third, personality variables are awkward to measure in applied settings. Traditional personality measures typically use 20 to 30 items to assess a single construct. Five or 10 personality variables require the administration of 100 to 300 items, which is too time-consuming, especially in populations with poor reading skills. Furthermore, the content of items is frequently quite personal, and respondents may find them to be invasive and irrelevant to the health service that they seek.

Given the above, why should health researchers use personality variables? The present chapter provides perspectives on these criticisms and highlights what we believe are reasonable research strategies for incorporating personality variables. We begin by discussing preliminary issues, namely, defining personality, specifying different types of behavioral criteria that may be of interest, and identifying major issues in the design of interventions. We next consider three ways in which personality variables may be used in STD intervention research: (i) to identify relevant determinants of STD-related behaviors; (ii) to identify methods by which interventions can be implemented effectively, given knowledge of behavioral determinants; and (iii) to identify target populations who are likely to exhibit risk behaviors in the future. We then discuss recent trends in personality research as well as selected measurement issues that may be of use to STD researchers. We will not consider in this chapter issues related to the effects of STDs on personality (e.g., the effects of knowledge of seropositive human immunodeficiency virus status on personality and the development of psychological disorders). Space constraints do

James Jaccard and Tracey Wilson – Department of Psychology, State University of New York at Albany, Albany, New York 12222.

not permit a sufficient analysis of the dynamics underlying such relationships. Nor will we provide a formal review of the empirical literature on personality and STDs, although several relevant studies will be mentioned. Generally speaking, personality research in the STD area has not yielded an integrated body of knowledge, and attempts at summary may be premature. Our focus in this chapter is on describing directions that future personality research can take.

PRELIMINARY ISSUES AND DEFINITIONS

Defining Personality

Personality has been defined in the context of several different theoretical systems, each with divergent epistemological assumptions. These systems include psychoanalytic theories, learning theories, developmental theories, trait theories, and cognitive theories, all of which have incorporated, to a greater or lesser extent, perspectives based on logical positivism, constructivism, and symbolic interactionism, to name a few. The major focus of this chapter is on dispositional conceptualizations of personality (which are typically associated with trait theories), primarily because such conceptualizations are used widely in health-related research.

Dispositional characterizations of personality have been diverse. Some theorists characterize dispositions in strict, behavioristic terms. A disposition is seen as an energizing force within the individual that is activated by certain stimuli in the environment. Once activated, the force is channeled, based on the individual's reinforcement history, into a given overt response. Critics of the trait approach tend to characterize dispositions in the extreme, portraying the individual as one who is at the mercy of the environment and these energizing forces. Stimulus events over which the individual has little control occur during everyday life, and these activate the energizing force. The response follows from this activated force, again with little control or conscious choice on the part of the individual. Such mechanistic characterizations of dispositions fail to capture the essence of traits as conceptualized by most trait theorists.

A more general characterization of dispositions has evolved recently. Over the course of life, an individual engages in a wide range of activities and interacts with the environment in diverse ways. Based on these interactions, he or she learns certain cognitive rules, strategies, and discourse for interpreting and dealing with the environment and other individuals in that environment. Dispositions represent residues or psychological summaries of these past experiences that, in turn, bias the individual to behave, interpret, and interact with the environment in consistent, systematic ways. Individuals who are characterized as dominant on the trait dimension of submissive-dominance, for example, are those whose past history and experiences (e.g., their childhood experiences, recent experiences, and so on) have biased them toward behaving in consistently dominant ways across a variety of situations.

This characterization of dispositions suggests several measurement strategies that can be used when studying personality variables. One strategy is to assess the more detailed cognitive strategies, heuristics, and discourse that people have derived in the context of their behavior on a given trait dimension. A second strategy is to assess only the overall behavioral tendency of the individual, without more detailed analyses of the underlying cognitive and affective mechanisms surrounding these tendencies. Measurement strategies among personality researchers have been predominantly focused on the latter. Such measures can be useful but are not sufficient. Again, because of the predominance of the overall-oriented measures in the field, we will focus our discussion on the more general assessment strategy. However, we will also note cognitive- and affective-based approaches that we believe hold promise for future research.

Most personality research focuses on three or four personality variables that the investigator believes are relevant to the domain of interest. There exists some controversy as to the utility of such an approach. Several personality theorists (15, 53) believe that one should first isolate the core dimensions of personality and then study these dimensions and their implications in an integrated fashion. For example, Costa and McCrae (10) have identified five major dimensions that they believe capture the vast majority of trait terms: extraversion (talkative, frank, adventurous, sociable versus silent, secretive, cautious, reclusive), agreeableness (good-natured, gentle, cooperative versus irritable, jealous, headstrong, negativistic), will to achieve/conscientiousness (responsible, scrupulous, perservering versus careless, undependable, unscrupulous, willing to quit), emotional stability (poised, calm, composed versus nervous, anxious, excitable), and openness to experience (intellectual, artistically sensitive, imaginative versus insensitive, narrow, crude, simple). Other personality theorists eschew such a position, noting that the hundreds of trait concepts proposed by social scientists cannot be captured adequately in a few fundamental dimensions. They suggest choosing one's trait concepts based on a careful analysis of the content domain and the behavioral criteria that are the focus of interest. By selecting concepts that are specific to the problem at hand, better predictive power should result (2, 21).

Our discussion treats personality variables in the abstract, without reference to their content (although specific variables are used when providing examples). This reflects our bias toward the specificity position in variable selection as well as our emphasis on broader conceptual issues. However, to provide context, we mention in Table 1 some of the more well developed and researched trait concepts in the personality field that may prove useful to STD researchers. The listing is illustrative, not exhaustive, and will be augmented in later sections of the chapter.

Conceptualizing Behavioral Criteria

When analyzing the relationship between personality and behavior, it is important to examine carefully the nature of the behaviors being predicted. In this section, we discuss three facets of behavioral measures: (i) the prediction of specific behaviors as opposed to behavioral patterns, (ii) specification of the dimensions of condom use, and (iii) the analysis of behaviors versus outcomes.

Table 1. Trait concepts

Concept	Brief description	Comments
Antisocial personality	Tendency in adolescents to perform a broad range of antisocial behaviors, including drug use, cigarette smoking, premarital sex, and alcohol consumption	See Jessor and Jessor (32); correlates with condom use and promiscuity (5)
Chronic self-destructiveness	Tendency to engage in a wide range of "self-destructive" or unhealthy, unsafe behaviors	See Kelley et al. (33, 34); correlates with condom use (K. Kelley and D. Streeton, unpublished data)
Erotophobia-erotophilia	Negative versus positive attitudes toward sexuality	See Byrne and Schulte (8); correlates with condom use (51)
Impulsivity	Tendency to act on the spur of the moment, without deliberation or careful thought	See Eysenck and Eysenck (16); correlates with inconsistent use of coital-dependent birth control methods (E. Koh, M.A. thesis, State University of New York at Albany, 1990)
Independence-conformity	Tendency to be independent of or to conform/acquiesce to the desires of others	See Moscovici (39)
Locus of control	Tendency to believe one can control outcomes in one's life, versus a view that outcomes depend on luck, fate, or chance	See Strickland (49); correlates with sexual risk taking (19)
Masculinity-femininity	Tendency to be characterized by instrumental (confident, outgoing, ambitious) versus expressive (warm, sensitive, empathic) traits or a combination of the two	See Spence and Helmreich (48) and Spence et al. (47)
Neuroticism-extraversion-psychoticism	Personality system of Eysenck and Eysenck that incorporates notions of impulsivity, sociableness, and emotional stability	See Eysenck and Eysenck (13, 14)
Risk taking	General tendency to take risks and to pursue choices that have a low probability of benefit	See Jackson et al. (31)
Self-efficacy	Beliefs about one's ability to deal effectively with tasks and problems	See Bandura (4)
Self-esteem	Self-acceptance and a positive attitude toward oneself; positive self-evaluations	See Higgins (24); correlates with diverse aspects of STD-related behavior (M. Gerrard, M. Kurylo, and T. Reis, unpublished data)

Continued on following page

Table 1—*Continued*

Concept	Brief description	Comments
Self-monitoring	Tendency to focus on the rules of appropriate behavior and on the demands of the immediate situation versus emphasizing one's true inner feelings and beliefs	See Snyder and Gangestad (44); correlates with number of casual sexual partners (46)
Sensation seeking	Need for varied, novel, and complex sensations and the willingness to take physical and social risks for such experiences	See Zuckerman (52)
Sex guilt	Affective and cognitive guilt about sexual behavior	See Mosher (40); correlates with aspects of condom use (20)
Social desirability	General desire to present oneself in the best possible manner so as to create favorable impressions	See Paulhus (41) and Snyder and Ickes (45)

Behavioral patterns

Behavioral criteria refer to the observed behaviors that the scientist is attempting to predict and/or understand. We have found it useful, following Fishbein (17), to characterize behavioral criteria in terms of a matrix, as illustrated in Fig. 1. The rows of the matrix represent different target behaviors that may be of interest to the investigator. For example, each row might represent a high-risk behavior for contracting an STD (e.g., sexual intercourse without the use of a condom, sexual intercourse with a casual partner whose sexual history is unknown). The columns of the matrix represent discrete time periods during which the behaviors are observed. For example, each column might reflect a 1-week period over the course of a 6-month interval, yielding a total of 26 columns. The cell entries represent behavioral scores for a given behavior during a given time period.

The matrix indicates different types of behavioral criteria that investigators can focus on. First, there is a *single act, single observation* criterion in which the investigator attempts to predict and understand a single behavior at a single point in time (1). Second, there is a *single act, multiple observation* criterion in which a single behavior is monitored over multiple time periods and an overall index of behavior is derived across these time periods (e.g., by summing within the row, across columns). For example, an investigator might be interested in condom use over a 6-month period. Measures of reported use are obtained at each weekly period designated by a column of the matrix, and these scores are then aggregated to yield an overall single act, multiple observation criterion. Alternatively, the investigator may obtain an independent estimate of the overall marginal score, without measuring the individual row cells. This is typified in the literature by self-report measures that ask individuals to report the consistency or frequency of condom use over an extended time period (e.g., 6 months). Even though only a single measure is obtained, conceptually, the behavioral criterion is a single act,

	Time 1	Time 2	Time 3	....	Time *p*
Behavior 1	R_{11}	R_{12}	R_{13}	....	R_{1p}
Behavior 2	R_{21}	R_{22}	R_{23}	....	R_{2p}
Behavior 3	R_{31}	R_{32}	R_{33}	....	R_{3p}
.					
.					
.					
Behavior *m*	R_{m1}	R_{m2}	R_{m3}	....	R_{mp}

Figure 1. Types of behavioral criteria. Time frames can be defined as narrowly as desired (e.g., 1 day), thereby focusing on highly specific situations. Similarly, the columns of the matrix can be characterized in terms of situational or environmental factors rather than (or in addition to) temporal criteria, leading to even more restrictive behavioral criteria.

multiple observation criterion that represents an (albeit imperfect) aggregation across multiple sexual encounters. A third criterion is a *multiple act, single observation* measure, in which an aggregate score across multiple behaviors is derived within a time period (i.e., within a column, across rows). This is characterized in the literature by measures of individual risk behaviors that focus on a relatively narrow time frame and that derive an overall score of behavioral risk taking by aggregating across behaviors. Individuals with high scores tend to exhibit a pattern of behaviors that is risky, while individuals with low scores tend to exhibit a pattern of behaviors that is low risk. Finally, one can derive a *multiple act, multiple observation* criterion, in which an overall index of behavior is calculated across behaviors and across time periods. Examples of this in the literature are self-report measures of various risk behaviors during extended time periods that are then aggregated to yield an overall behavioral risk-taking index.

Although there are ambiguities in the above analysis, the general sense of the four types of behavioral criteria is important theoretically. Research in social and personality psychology suggests that the kinds of variables that are relevant for predicting and understanding behavior are different depending on the type of behavioral criterion one is using (25). This is particularly important for personality variables, because they typically represent broad-based dispositions that should be predictive of behavioral patterns across time (i.e., single act, multiple observation criteria; multiple act, single observation criteria; and multiple act, multiple observation criteria) as opposed to highly specific, single act, single observation criteria. This has been demonstrated empirically in numerous studies (12, 25).

The mechanisms underlying the ability of personality to predict multiple act or multiple observation criteria involve distinctions between enduring influences on behavior as opposed to transitory, situational influences. Consider a criterion such as the consistent use of condoms at each act of intercourse over a 6-month period.

During any given sexual encounter, there will be at least two classes of factors influencing condom use. One set of factors will be relatively stable, enduring variables (such as personality) that will be biasing the individual toward (or away from) condom use in each sexual encounter. The influence of these variables will be constant (i.e., stable) across occasions. The other set of factors will be more transitory variables that, on some occasions, bias behavior toward condom use (e.g., a partner who is favorable toward using condoms) and on other occasions bias behavior away from condom use (e.g., a different partner who is opposed to using condoms). When behavioral scores are aggregated across occasions, the constant influence of the general variables is reflected in the aggregate index, whereas the more specific situational influences cancel each other (thus representing error variance) and fail to reveal any systematic relationship with the overall score. This is not to imply that situational variables are unimportant in STD research. It only illustrates the idea that more stable, enduring variables will tend to be more highly correlated with multiple act or repeated observation behavioral criteria than with single act, single observation criteria. One reason why personality variables have tended to exhibit poor predictive power in health settings is that they have usually been used to predict relatively restricted behaviors as opposed to behavioral patterns.

The facets of condom use

Condom use is a major behavioral variable of interest in STD research. However, "condom use" is a somewhat ambiguous concept that requires further distinctions. Jaccard et al. (28) have identified four major facets of contraceptive behavior. First, the individual must decide whether to use a contraceptive method in general, and if so, he or she must decide what method to use as the major method of protection. This is referred to as *contraceptive choice*. A second aspect of contraceptive behavior is the consistency of contraceptive use. Many individuals rely on coital-dependent methods, and as a result, individuals may not use a birth control method each time they engage in sexual intercourse. Consistency refers to the proportion of times that an individual uses a given method relative to the total number of times he or she engages in sexual intercourse over a specified time period. A third aspect of contraceptive behavior is the accuracy with which birth control methods are used. An individual may use a given method every time he or she engages in sexual intercourse but may not use the method correctly. A fourth aspect of contraceptive behavior focuses on continuity. At any given point in time, individuals will have a most preferred method of contraception that they will identify as their "major" method. Although they may not always use this method, they will use it most often and will generally prefer its use to other methods. Over time, the individual's major method of birth control may change. Of interest is the identification of factors that lead to such switching.

Our own research on these four facets of contraceptive behavior has revealed that explanatory variables that are predictive of one facet are not necessarily relevant to other facets. For example, knowledge about how to correctly use the condom is a necessary but not sufficient condition for the prediction of accurate use of the condom. However, such knowledge has no relevance to the consistent use of condoms, nor does it exhibit explanatory power in the prediction of condom choice or switching from the condom to another method of birth control. Similarly, the facets differ in the extent to which they reflect behavioral patterns across situations and thus may be differentially predictive from personality variables. Whereas consistency and accuracy of use tend to reflect behavioral patterns as defined by single act, repeated observation criteria, contraceptive choice and continuity tend to reflect general decisions about one's overall contraceptive strategy. As such, these latter two facets are not characterized by an aggregated behavioral index. One might therefore expect personality variables to be more predictive of accuracy and consistency to the extent that these measures invoke assessments of behavioral patterns across time.

There are additional complications. Our review of the literature has shown that consistency and accuracy of a birth control method are not always defined and measured in terms of behavioral patterns. For example, some investigators measure consistency by obtaining self-reports of condom use over a 6-month period, whereas other investigators operationalize consistency by measuring whether condoms were used at the last sexual encounter. In the former case, the criterion is a single act, repeated observation measure, whereas in the latter case, it is a single act, single observation measure. These measures may be differentially predicted by personality variables, as indicated by our own research. Some investigators obtain measures of consistency only among condom users (i.e., individuals who have declared the condom as their major method of contraception in the context of the choice facet), whereas other investigators assess consistency of use in the population in general, independent of the overall method of choice. The latter strategy confounds the facets of choice and consistency in a complex way and may obscure the explanatory power of personality (and other) variables. The social-psychological profile of an individual who has decided to use condoms in general but then does so on a highly inconsistent basis may be quite different from that of an individual who decides to use another method of protection (e.g., withdrawal, the diaphragm) and hence exhibits low condom use.

Behavior and outcomes

One additional distinction in defining behavioral criteria should be noted, namely, the distinction between behavior and outcomes. Having an STD is not a behavior per se that an individual performs; rather, it is a physical state that is the outcome of performing certain behaviors (e.g., having unprotected sexual intercourse with an infected partner). There is not necessarily a one-to-one correspondence between a given risk behavior and the presence or absence of an STD. Two individuals may be equally inconsistent users of condoms, but one individual may fail to contract an STD because he or she always has intercourse with noninfected partners. Whereas a personality variable (or any explanatory variable for that matter) may bias a given behavior, such as condom use, and thereby exhibit a systematic relationship with that behavior, the same variable may not be related to the presence or absence of an STD because of the less than perfect correspondence between the behavior and the outcome. This distinction is important in understanding inconsistent results in the literature on personality variables when different behaviors and outcomes are used as dependent variables.

The Design of Interventions

Jaccard et al. (29) have discussed different facets of designing effective behavioral interventions. The present chapter focuses on the potential utility of personality variables for three facets of program design. First, personality variables can be used in the context of theoretical frameworks designed to identify the determinants of a target behavior, so that program designers will know the kinds of variables that must be changed to effect changes in the target behavior. This appears to be the most common motivation for personality research with regard to STDs. Second, personality variables can be used to identify the best strategies for changing behavioral determinants, once those determinants have been identified. For example, a research program may indicate the importance of educating people about the risks of contracting STDs and the serious consequences that can result if STDs are untreated. These cognitive-informational variables may then become the focus of an intervention. Individuals at risk in the target population may also tend to score high on Snyder and Gangestad's self-monitoring scale (44), a personality orientation that reflects an individual's relative concern with other peoples' approval of his or her behavior as opposed to concern with expressing one's true inner attitudes and values, independent of how others view those expressions. DeBono and Harnish (11) have shown that individuals high in self-monitoring, when exposed to educational messages, tend to be more influenced by sources who are attractive peers rather than experts. The reverse is true of individuals who are low in self-monitoring. If the target audience of an intervention tends to be high self-monitors, then the choice of who delivers an educational message may be guided by these personality concerns (e.g., appeals would be delivered by attractive peer-role models). There is ample evidence that segments of the population (as defined by such variables as age, class, and risk status) differ in personality dimensions (37, 45). Such differences may be important in designing interventions. Finally, personality variables can be used as predictors of target populations who are likely to need intervention because of probable problem behavior in the future. For example, Hammond, et al. (23) correlated measures of psychoticism, extroversion, neuroticism, and social desirability tendencies with the patient's attendance or nonattendance at the first review appointment at an STD clinic. Psychoticism was found to discriminate attenders from nonattenders. Hammond et al. (23) suggested that the scale be used as a way of identifying women who need special counseling about the importance of keeping their first review appointment. We will discuss issues for each of these uses of personality variables.

IDENTIFYING BEHAVIORAL DETERMINANTS

Causal Model Perspectives on Personality Variables

Formal causal modeling has become an increasingly popular tool for expressing and testing theoretical frameworks about systems of variables. We will use causal modeling principles to organize the present discussion. There are six types of relationships that can occur within a causal model, as illustrated in Fig. 2. A *direct* causal relationship is one in which a variable, *X*, is a direct cause of another variable, *Y* (i.e., it is an immediate determinant of *Y* within the context of the theoretical system). An *indirect* causal relationship is one in which *X* exerts a causal impact on *Y*, but only through its impact on a third variable, *Z*. A *spurious* relationship is one in which *X* and *Y* are related, but only because of a common cause, *Z*. There is no formal causal link between *X* and *Y*. A *bidirectional* or *reciprocal* causal relationship is one in which *X* has a causal influence on *Y*, which in turn has a causal impact on *X*. An *unanalyzed* relationship is one in which *X* and *Y* are related, but the source of the relationship is unspecified. Finally, a *moderated* causal relationship is one in which the relationship between *X* and *Y* is moderated by a third variable, *Z*. In other words, the nature of the relationship between *X* and *Y* varies depending on the value of *Z*. Most personality research in the STD area has focused on simple models positing direct relationships between three or four personality variables and a given outcome. Such models do not do justice to the complex interplay among personality, social, demographic, and cognitive variables that impinge on STD behavioral criteria. In this section, we consider the use of personality variables in the context of direct, moderated, indirect, and spurious relationships and then discuss the advantages of developing theoretical networks that combine these types of relationships.

Direct relationships

Most research on direct personality correlates of STD-related behaviors has used simple linear models to isolate potential personality determinants of risk behaviors. A wide range of personality dimensions has been explored, including "normal" traits such as risk taking and locus of control, to more clinical-psychopathological determinants, such as antisocial personality syndromes and the facets of the Minnesota Multiphasic Personality Inventory. Overall, the magnitude of the relationships has not been particularly impressive, in part because of the way in which behavioral criteria have been defined as well as for reasons which will be discussed below. The continued reliance on linear models for describing the relationship between personality variables and behavior may mask the relevance of personality. Certainly, other model forms can be explored. For example, consider an extremity-threshold model (28) for a personality measure of risk aversiveness versus risk seeking as applied to the analysis of inconsistent condom use among a group of condom users. Risk-aversive individuals are people who generally avoid taking risks, whereas risk-seeking individuals are people who tend to seek out risky situations. Many variables affect consistent condom use over time, including such factors as perceptions of the adverse effects of condom use on sexual spontaneity and pleasure, partner attitudes toward the condom, alcohol consumption, and so on. It may be the case that condom users who are highly risk averse are consistent users of the condom because of their strong risk-averse orientation. Some of these individuals may believe that condoms adversely affect sexual spontaneity and pleasure and may also have sexual partners who oppose the condom, but their strong aversion to risk overrides these factors and biases their behavior toward

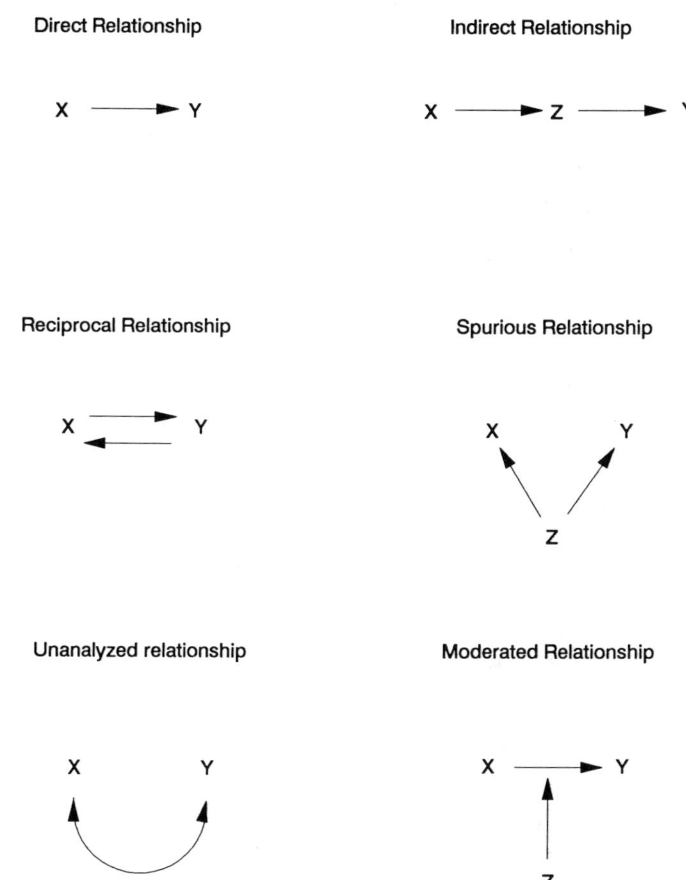

Figure 2. Types of causal relations.

highly consistent use. By contrast, individuals who are less risk averse may be more susceptible to the influences of partner orientations, alcohol consumption, and not wanting to interfere with sexual pleasure. For these individuals (who score below a certain threshold of risk aversiveness), such variables may influence consistent condom use, thereby creating error variance in the relation between condom use and risk aversiveness. The result is a function between risk aversiveness and use consistency that appears random below the threshold and uniformly high above the threshold. A simple correlation between the two measures would be nondiagnostic of the underlying mechanisms. Other models that may be applicable and that are nonlinear in nature are described by Jaccard (25). Even if personality researchers are successful in isolating direct causal links between personality and risk behavior, there remains the question of the utility of such knowledge for designing interventions to reduce STDs. As noted above, personality variables are notoriously difficult to change and hence may not be easily influenced in short educational campaigns. In addition, there may be ethical ramifications of changing personality, because such changes may affect other aspects of the individual's life, perhaps in adverse ways. One way of confronting this problem is not to change the individual's personality but rather to negate the influence of the personality variable in the specific target domain of interest. For example, in our research on social problems in other domains (e.g., drunk driving), we have found that an effective strategy is to make the individual aware of the relevant variables that may influence his or her behavior and to encourage the individual to think about their impact on his or her own life. In essence, we teach individuals about the social psychology of the phenomenon in question and urge them to think about their own situation in light of this. For example, we have found that locus of control is related to drunk driving tendencies in some adults. Locus of control is not a construct that is easily changed in brief educational settings. Furthermore, few individuals have even heard of the concept of locus of control, much less thought about the implications of such a construct for their own behavior. Our educational material carefully explains the construct to them, illustrates how it can influence their decision to drive drunk, encourages the individual to reflect on his or her own orientations in terms of an internality-externality dimension, and then provides some behavioral heuristics for overcoming the impact of locus of control in the drunk driving situation. At no time is it necessary to assess the individual's locus of control, nor do we try to change it. Rather we attempt to negate its effects in the particular situation by making people aware of it and by providing behavioral heuristics to counter its impact. The same type of strategy might be effective in an STD context with personality variables. A pamphlet could be prepared discussing each of the relevant variables and its impact on risk behavior. Individuals would be encouraged to think about their own orientations on each variable and then, when possible, would be provided behavioral strategies or heuristics to help overcome the negative influence of the variable. Alternatively, a videotape might be prepared that covers the same material, and individuals can be offered the opportunity to watch the video when attending a clinic. At this point, we do not know whether such an approach would be effective in the STD domain, but it seems to warrant further attention.

Moderated relationships

Personality variables can also be used to clarify the relationship between cognitive-informational variables and STD behavioral criteria via moderated relationships. Consider an example in which an investigator identifies three types of cognitive variables thought to be related to condom use: (i) perceptions of the effects of condom use on sexual spontaneity, (ii) perceptions of the efficacy of condoms in preventing STDs, and (iii) perceptions of partner opposition to using condoms. In a correlational study, measures of each type of belief are obtained and a regression analysis is performed regressing the measure of condom use onto the three belief measures. Suppose that, unbeknownst to the investigator, there are actually three distinct segments of the study population. In one segment, condom use is determined primarily by perceptions about spontaneity; in another segment, condom use is determined primarily by perceptions of partner opposition; and in the third segment, condom use is determined about equally by perceptions of spontaneity and efficacy in preventing STDs. Stated another way, the linear equation relating condom use to the cognitive variables differs in each segment of the population. If the analysis is conducted across segments, ignoring this segment heterogeneity, then it is possible (depending on the joint distribution of variables) for all three variables to yield zero or very low correlations and regression coefficients with the criterion. The investigator may dismiss the variables as being unimportant when, in fact, they are the primary determinants of condom use. The relationships of the variables with condom use, however, are obscured by individual differences in the relative importance of the three variables in influencing condom use (see reference 27 for elaborations). The problem of segment heterogeneity is important because major segments of the population are likely to differ in their reasons for not using condoms. To the extent that variables can be identified that permit the investigator to systematically segment the population as a function of differential weighting schemes, then misleading inferences will be lessened by incorporating such variables as interaction terms in the estimating equations (see reference 30 for a discussion of interaction analyses in multiple regression and structural equation models). Personality variables may represent an important source of such moderator variables. For example, individuals who score high on the trait of self-monitoring may give greater emphasis to partner desires when making decisions about condom use, whereas low self-monitors may give greater emphasis to personal consequences, such as possible STD infection and sexual spontaneity. By incorporating such moderator variables into one's theoretical framework, the relationships between cognitive variables that are amenable to change and behavioral outcomes may be clarified. The problem of heterogeneity of weights also is relevant to the observation of weak direct relationships between personality and behavior. If different personality traits are relevant to behavior for different segments of the population (i.e., the regression coefficients in the linear equations for a set of personality predictors differ for segments of the population), then combining these heterogeneous segments in a single analysis may attenuate the predictive power of personality measures (27).

Indirect relationships

Indirect relationships between personality variables and risk behavior also may be of interest. There currently exist numerous social-psychological models that identify cognitive factors that impinge on STD-related behaviors. For example, expectancy-value models of attitudes (18) suggest that an individual's decision to use condoms is influenced, in part, by his or her beliefs about the advantages and disadvantages of condom use. Individuals possess multiple beliefs about condoms (e.g., condoms are embarrassing to buy, condoms interfere with sexual pleasure, condoms are messy, condoms are difficult to use, condoms prevent STDs, condoms are ineffective in preventing pregnancy). Any given belief has two components, a certainty component and an evaluative component. The certainty component refers to how certain the individual is that using the condom does, in fact, lead to the advantage or disadvantage in question. The evaluative component refers to how positive or negative the advantage or disadvantage is perceived as being. Expectancy-value theorists have developed methods for isolating sets of beliefs that underlie attitudes and behavior. To change behavior, one or more of the beliefs is selected as a target for educational intervention. At issue is which of the many beliefs, and which component of a belief, one should focus the intervention efforts upon. One possible criterion uses the analysis of indirect relationships between personality and behavior, in which beliefs are conceptualized as the mediating variable. Some beliefs that are related to behavior derive from more fundamental aspects of the individual's personality, whereas other beliefs may be unrelated to personality. It is probably the case that beliefs that are rooted in fundamental personality dimensions are more difficult to change (and/or to sustain change) than beliefs that are independent of personality. Thus, the selection of target beliefs might focus on identifying beliefs in which indirect relationships with personality variables are absent compared with beliefs in which indirect relationships are present.

Spurious relationships

Personality variables also can be used effectively for the analysis of spurious relationships. One area of application is the control of response sets in the context of measurement error. Many studies rely on self-reports of risk behaviors, and it is well known that such measures may be subject to good impression or social desirability biases. Research also documents that there exist individual differences in the desire to please others and to respond on inventories in ways that will present oneself in the best possible light. Not only may measures of behavioral criteria be influenced by such tendencies, but so too may cognitive and attitudinal measures about STDs. To the extent that general social desirability tendencies are a common cause of responses to cognitive measures and behavioral measures, then a spurious relationship exists between the measures. Personality variables can be included in statistical analyses and causal models to control for this source of measurement error. In addition to social desirability, scales have been developed to assess chronic lying tendencies, tendencies to respond randomly in assessment situations, and acquiescence response sets.

Integrated causal relationships and personality variables

The above sections make evident our sentiments toward building complex models of the relationships among personality, cognitive, attitudinal, and behavioral variables. By formally linking such variables, the importance and dynamics of all of them can be clarified. As one illustration, consider the behavior of taking a human immunodeficiency virus antibody test. According to theoretical work in social psychology, a person's test-taking behavior at any given time should be influenced by his or her intention to perform that behavior. This rather simple proposition (that people do what they intend to do) reflects a direct relationship between two variables, a behavioral intention and a behavior. It is also known that behavioral intentions are not always predictive of behavior and that there are variables that moderate the intention-behavior relationship. For example, a person may intend to take a human immunodeficiency virus test but not know how to go about obtaining one. Knowledge of how to enact the behavior is a variable that moderates the relationship between behavioral intention and behavior. Social psychologists (18, 26, 29) have identified over half-a-dozen variables that moderate intention-behavior relationships and that must be considered when predicting certain types of behavioral criteria. Because of such moderators, positive behavioral intent is usually found to be a necessary but not sufficient condition for behavioral performance. Personality variables, such as locus of control or general perceptions of behavioral efficacy, may have direct effects on behavioral intentions (or people's conscious decisions to perform a given behavior) but only may be related to behavior in a complex way through behavioral intentions and their moderators. The value of the personality variables would not be diagnosed by simple correlations between personality and behavior and would only be evident in the richer theoretical network.

DESIGNING INTERVENTIONS GIVEN KNOWLEDGE OF BEHAVIORAL DETERMINANTS

A researcher who identifies the behavioral determinants that are to be the focus of an intervention must then develop educational materials that can be used to bring about change in those determinants. One framework in social psychology that has been used to analyze this problem is called the persuasion matrix (37), a version of which is presented in Fig. 3. The rows of the matrix represent basic psychological processes in the persuasion process. For an educational message to be effective, an individual must attend to the message, comprehend its contents, and, once understood, accept the basic tenets of the message. If the focus is on long-term change, then a fourth parameter is important, namely, retention of the immediately induced change. According to several theories (42), acceptance of a message is determined in large part by whether and how individuals counterargue the contents of the message. The columns of the matrix represent classes of independent variables that can affect each of these processes. Educational messages can vary in terms of source characteristics (e.g., the attractiveness of the source, the age of the source, the expertise of the source, the gender of the source), message structure (e.g., speed of delivery, the use of figurative language, the use of implicit versus explicit conclusions, ignoring versus dealing with opposition arguments, the ordering of arguments within a message), channel media (e.g., radio, television, pamphlets, videos), and who the audience is that the messages are directed toward (e.g., audiences may vary in gender, education, intelligence, personality). Each of these classes of independent variables may affect attention, comprehension, acceptance, and retention, sometimes differentially so. McGuire (37) has reviewed research trends in each cell of the persuasion matrix.

One way in which personality variables can be important for designing effective interventions is in terms of identifying aspects of the educational process that must be considered, given the personality characteristics of the target population. For example, research has explored the relationship between persuasion and

	Source Variables	Message Variables	Channel Variables	Audience Variables
Attention				
Comprehension				
Acceptance				
Retention				

Figure 3. Persuasion matrix.

need for cognition (NC), a personality measure that assesses an individual's tendency to engage in effortful cognitive processing when exposed to educational materials (9). Individuals high in NC tend to attend carefully and think about the content of the message, whereas those who are low in NC tend to rely on non-content-relevant cues for acceptance (e.g., the overall conclusion made by the message, the characteristics of the source of the message, such as the source's attractiveness, and so on). If one's target population consists primarily of individuals who are low in NC, a different educational strategy might be used than if the target population is primarily high in NC. For example, with high-NC individuals, the educational materials might place greater emphasis on developing in-depth arguments and reasons for recommended actions, whereas such detail might be countereffective for low-NC individuals. Current research on personality and persuasion can thus inform the design of educational materials, given that the personality characteristics of the target population are known. Personality variables that have been studied in a persuasion context include self-esteem, involvement, anxiety, and self-monitoring. The vast majority of personality research in the STD area is correlational in nature and focuses on the prediction of behavioral criteria. The present section underscores the need for experimental research in which the relationship of personality to fundamental processes such as attention, comprehension, acceptance, and retention of educational materials is explored.

IDENTIFYING TARGET POPULATIONS

A third use of personality variables is as a predictive tool to identify individuals who may exhibit problematic behavior in the future and who may need special attention as a result. This use is illustrated by the research of Hammond et al. (23) as discussed earlier. Although personality variables may be good predictors in some cases, there exist difficulties that must be confronted. Personality measures are typically lengthy and invasive and hence are not well suited to quick administrations in health settings. This can be overcome by using specially developed short forms of the personality inventories or by developing proxy measures (e.g., using demographic or social variables) that can take the place of traditional measures. Most STD research that has pursued the use of personality variables as screening criteria has not employed standard prediction paradigms for developing prediction equations. Issues of variable selection, methods for defining prediction weights (e.g., least-squares estimators versus ridge estimators versus unit weights), issues of cross-validation, and different classification criteria have not been effectively exploited. For an overview of these issues, see reference 29.

SELECTED MEASUREMENT ISSUES

Inclusion of personality measures in health surveys is usually problematic because of the time demands of lengthy inventories. There are at least two approaches that an investigator can adopt when faced with limited time. First, a list of relevant personality variables can be prioritized, and only the two or three most important variables can be included in the survey. Second, the investigator can include a broader range of variables, using a short version of each measure by randomly selecting subsets of items from the original inventories. In doing so, the reliability and validity of the original instrument may be decreased, although initially high-quality measures may not be affected too adversely. The decision to emphasize breadth versus depth in the use of personality measures will ultimately depend on the purposes of the research and the quality of measures available. It should be possible through the creative use of proxies, short forms, and pilot work to include a range of personality variables in health surveys. Werner and Pervin (50) have reviewed major personality inventories and noted four facets of item content: (i) the area of psychological functioning addressed (cognitive, preferences, feelings, behavioral), (ii) the degree of reference to situational factors, (iii) the degree of reference to response frequency, and (iv) the nature of reference to time. Werner and Pervin (50) suggest guidelines for developing measures using these four facets (or, as another possibility, selecting subsets of items from a larger inventory) so as to maximize the relevance of the measure to the dependent variables of interest. Many personality measures have been developed for homogeneous populations (e.g., college students, white middle-class adults). It is crucial that such measures be subjected to pilot research when applied to populations that are distinct from the derivation samples. This includes not only basic assessments of reliability and validity but also linguistic and cultural differences that may affect item interpretation. Personality measures are subject to measurement error. Measurement error can bias parameter estimates in model evaluations and model tests. When possible, analytic strategies should be adopted that incorporate error theories into model estimation (e.g., confirmatory factor analytic approaches such as LISREL and EQS). Failure to incorporate error theories is tantamount to assuming perfectly reliable measures, an assumption that is patently untrue.

ADDITIONAL PERSONALITY APPROACHES

Our comments in this chapter have been restricted to traditional conceptualizations of personality in the context of trait theories. There are other approaches to personality that STD researchers might find of use. An extremely rich cognitive approach to personality has evolved in the context of personal construct theory (1, 35). A related cognitive approach has been described by Hamilton (22). These theories emphasize the conceptualization and measurement of the cognitive underpinnings of dispositions and go well beyond traditional conceptualizations of traits. Byrne and Schulte (8) describe a behavior sequence analysis of personality variables that represents a useful broad-based approach to personality analysis. Buss and Craik (7) describe a cognitive categorical approach to personality that is intriguing. Numerous studies have explored the role of self-schemata in the analysis of personality (6, 36), and these constructs also may prove fruitful in STD research. Aronoff and Wilson (3) describe approaches that emphasize the function of both enduring and situational influences on social perception, information processing, interpersonal attraction, and group dynamics. Bandura's (4) classic work on self-efficacy and its integration with cognitive variables is also noteworthy. Finally, Sherman and Fazio (43) have described parallels between attitude research and personality research and have highlighted numerous issues that personality researchers can profitably explore. This list of promising approaches is not intended to be exhaustive but certainly represents a diverse set of viewpoints on personality.

CONCLUSIONS

It is our belief that personality variables can be of use in the development of STD interventions but that there is a need for more complex theoretical models to guide personality research. We have highlighted directions and relationships that such models might explore. In doing so, we have elucidated a number of factors that may explain relatively weak observed relationships between personality and outcomes. These include (i) the focus on highly specific behavioral criteria as opposed to behavioral patterns; (ii) the confounding of distinct behavioral constructs (e.g., contraceptive choice and contraceptive consistency); (iii) the failure to distinguish outcomes from behaviors; (iv) the focus on simple linear models of the relationship between personality and behavior, when nonlinear models may be more appropriate; (v) the assumption of homogeneity of predictor weights across individuals when heterogeneity is likely; (vi) the failure to include mediating variables (e.g., behavioral intentions) that may be systematically related to personality but that reveal complex relationships to behavior through the presence of moderator variables; and (vii) problems with the measurement of personality constructs. We have also indicated ways in which personality variables can be used in intervention research other than as a focus of change. These include the use of personality variables for choosing cognitive and informational variables as targets of an intervention, the use of personality variables for designing educational materials and intervention implementation strategies, and the use of personality variables to develop prediction equations for the identification of target populations. Future research awaits such applications.

Acknowledgments. Preparation of this chapter was facilitated by Public Health Service grant HD24820 from the National Institutes of Health. We thank David Brinberg for his comments on a previous draft.

LITERATURE CITED

1. **Adams-Webber, J., and J. C. Mancuso.** 1983. *Applications of Personal Construct Theory.* Academic Press, Inc., New York.
2. **Ajzen, I., and M. Fishbein.** 1977. Attitude-behavior relations: a theoretical analysis and review of empirical literature. *Psychol. Bull.* **84:**888–918.
3. **Aronoff, J., and J. Wilson.** 1985. *Personality in the Social Process.* Erlbaum, Hillsdale, N.J.
4. **Bandura, A.** 1988. Perceived self-efficacy: exercise of control through self-belief. *In* J. Dauwalder, M. Perrez, and V. Hobbi (ed.), *Annual Series of European Research in Behavior Therapy.* Swets and Zietlinger, Lisse, The Netherlands.
5. **Biglan, A., C. W. Metzler, R. Wirt, D. Ary, J. Noell, L. Ochs, C. French, and D. Hood.** 1990. Social and behavioral factors associated with high risk sexual behavior among adolescents. *J. Behav. Med.* **13:**245–261.
6. **Burke, P. A., R. E. Kraut, and R. H. Dworkin.** 1984. Traits, consistency, and self schemata: what do our methods measure? *J. Pers. Soc. Psychol.* **47:**568–579.
7. **Buss, D. M., and K. Craik.** 1983. The act frequency approach to personality. *Psychol. Rev.* **90:**105–126.
8. **Byrne, D., and L. Schulte.** 1990. Personality dispositions as mediators of sexual responses. *In* J. Bancroft (ed.), *Annual Review of Sexual Research.* Society for the Scientific Study of Sex, Philadelphia.
9. **Cacioppo, J. T., R. E. Petty, C. F. Kao, and R. Rodriguez.** 1986. Central and peripheral routes to persuasion: an individual difference perspective. *J. Pers. Soc. Psychol.* **51:**1032–1043.
10. **Costa, P., and R. R. McCrae.** 1985. *The NEO Personality Inventory Manual.* Psychological Assessment Resources, Odessa, Fla.
11. **DeBono, K., and R. J. Harnish.** 1989. Source expertise, source attractiveness, and the processing of persuasive information: a functional approach. *J. Pers. Soc. Psychol.* **55:**541–546.
12. **Epstein, S.** 1979. The stability of behavior. I. On predicting most of the people much of the time. *J. Pers. Soc. Psychol.* **37:**1097–1126.
13. **Eysenck, H., and S. Eysenck.** 1969. *Personality Structure and Measurement.* Routledge and Kagan, London.
14. **Eysenck, H., and S. Eysenck.** 1976. *Psychoticism as a Dimension of Personality.* Hodder & Stoughton, London.
15. **Eysenck, H. J.** 1986. Can personality study ever be scientific? *J. Soc. Behav. Pers.* **1:**3–19.
16. **Eysenck, S., and H. Eysenck.** 1977. The place of impulsiveness in a dimensional system of personality description. *Br. J. Soc. Clin. Psychol.* **16:**57–68.
17. **Fishbein, M.** 1973. The prediction of behavior from attitudinal variables. *In* C. D. Mortensen and K. Soreno (ed.), *Advances in Communication Research.* Harper and Row, Publishers, Inc., New York.
18. **Fishbein, M., and I. Ajzen.** 1975. *Beliefs, Attitudes, Intentions, and Behavior.* Addison-Wesley Publishing Co., Inc., Reading, Mass.
19. **Foreit, J. R., and K. G. Foreit.** 1981. Risk-taking and contraceptive behavior among unmarried college students. *Popul. Environ.* **4:**174–188.
20. **Geis, B. D., and M. Gerrard.** 1984. Predicting male and female contraceptive behavior: a discriminant analysis of groups high, moderate and low in contraceptive effectiveness. *J. Pers. Soc. Psychol.* **46:**669–680.
21. **Gergen, K. J., A. Hepburn, and D. Fisher.** 1986. Hermeneutics of personality description. *J. Pers. Soc. Psychol.* **50:**1261–1270.
22. **Hamilton, V.** 1983. *The Cognitive Structures and Processes of Human Motivation and Personality.* John Wiley & Sons, Inc., New York.

23. **Hammond, D., R. D. Maw, and M. Mulholland.** 1989. Personality types of women attending an STD clinic: correlation with keeping first interview appointments. *Genitourin. Med.* **65:**163–165.
24. **Higgins, E. T.** 1987. Self-discrepancy: a theory relating self and affect. *Psychol. Rev.* **94:**319–340.
25. **Jaccard, J.** 1974. Predicting social behavior from personality traits. *J. Res. Pers.* **7:**358–367.
26. **Jaccard, J.** 1975. A theoretical analysis of selected factors important to health education strategies. *Health Educ. Monogr.* **3:**152–166.
27. **Jaccard, J., and P. Dittus.** 1990. Idiographic and nomothetic perspectives on research methods and data analysis. *In* C. Hendrick and M. Clark (ed.) *Review of Personality and Social Psychology.* Sage Publications, Beverly Hills.
28. **Jaccard, J., D. Helbig, C. K. Wan, M. Gutman, and D. C. Kritz-Silverstein.** 1990. Individual differences in attitude-behavior consistency: the prediction of contraceptive behavior. *J. Appl. Soc. Psychol.* **20:**575–595.
29. **Jaccard, J., R. Turrisi, and C. Wan.** 1989. Implications of behavioral decision theory and social marketing for designing social action programs. *In* J. Edwards, R. Tindale, L. Heath, and E. Posavac (ed.), *Social Influence Processes and Prevention.* Plenum Press, New York.
30. **Jaccard, J., R. Turrisi, and C. Wan.** 1990. *Interaction Effects in Multiple Regression.* Sage Publications, Beverly Hills.
31. **Jackson, D., L. Hournay, and N. Vidmar.** 1972. A four dimensional interpretation of risk. *J. Pers.* **40:**83–501.
32. **Jessor, R., and S. Jessor.** *Problem Behavior and Psychological Development: a Longitudinal Analysis.* Academic Press, Inc., New York.
33. **Kelley, K., D. Byrne, D. Pryzbyla, C. Eberly, B. Eberly, V. Greenlinger, C. K. Wan, and J. Gorsky.** 1985. Chronic self-destructiveness: conceptualization, measurement, and initial validation of the construct. *Motiv. Emotion* **9:**135–151.
34. **Kelley, K., F. Cheung, P. Rodriquez-Carrillo, R. Singh, and C. K. Wan.** 1986. Cross-cultural generality of chronic self-destructiveness. *J. Soc. Psychol.* **126:**573–577.
35. **Mancuso, J. C., and M. Shaw.** 1988. *Cognition and Personal Structure.* Praeger Publishers, New York.
36. **Markus, H.** 1977. Self-schemata and processing of information about the self. *J. Pers. Soc. Psychol.* **35:**63–78.
37. **McGuire, W. J.** 1985. Attitudes and attitude change. *In* G. Lindzey and E. Aronson (ed.), *Handbook of Social Psychology.* Random House, New York.
38. **Mischel, W.** 1968. *Personality and Assessment.* John Wiley & Sons, Inc., New York.
39. **Moscovici, S.** 1985. Social influence and conformity. *In* G. Lindzey and E. Aronson (ed.), *Handbook of Social Psychology.* Random House, New York.
40. **Mosher, D. L.** 1979. Sex guilt and sex myths in college men and women. *J. Sex Res.* **15:**224–234.
41. **Paulhus, D.** 1989. Socially desirable responding: some new solutions to old problems. *In* D. Buss and N. Cantor (ed.), *Personality Psychology.* Springer-Verlag, New York.
42. **Petty, R. E., and J. T. Cacioppo.** 1986. The elaboration likelihood model of persuasion. *In* L. Berkowitz (ed.), *Advances in Experimental Social Psychology.* Academic Press, Inc., New York.
43. **Sherman, S. J., and R. H. Fazio.** 1983. Parallels between attitudes and traits as predictors of behavior. *J. Pers.* **51:**308–345.
44. **Snyder, M., and S. Gangestad.** 1986. On the nature of self monitoring: matters of assessment, matters of validity. *J. Pers. Soc. Psychol.* **51:**125–139.
45. **Snyder, M., and W. Ickes.** 1985. Personality and social behavior. *In* G. Lindzey and E. Aronson (ed.), *Handbook of Social Psychology.* Random House, New York.
46. **Snyder, M., J. A. Simpson, and S. Gangestad.** 1986. Personality and sexual relations. *J. Pers. Soc. Psychol.* **51:**181–190.
47. **Spence, J., K. Deaux, and R. Helmreich.** 1985. Sex roles in contemporary American

society. *In* G. Lindzey and E. Aronson (ed.), *Handbook of Social Psychology*. Random House, New York.
48. **Spence, J., and R. Helmreich.** 1978. *Masculinity and Femininity: Their Psychological Dimensions, Correlates, and Antecedents*. University of Texas Press, Austin.
49. **Strickland, B. R.** 1989. Internal-external control expectancies: from contingency to creativity. *Am. Psychol.* **44:**1–12.
50. **Werner, P., and R. Pervin.** 1986. Analysis of personality inventory items. *J. Pers. Soc. Psychol.* **52:**222–232.
51. **Yarber, W. L., and W. A. Fisher.** 1983. Affective orientation to sexuality and venereal disease preventive behaviors. *Health Values* **7:**19–23.
52. **Zuckerman, M.** 1979. *Sensation Seeking*. Erlbaum, Hillsdale, N.J.
53. **Zuckerman, M., D. M. Kuhlman, and C. Camac.** 1988. What lies beyond E and N? Factor analyses of scales believed to measure basic dimensions of personality. *J. Pers. Soc. Psychol.* **54:**96–107.

Approaches to Changing Human Behaviors

Implications for Design of Interventions for Control of Sexually Transmitted Diseases Including HIV Infection

Alternative Models of Behavior Change

Robert Hornik

Why is it that some people learn about sexually transmitted diseases (STDs) and about ways to avoid them, yet don't initiate and maintain new behaviors that will reduce risk? Professional educators and information campaign developers know how to diffuse knowledge and skills, if they are given the resources. It is much less clear that they know how to ensure that knowledge and skills, once achieved, produce appropriate practice.

This chapter focuses on the question of turning knowledge into behavior, why some people readily adopt new practices when they learn "the facts" and other people do so more slowly or not at all. There are many different answers available, many models of behavior change proposed. The goal for this chapter is to sort through them, admitting that this sorting will produce no definitive answer. The existing research is surely insufficient, and more than that, there is no one answer. The answer depends on the behavior; it depends on the context; it depends on the individual. However, this chapter does two things: (i) it describes alternative behavior change models typically offered, with examples, and (ii) it discusses the implications for program design of each behavior change model.

The consideration of alternative answers or models of behavior change has a constraint, however. There is a need to be practical, since this is a chapter and a book about STD interventions. It is interesting to know what explains current behavior; however, the immediate task is to suggest promising routes to intervene in that behavior. An explanation that fails to suggest what might work, or what won't work, to effect behavior change is valued less. Thus, knowing that occupational role accounted for 10% of the variance in the frequency of genital self-examination may have no direct programmatic implications. No STD program can affect occupational role; the result doesn't indicate what intervention strategy should be followed. A model of behavior may be enriched by such a result; it doesn't help to create a model of behavior change. That is the task for this chapter and for STD behavioral researchers.

Also, this chapter presents the logic of each approach in its own terms and within a common framework. However, it is not a critique of research. It does not review specific empirical studies or evaluate the established utility of each of the models for STD work. Such a critique would be instructive but is ruled out on three grounds: (i) there is relatively little research that applies specifically to STD-related practices; (ii) a broad review would require extended methodological discussion about the way research is done under each approach as well as the synthesis of widely varying results, for which there is no space; and (iii) the end result would

Robert Hornik – The Annenberg School for Communication, University of Pennsylvania, Philadelphia, Pennsylvania 19104-6220.

be far from definitive. None of the models would be shown to be invariably inappropriate. All would be worth some consideration in some contexts.

There is one final introductory point: all behavior change programs operate under a behavior change model. Sometimes those models are explicit; more often they are implicit: they can be read only from observing just what it is that implementers of programs do. For example, a program that focuses its efforts on diffusing the message that human immunodeficiency virus is transmitted by sexual intercourse, with the expectation that condom use will increase, has a particular model of change, although perhaps no one has made it explicit. Indeed, none of the staff might endorse it were they forced to make it explicit. The model is that if people just know that human immunodeficiency virus is spread sexually, they will make use of condoms; the program staff are then assuming that knowledge of the facts will lead to new behavior, universally.

When such programs fail to produce the desired behavior change, there is often recrimination—the education solution is rejected as unsuccessful. Yet all that may have been shown is that one model of behavior change, and a particularly crude one, has failed. If program designers were to read the behavior change literature and consider the alternative models it presents, they might question such a simple model a priori. This chapter may serve as an introduction to those alternative models.

This presentation is quite brief and does little justice to the richness of each intellectual tradition represented. See Selected Readings, below, for additional references that will help to examine the relevant approaches in greater detail.

CLASSES OF EXPLANATION

It is useful to divide models of behavior change into six broad categories: (i) community-level structural models; (ii) social expectation models; (iii) individual-level structural models; (iv) cognitive models, including expectancy-value models and perceived self-efficacy models; (v) drive or trait models; and (vi) behaviorist models. This section presents brief descriptions of each of the models, with hypothetical examples, and provides comparisons among them. There is an attempt to put them in a common framework to make those comparisons easier, but this is a slippery business. The categories are not mutually exclusive; all the major researchers in each category admit to the relevance of some, if not all, of the other major models. Also, the models are not perfectly parallel (e.g., the cognitive and drive or trait models may be seen as explanations for how the first three models might work). Nonetheless, it is useful to present them as distinct models because in that form they direct the thinking of intervention developers.

Each model derives from the social science health behavior literature, reflecting work either from a particular source or sources or from the broader discussions typical in this literature. Much of the formal framework has appeared elsewhere (2), but much of its argument would be familiar to medical anthropologists and sociologists and public health educators or communication specialists.

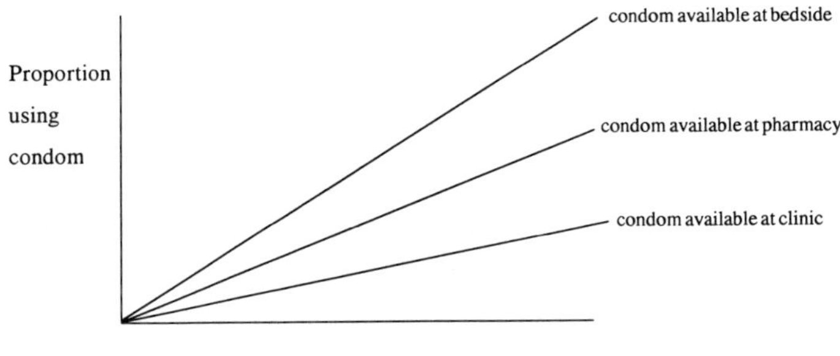

Figure 1. Community structure: knowledge, behavior, and condom availability.

Community-Level Structural Models

In simple form, community-level structural models suggest that environmental forces beyond the control of the individual constrain or help the knowledge-behavior link. Common examples include the presence or absence of legal restrictions on availability of condoms, wage scales that define what proportion of people will have the resources to purchase STD medication, or access to clinics capable of diagnosing and treating STDs. Each of these would make it either harder or easier for an individual who learned about a practice to realize it.

Consider, for example, the case of using condoms with partners other than a spouse. One might hypothesize that access to condoms will affect the likelihood of turning knowledge about the utility of condoms for protecting against STDs into actual practice. One can compare three situations. In the first, national policy requires that every hotel make condoms available at bedside. In the second, condoms are openly available but must be purchased at pharmacies. In the third, condoms can only be distributed through family planning clinics. One might expect a result like that pictured in Fig. 1. Those with easiest access (at bedside) would be more likely to turn their knowledge into behavior. The slopes decrease for each level of access.

This view of behavior change is common enough in the United States but has been particularly influential in Europe and some developing countries. The view (called health promotion in Europe) suggests that while individual education may be one strategy for achieving behavior change, change in society-level structures (like easing access to condoms) may be a more effective point of intervention. In another health arena, it argues that lobbying for legislation that mandates smoke-free airplanes and workplaces and forbids cigarette vending machines may have a larger impact on smoking behavior than individual antismoking education.

Implicit in this view is sometimes a willingness to accept a diminution in individual decision-making. In the case of increasing access to condoms by requiring them to be in every bedside table, one risks offending some visitors to the hotel (while giving others more opportunity to choose, of course). In forbidding cigarette sales by vending machines, one reduces the ability of individuals to choose whether or not to smoke. Educational strategies may be less restrictive of individual choice than structural modification strategies to the extent that they are attempts to allow a more informed choice. However, societies make rules restricting individual choice (or creating incentives or disincentives for it); whether or not a particular health practice will be subject to such societal incentives or disincentives will be the outcome of political debate. However, as STD interventionists compare potential strategies, they will need to consider not only their respective efficacy in achieving behavior change but their ethical implications as well, particularly with regard to restrictions on individual choice.

Social Expectation Models

Social expectation models suggest that behavior that appears to be individual (a decision to use a condom, a change in patterns of partner choice) can be viewed as social behavior instead. Individual practices are substantially the result of conformity to the expectations of others. Thus, sexual behavior may appear to be the most private of decisions, shared only with the partner involved. Yet it may be that in the aggregate, there is substantial homogeneity in such practices within social networks.

There are at least two paths through which private acts may be socially influenced. One way is through direct experience. An individual defines for himself or herself expected and acceptable sexual practices through sexual experience with particular partners. However, those partners have also defined their boundaries and expectations through experience with others. Thus, the social network communicates the private experience.

Also, social expectations for sexual practice may be communicated outside of direct sexual experience. Conversation among those in a social network, mass media presentations, books, and observations of others' behavior when it is accessible all may provide important cues as to what is or is not expected or acceptable in private sexual interactions.

This process of influence may occur without any requirement that people make complex cognitive judgments about the practice. Users may be no more able to cite the benefits of condom use than others who do not use condoms. They use condoms because they know they are expected to use condoms in a particular context and know it would be unacceptable to do otherwise. This socially influenced action may reflect a quite conscious conformity with others' expectations. It may be possible for people to describe what other people expect from them and indicate their own need to conform to those expectations. Their conformity is a response to a conscious awareness of social norms.

However, there may be a social influence process regardless of people's ability to articulate that influence as the source of their behavior. It may be that people are unable to articulate why they use condoms, they just do it. Some social models suggest that such habitual behavior reflects external expectations; people come to act habitually in a way that is consistent with the way that others act and expect

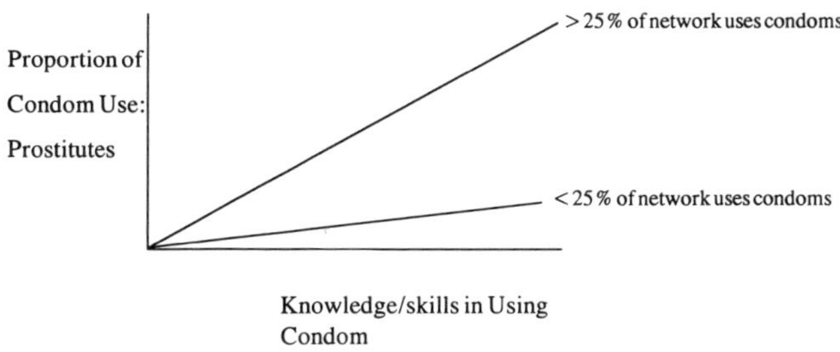

Figure 2. Social: knowledge, behavior, and social behavior.

them to act. Their conformity reflects the demands of their social network without any reflective process producing awareness of those demands.

Whether or not one believes that individuals can or cannot articulate the social sources of their behavior, the underlying theoretical argument is the same. Much behavior can be understood at a social group level rather than at an individual level. The applied question of interest should be "How do groups change their behavior?" rather than "How do individuals change their behavior?" Figure 2 illustrates this class of model. Assume that the practice of interest is condom use among female sex workers. Even if an individual has the knowledge and skills to make use of condoms effectively, will she do it? A social model would suggest that she is more likely to turn that knowledge into practice if she knows that those in her social network expect her to do so. Perhaps the ability of one sex worker to demand that her clients use condoms depends on the willingness of other sex workers to make a similar demand. In that case, one would expect that the slope between knowledge and behavior would be considerably greater among social networks in which relatively more of the sex workers were making such demands than among sex workers among whom the demands were less commonly made.

In Fig. 2, the extent to which other sex workers were demanding that their clients use condoms would be measured by the frequency of condom use. In this hypothetical case, few of the individual sex workers are affected by their knowledge about the use of condoms to avoid infection if few of their coworkers are using condoms. Knowledge is much more sharply related to practice among sex workers whose coworkers are using condoms.

This example assumes that there are strong norms about condom use, either positive or negative. It says that only when norms are consistent with knowledge will individual knowledge have an effect. However, another perspective might focus not on the direction of social norms but on their strength. This view suggests that when there are strong social norms about condom use, individual knowledge will make little difference. Knowledge would only be relevant when norms are weak and thus there would be greater freedom to ignore social expectations.

These first two classes of explanation (community structural and social expectation models) focus outside the individual—they argue that people turn knowledge into behavior depending on external influences and that those influ-

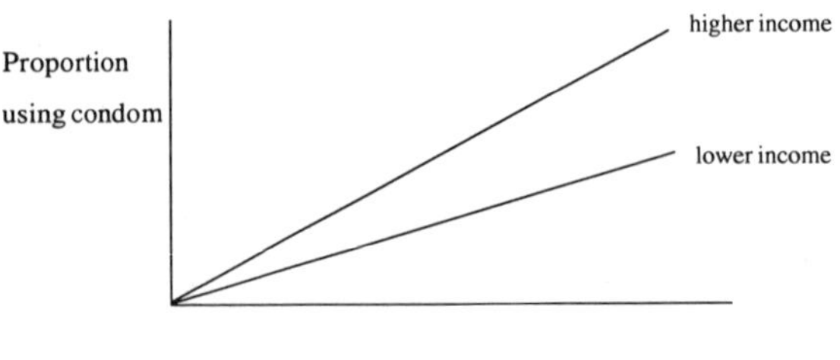

Figure 3. Individual structure: knowledge, behavior, and disposable income.

ences have their effects on aggregates larger than the individual. The next four models shift the focus to the individual, although the first of them maintains the concern with external influences.

Individual Structural Models

The community-level structural model suggested that there are forces constraining or supporting STD-preventive behavior at the community level. A parallel argument can be made about individuals. They learn about safer practices, but their individual material circumstances make it easier or more difficult for them to adopt such practices.

Those circumstances may have to do with a social role restriction; for example, married women may be prevented from demanding that their husbands use condoms even though the women know the husbands have outside partners. The woman may suffer a loss of income or risk physical harm or simply not have the physical ability to refuse intercourse.

The circumstances may also reflect occupational role. A sex worker may be unable to demand that her clients use condoms if she cannot afford the loss of customers were they to go elsewhere.

The circumstances may be defined by low or high income. A poor man who knows about condoms is unable to purchase them; the wealthier woman who knows about the risks of untreated STDs can afford to buy the medication that will cure the STD. Figure 3 presents the hypothetical example of men with different income levels, with contrasting slopes representing their different abilities to turn knowledge about condoms into practice.

As an additional note, often a behavior seen from one perspective as embedded in individual structural circumstance can be seen from another as embedded in community structural circumstance. Thus, a person's failure to use condoms can be attributed to low income, or the same failure can be attributed to the community's failure to provide access to condoms at a low price. It is the same behavior and the same causal process, but it can be seen from different aspects.

This is a problem if one is using the model categories as a guide for interventions. Insofar as one sees a problem as individual, there also may be a temptation to see solutions as individual also. Consider the problem of the sex worker accepting clients without condoms. If her poverty is the focus of the explanation, then the temptation is to create an individual solution; this solution may be to find her another job or to convince her to make a decision to rethink the issue and accept the need to sacrifice short-term profit for long-term survival. If, in contrast, one sees the problem as embedded in the community of clients and of the sex worker industry as a whole, the types of interventions open for consideration may be quite different; here the possibilities include mass client education to stimulate norm change so that clients do not reject condom use or the organizing of sex workers to provide solidarity around issues of self-protection.

Cognitive Models

These explanations for behavior change all focus on things that go on inside people's heads: their knowledge, beliefs, attitudes, and perceptions of others. These explanations have dominated discussions about health behavior change in the United States. While there are many varieties of such theories and many contributors to the literature about each one, three theoretical perspectives have been the most discussed. The theory of reasoned action (see Chapter 14) and the health belief model (4) both are expectancy-value theories. The third perspective accepts many of the concepts discussed in the other two but adds to them an additional concept, perceived self-efficacy (1).

The theory of reasoned action

The theory of reasoned action incorporates three elements: it has an overarching theoretical perspective shared by all of this class of model, that much of behavior is cognitively determined; it has a prescription as to what elements of cognition are worth examining for their power to predict behavior; and it has a methodology for doing that examination. Figure 4 presents the basic model, which incorporates several propositions.

First, as Fig. 4 outlines, behavior is substantially a reflection of behavioral intentions. There are several caveats to that proposition. The theory only addresses behaviors said to be under volitional control. If a behavior is beyond an individual's control, one cannot expect an association between intention and behavior (e.g., "I will get an STD checkup tomorrow" isn't under my control if there is no facility open tomorrow).

Also, behaviors and behavioral intentions are linked to the extent that one is dealing with highly specific behaviors and exactly matching behavioral intentions. A generalized intention to practice safer sex may be minimally related to condom use. A specific intention to use a condom tomorrow when one has intercourse with a sex worker is expected to be related to that specific behavior.

In its second proposition, the model suggests that behavioral intentions reflect two types of cognitions: attitudes toward the behavior, and perceived social norms. One intends to behave in a specific way partly as the result of what one thinks about the behavior oneself and partly as a function of what others expect one to do.

The third proposition is that attitude toward the behavior is a function of a

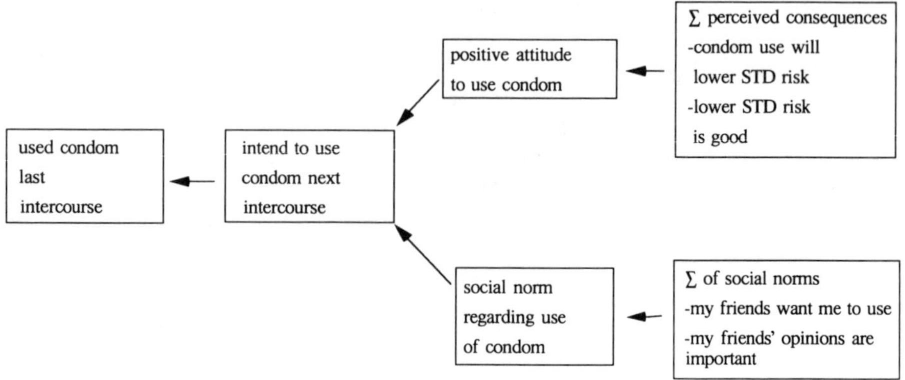

Figure 4. Theory of reasoned action.

weighted sum of a set of the products of perceived consequences of practicing the behavior and the subjective value of each of those consequences. The attitude toward using condoms might reflect such perceived consequences as the efficacy of condoms in reducing STDs, the effects of condom use on sexual pleasure, embarrassment at having to purchase condoms at a pharmacy, and extending the time to male orgasm. The matching subjective values for each consequence include the value of reducing risk for STDs, the value of avoiding reduction in sexual pleasure, the value of avoiding embarrassment, and the value of extending the time to orgasm.

The fourth proposition is that perceived social norms are also a function of a composite of other people's expectations. That composite is the weighted sum of the product of perceptions of each of a set of external social actors and one's motivation to comply with those actors. Thus, the degree of one's agreement with a statement like "Most of my friends think I should use condoms when I have sex with prostitutes" is multiplied by one's response to a statement like "I want to do what my friends think I should do."

The theory of reasoned action provides positive guidance about how to think about cognitive influences on behavior change. The approach makes no prediction about whether attitude toward the behavior, on the one hand, or social norms about the behavior, on the other, will most influence a particular behavior. It assumes that the answer will vary for different behaviors and different populations. Similarly, the approach makes no prediction about which perceived consequences will most influence the overall attitude toward the behavior. At its core, the theory assumes that cognitions matter but leaves it as a matter of investigation as to which will matter in a specific case. It directs the search for such cognitions but doesn't predict the outcome.

In numerous instances, the predictive power of each of the model's propositions has been supported. Behavioral intentions have been shown to correlate with behavior; attitudes and social norms have been shown to predict behavioral

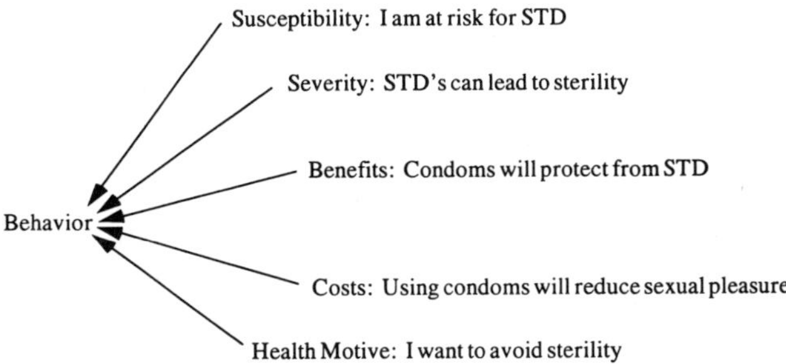

Figure 5. Health belief model.

intentions. However, for intervention developers the issue is cause, not prediction, of behavior. The implication of the theory is that if a perceived consequence (e.g., agreement with the statement "Regular use of condoms will reduce my risk of STDs") is predictive, then it is a cause of the behavior. If that is true, then one ought to be able to focus an intervention on changing that perception and have an expectation that behavior subsequently will change. Thus, if perception of the degree to which condom use reduces one's risk of STDs is a strong predictor, then one might want to do a public education program focused on increasing that perception. If the perception changed, one would expect a subsequent increase in condom use. The question of whether the theory of reasoned action can serve this function remains open.

The health belief model

The health belief model (4) offers a less elaborate approach but has much in common with the theory of reasoned action. The health belief model is an expectancy-value theory in that it assumes that people's behavior is guided by their expectations of consequences of adopting new practices. In contrast to the theory of reasoned action, health belief models largely ignore issues of social norms and view the effects on behavior as much more direct. There are four essential constructs, each of which is seen as directly affecting behavior. (i) The first construct is susceptibility. Does one perceive oneself as vulnerable to the disease? This might be measured by one's agreement with a statement like "I am at risk for STDs." (ii) The second construct is severity. Does one perceive that getting the disease has worrisome consequences? "STDs can lead to sterility." (iii) The third construct is benefits minus costs. What positive and negative effects does one expect from adopting the new practice? "Regular use of a condom will reduce my risk of STDs" and "Using condoms reduces sexual pleasure." (iv) The final construct is health motive. Is there concern about the consequences of contracting the disease? "I want to avoid sterility." The theory relies heavily on the assumption that cognitions matter. Figure 5 summarizes the essential features of the model.

Neither Fig. 4 nor Fig. 5 follows the graphic method used to present the first three classes of explanation. They depart from the underlying framework (What causes knowledge to turn into behavior?) of those earlier models and of the ones to be presented subsequently. This reflects a respect for the way the authors of these approaches present their work. Nonetheless, both the health belief model and the theory of reasoned action can be presented as parallel to the others, although this does some injustice to the authors' views.

Assume that one can separate basic knowledge and skills in condom use from other attitudes and beliefs in each model. One might hypothesize that the relationship between those basic types of knowledge and skills and behavior is conditioned by the other complex cognitive variables. Thus, for the theory of reasoned action, basic knowledge would be more likely to produce behavior if the composite attitude toward the behavior were supportive or if perceived social norms were supportive. Rather than expecting only additive main effects for both social norms and attitudes, one would expect an interaction of knowledge with norms and/or attitudes in their joint effects on behavior (or behavioral intentions).

The health belief model might be reconceptualized in a similar way. The basic knowledge elements (some of which will be captured by the benefits construct) will more readily turn into behavior if one believes oneself at more risk versus less risk, that the consequences are more severe rather than less severe, and that the costs are lower rather than higher, and if one is more motivated to protect oneself from given consequences rather than less motivated. The graphic presentation would feature differently sloped lines for each pair of contrasting groups.

It is unclear whether such a reconceptualization of either theory would be at all productive empirically, or whether it merely serves the immediate purposes of this presentation. The test would be whether the interaction between knowledge and other variables produces a more powerful explanation for behavior than do main effects alone.

Social cognitive models

Bandura's (1) work on this subject has addressed many issues about learning and performing new skills that are not within the focus of this chapter. His own theories of behavior change also incorporate many elements corresponding to the other cognitive theories. Indeed, Rosenstock and his colleagues (4) have argued that most constructs in Bandura's view of behavior are roughly equivalent to the major constructs of the health belief model, with one central addition: the concept of self-efficacy with regard to the performance of a particular behavior. This concept reflects the actual capacity to perform a behavior and the self-confidence that one can actually perform it.

Bandura (1) frequently cites a study that suggests that math ability turns into math performance when one has self-confidence in those abilities. He argues that the same is true for many areas of performance. It is easy to see the relevance of self-efficacy in the context of STD-related practices. Consider the case of someone who knows about condoms and their utility in preventing STDs but fails to use them in a specific context. One explanation for that failure may be lack of perceived self-efficacy. One does not believe that one can negotiate the use of a condom in that context. Figure 6 illustrates that hypothetical relationship. Those with a greater

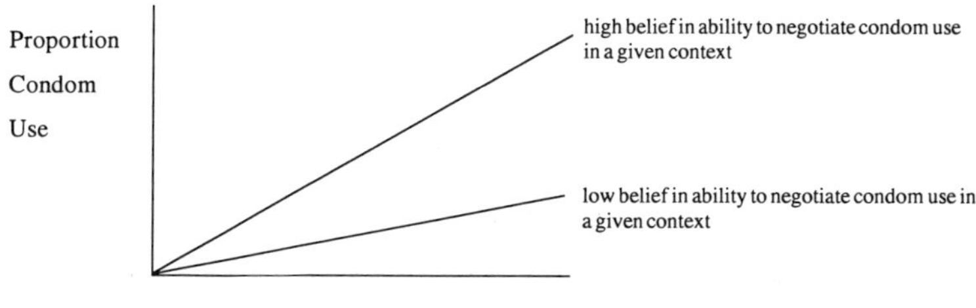

Figure 6. Self-efficacy: knowledge, behavior, and belief in ability to negotiate condom use in a given context.

sense of self-efficacy are more likely to turn knowledge into behavior than those with lower self-efficacy.

There is one additional parallel between Bandura's approach (1) and that of the theory of reasoned action. Fishbein (Fishbein et al., this volume) claims the theory of reasoned action applies when one is dealing with specific behavior and behavioral intentions. Similarly, social cognitive theory applies the concept of self-efficacy in quite specific situations. It is not an enduring personality characteristic like self-esteem or locus of control or other psychological orientations that are said to affect a broad range of behaviors. It is the self-confidence to perform a specific behavior in a specific context.

Drive or Trait Models

Drive or trait theories suggest that enduring elements of human personality influence behavior. Some people have stronger drives or more of one trait or another than other people that influence them to act in a particular way. A straightforward example appears in Fig. 7. One might hypothesize that there exists a personality trait called openness to change or innovativeness (3). Then one might expect that the effect of knowledge on behavior would vary sharply with that trait. Those who were more innovative would readily turn knowledge into behavior; those more closed by dint of personality would show less of a knowledge-behavior link.

Drive and trait models often are used in popular discussion to explain failures to change behaviors. For example, people say "He is just stubborn" or "She is always willing to try something new." Implicitly, they blame or credit change to enduring elements of character. Other examples might focus on particular drives: as people vary in their sex drives or in their drive to reduce fear, they will vary in the effects of knowledge on behavior. These are certainly common "folk" explanations for behavior. Nonetheless, empirical work that relies on traits or drives as explanations for health behavior change is rarer. One might suggest several reasons for the scarcity. (i) It is difficult to measure personality traits or drives with any reliability. (ii) There is the subjective preference of many researchers to look

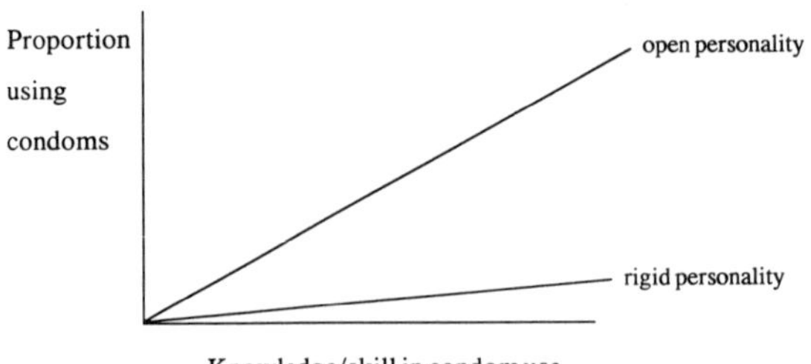

Figure 7. Trait model: knowledge, behavior, and "openness."

elsewhere. "They wouldn't change because they were just too rigid" sounds more like a rationalization for a failed program than an explanation. (iii) There is a concern that these models, even if they are powerful, have no positive practical implications. Personality traits are enduring, assumed not to be open to intervention. What can one say to a practitioner if one attributes behavior to an unchangeable trait except "You might as well go home." Most people who do research on behavior change want to influence practice; a research path whose success leads to going home may not be a favored path.

Behaviorist Models

In the broadest terms, behaviorist models suggest that behavior is shaped by its antecedents and its consequences. In crude terms, if one engages in a practice that is rewarded, it is likely to be repeated. The argument denies that cognition is essential. There is no need to call on or describe an intermediate thinking process through which individuals recognize the rewards and decide to maintain desirable behavior. It is enough to know whether the performance of the behavior was associated with a reward (or punishment) to expect an outcome.

Figure 8 illustrates a hypothetical example. Will repeat visits to an STD clinic reflect knowledge about the services offered at the clinic? Yes, the behaviorist model says, insofar as previous visits have been rewarding (either in terms of outcome or in terms of the pleasantness of the experience).

The typical application of behaviorist models to other areas of health behavior change has been to link the performance of desired behavior to immediate rewards or of undesired behavior to immediate punishments. For example, vaccination programs have given a special certificate to mothers whose children have obtained all required vaccinations, or alcoholics have been given the drug Antabuse so that consumption of alcohol produces nausea.

IMPLICATIONS FOR PROGRAM DESIGN

These models are intrinsically interesting. However, they become useful only insofar as they support specific implications for program design. What program designs should be adopted if one accepts a particular model? Here, each model is

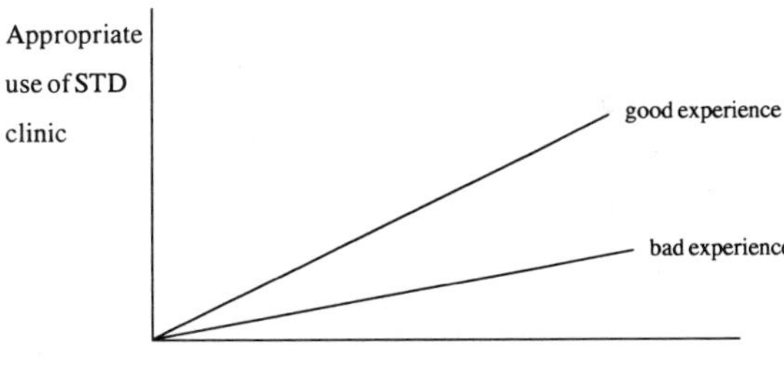

Figure 8. Behaviorism: knowledge, behavior, and experience and STD clinic.

examined briefly to answer the question "Well, if the data fit this model, how would I intervene?" Since more than one model may fit the data, it may be appropriate to consider more than one set of implications. To some extent, this section summarizes points implied or made explicitly earlier.

Community-Level Structural Models

Assume that one had evidence that community structural variables (like availability of STD services) substantially constrain the effects of knowledge in producing behavior. For example, people don't obtain STD diagnosis and treatment even though they know about them because the services are not offered at public clinics. These results might support two complementary implications. The first is that program designers ought to address structural arrangements before diffusing new knowledge meant to produce individual behavior change. They ought to change those structural limitations if at all possible (e.g., by influencing public policies that restrict STD services). The second implication comes into play if they are unable to resolve such structural limitations. Program designers would then need to limit their behavior promotion activities to audiences for whom the new behaviors were feasible. For example, they would need to consciously limit the reach of their STD service promotion messages to audiences for whom such services were actually available. In doing so, they would greatly reduce their expectations for a broad effect.

Social Expectation Models

Two versions of this logic were presented. One assumed that influence flowed from the social environment's expectations for one's behavior, regardless of whether one perceived or could articulate that interest. The second focused on the influence of perceptions of other people's expectations on behavior. Under most circumstances, one would anticipate that perceptions of others' expectations and their actual expectations would be closely related. Nonetheless, in thinking about possible intervention paths, it may be worthwhile separating them.

To the extent that social network influence is powerful and is defined by the actual behavior of the network, a program planner may need to adopt a long-term perspective on change. In this model, people change their behavior in response to the true expectations of others more than through changes in individual beliefs or attitudes. It suggests that short of a shift in social norms, individuals won't change. In this situation, the intervention plan would ensure that all channels reaching the network contain the same message to increase the perception that the new practice has wide support. Second, one might use approaches that increase the level of community discussion on the assumption that such discussion will accelerate the process of social norm diffusion. Finally, one would expect that the pace of change will be slow and that it will be necessary to maintain an intervention for an extended period.

A somewhat easier path might open if evidence suggested that what mattered was the perception of others' expectations rather than their actual behavior. An intervention that focused on increasing the perception that others were changing might have an effect even if it exaggerated the degree of actual change. Thus, the French AIDS campaign had attractive young people declaring their social solidarity and commitment to new protective behavior. (The catch phrase in the commercials referred to human immunodeficiency virus and said "It won't get by me.") The message seems to imply a well-established social solidarity. One might speculate that the message, broadcast quite early in the epidemic, exaggerated the actual degree of social solidarity. It appears to be based on the hope that the perception of such collective unity would accelerate adoption of protective behavior.

Individual-Level Structural Models

Assume that individual structural variables constrained the effects of knowledge on behavior. For example, people learn about the utility of condoms from an educational campaign, but the degree to which the new knowledge affects their use of condoms depends on their degree of disposable income. The program implications of these results are parallel to those described under the community-level structural models, unsurprisingly. Either intervention planners would have to address individual structural factors directly (by subsidizing condoms, for example), or if that was beyond their resources, they would have to limit the target audience for educational programs to those for whom the recommended practice was feasible.

Cognitive Models

Theory of reasoned action

The social norms side of this model was discussed above. The attitude side would demand that one locate areas of beliefs that were strongly related to behavioral intentions and about which a substantial segment of the audience held nonoptimal views. Assume that while a belief that STDs could lead to sterility was substantially related to behavioral intention, the majority of respondents did not believe that this was true. The model suggests that this message would be a powerful leverage point to change behavior. It would encourage an educational program to address it.

Health belief model

The implications from this model are analogous to (and sometimes identical to) those from the theory of reasoned action. Program planners would identify beliefs about severity or susceptibility or benefits or costs or health motive that are substantially related to behavior. They would then mount educational campaigns to address those beliefs.

Self-efficacy

Assume that knowledge turns into behavior when a perception of self-efficacy to perform that practice exists. For example, young women use condoms with their partners more often when they both have the skills and believe they are more able to negotiate with their partners about such use. The needed intervention would be to train the audience (in this case, the young women) in the skills of negotiation and, at the same time, develop their confidence that they can perform the behavior. Bandura (1), in material not addressed in this chapter, suggests a number of approaches for transferring such skills: guided trial, vicarious or observational learning, and persuasion.

Drive or Trait Models

At first glance, drive or trait models seem closed to intervention, by definition. After all, they attribute behavior to stable characteristics of individuals. Nonetheless, some programs do make use of the assumed existence of drives. For example, fear arousal programs make use of the assumption of a drive toward fear reduction; they arouse fears and then provide a means to reduce the fear: "AIDS kills—celibacy saves." Similarly, if program planners were able to establish that a particular segment of their audience was more closed to innovation than another, they might either (i) ignore that audience in favor of one more easily influenced to maximize cost-effectiveness or (ii) expend extra resources in trying to reach that more closed audience, if that audience was of particular concern.

Behaviorist Models

Assume that the rewards associated with the performance of a practice substantially determine its continuation. The task for the program designer is either to get the behavior to happen so that it can be rewarded or, at the very least, to be sure that when the behavior does happen, it is rewarded. In practice, this may involve a detailed analysis of exactly what the desirable behavior entails so as to locate opportunities to reward good practice. If the behavior is attendance at an STD clinic at the first sign of an STD, then all the steps in performing that behavior would be examined: missing work or other normal activity, the trip to the clinic, the wait to be seen, the medical examination, posttreatment interactions, following the treatment regimen, and resolving the STD, etc. The steps would be examined to see what pain or pleasure was associated with each, with the intention of developing ways of eliminating the pain and exaggerating the pleasure.

CHOOSING THE APPROPRIATE MODEL

This chapter presents a set of alternative or complementary views of the process that underlies behavior change. Each has some implications for how one approaches the task of designing interventions. The discussion may help systematize thinking about ways to design STD interventions. There is no illusion that it answers the questions about what is the best approach. It is but a guide to thinking about some of the issues.

The separate presentation of each model exaggerates the distinctions among them. It is likely that many of them or even all of them operate simultaneously. Program designers should not assume that separate presentation implies that just one must be accepted and acted upon. Each may provide insights that will help direct program design. It may be worthwhile to rearrange access to condoms, *and* educate women about the link between STDs and sterility, *and* address broad social norms about condom use, *and* be sure that people are confident that they can negotiate condom use with new partners, *and* associate newly practiced behaviors with rewards. The goal won't be to select one strategy in isolation but to select a set of strategies that together promise to achieve the desired goals.

How then does one choose among models? First, there is judgment. Through discussions among expert informants, examination of prior research, or group discussions with target audience members, one generates a restricted list of the models and the particular versions of them most likely to operate in a specific context.

Then there is research. Within the limits of the resources at hand (of time, money, and skill), one can undertake research within each promising model to see which of them fit the data and which do not. This will help further narrow the search, but it will not provide definitive answers. There will be a limited number of versions of each model that are tested; each piece of research will reduce uncertainty but not eliminate it; strong prior judgments may survive justifiably even if the data are only mildly supportive. So, third, there is judgment again. Program designers will have to consider their specific audience, their specific behavior, and their specific context and then, guided by available research, make their best assessment. Ongoing pretesting, monitoring, and evaluation may help them correct their mistakes.

In sum, what does this chapter suggest? Rarely does the literature say that knowledge is enough. While inexperienced practitioners may be taken aback at the finding that simple knowledge doesn't define behavior, neither experience nor theory suggests that it would. Indeed, one view of the question common to all of the models is "What are the conditions under which knowledge leads to behavior?" That is a question that assumes that often knowledge won't lead to behavior and that the research task is to find out when it does.

Project designers may or may not test alternative models before they launch their programs. However, whatever the degree of research they undertake, at least the process of thinking through the model(s) under which they operate should help refine their designs. Why is it that people do what they do now? How is it that the intervention they will undertake will produce behavior change? A careful review of these alternative models of behavior change should ease that process of elaboration of how a particular intervention is meant to produce its change. Such a step-by-step review will judge some proposed interventions as naive and enrich other program designs whose underlying models survive the process of being made explicit.

This explicit incorporation of theory in the program development process is, in the view of this chapter, an eminently practical activity. Program designers have a great variety of choices open to them. They need devices that help them understand what the many choices are; they need devices that allow them to choose among those alternatives. Both of those tasks are likely to be eased by the systematic consideration of program strategies in the light of alternative models of behavior change.

Acknowledgments. I am grateful to many people who read and made helpful suggestions about an earlier draft of this chapter. They are not responsible for material that I have failed to modify despite their best advice. They include Martin Fishbein, Robert Jones, Dan Romer, Susan McCombie, Judith McDivitt, Lorraine Ritacco, William Smith, and Stanley Yoder.

LITERATURE CITED

1. **Bandura, A.** 1986. *Social Foundations of Thought & Action: A Social Cognitive Theory.* Prentice-Hall, Inc., Englewood Cliffs, N.J.
2. **Hornik, R.** 1989. The knowledge-behavior gap in public information campaigns: a development communication view, p. 113–138. *In* C. T. Salmon (ed.), *Information Campaigns: Balancing Social Values and Social Change.* Sage Publications, Inc., Newbury Park, Calif.
3. **Rogers, E.** 1983. *Diffusion of Innovations,* 3rd ed. The Free Press, New York.
4. **Rosenstock, I., V. Strecher, and M. Becker.** 1988. Social learning theory and the health belief model. *Health Educ. Q.* **15:**175–183.

SELECTED READINGS

Ajzen, I., C. Timko, and J. White. 1982. Self-monitoring and the attitude-behavior relation. *J. Pers. Soc. Psychol.* **42:**426–435.

Fishbein, M. 1972. Toward an understanding of family planning behaviors. *J. Appl. Soc. Psychol.* **2:**214–227.

Fishbein, M., and I. Ajzen. 1981. On construct validity: a critique of Miniard and Cohen's paper. *J. Exp. Psychol.* **17:**340–350.

Hewstone, M., and L. Young. 1988. Expectancy-value models of attitude: measurement and combination of evaluations and beliefs. *J. Appl. Soc. Psychol.* **18:**958–971.

Hornik, R. 1988. *Development Communication: Information, Agriculture, and Nutrition in the Third World.* Longman, New York.

Janz, N., and M. Becker. 1984. The health belief model: a decade later. *Health Educ. Q.* **11:**1–47.

Leviton, L. 1989. Theoretical foundations of AIDS-prevention programs, p. 42–90. *In* R.

Valdiserri (ed.), *Preventing AIDS: The Design of Effective Programs.* Rutgers, The State University, New Brunswick, N.J.

Maslow, A. 1970. *Motivation and Personality,* 2nd ed. Harper and Row, Publishers, Inc., New York.

Petty, R., and J. Cacioppo. 1986. *Communication and Persuasion: Central and Peripheral Routes to Attitude Change.* Springer-Verlag, New York.

Rice, R., and C. Atkin (ed.). 1989. *Public Communication Campaigns.* Sage Publications, Inc., Newbury Park, Calif.

Organizing Large-Scale Interventions for Sexually Transmitted Disease Prevention

William A. Smith

The previous chapter set out some useful theories that can inform sexually transmitted disease (STD) and human immunodeficiency virus (HIV) prevention programs. However, those theories are only useful to the extent that they help managers make decisions. If we are to have a major impact on the problems with which this book is concerned, we must develop more efficient and effective behavior change programs. Experience in a wide range of such programs has demonstrated that social marketing constitutes an extremely powerful framework for helping managers make both strategic and tactical decisions to bring about rapid and lasting behavior change. It is a framework that helps translate the behavior change theories and concepts introduced by Hornik (this volume) into specific plans and actions that program managers can undertake.

This chapter focuses on program design. In the real world, most action programs are eclectic. They are influenced first by the characteristics of the problems being addressed (improve STD treatment coverage, promote risk self-assessment, reduce unprotected high-risk sex, etc.); second, by the nature of the audiences targeted (women, men, poor, affluent, rural, urban, etc.); and third, by the character and experience of the program manager (anthropologist, psychologist, advertising executive, epidemiologist, clinician, etc.). Each of these influences interacts with the availability of resources to produce programs that range in size from huge national mobilizations to small community service projects.

The chapter begins by describing three popular approaches to action programs: public communication campaigns, structural interventions, and behavioral analysis interventions. These approaches combine in various ways, with varying emphasis, the different theoretical models described by Hornik (this volume). The labeling and selection of the three approaches (campaigns, structural interventions, behavioral analysis) are somewhat arbitrary and are focused on demonstrating that while organizing systems often draw on similar theoretical roots, they look quite different from each other when translated into action programs. In fact, each approach tends to be characterized by a dominant paradigm drawn from one or two of the theoretical models described by Hornik.

The first part of this chapter seeks to demonstrate that today's STD program manager faces a formidable array of positive action alternatives. The manager's dilemma is in deciding which approach is best suited to a particular set of resources, staff, program objectives, and audiences. The second part of the chapter

---

William A. Smith – The Academy for Educational Development, Washington, D.C. 20037.

briefly describes social marketing and argues that social marketing provides a systematic and comprehensive program-planning process to address this need. It argues that STD prevention is influenced by multiple behaviors of different quality and complexity. For example, behaviors as distinct from each other as compliance with STD treatment regimens; risk self-assessment and voluntary testing; reduction in the number of sexual partners; increased use of condoms, lubricants, and nonpenetration; and delayed initiation of sexual activity constitute a wide variety of behavioral challenges facing the STD-HIV program manager. Therefore, single approaches are often inadequate as large-scale organizing systems for effective interventions. Social marketing, however, offers the program manager a practical system for selecting and organizing various theoretical approaches in a way that ensures that the salient variables are (i) identified, (ii) balanced against each other, and (iii) shaped into programs that meet the needs of a particular target audience, a particular kind of behavior, and a particular program manager. The greatest strength of social marketing is its tenacious focus on the consumer, the user, and the audience to be influenced as the organizing principle for program planning.

THREE ORGANIZING MODELS FOR LARGE-SCALE BEHAVIORAL INTERVENTIONS

This section describes three of the many organizing models available to STD program managers today: public communication campaigns, structural interventions, and behavioral analysis interventions. To distinguish these three approaches from each other, it is useful to focus first on their dominant paradigm. Table 1 classifies specific actions from the various program examples presented throughout this chapter as representative of the theoretical models presented by Hornik (this volume). Boldface terms represent the dominant paradigm characteristic of each example. Note that the three organizing models share theoretical roots but that the dominant paradigms are different.

The dominant paradigm of most public communication campaigns focuses on the ability to address cognitive factors (knowledge and attitudes) and influence social norms on a large scale. Structural interventions such as counseling, community organization, and service delivery programs often focus on external obstacles such as service availability, income, job status, or discrimination and/or on internal obstacles such as self-esteem and self-efficacy. Behavioral analysis programs contribute a system to identify, organize, and monitor behavioral consequences as a primary means to influence behavior. Each of these uniquely identifiable strengths is described in the following examples.

Public Communication Campaign

The public communication campaign is an organized process of large-scale behavior change designed to influence the knowledge and/or attitudes of a specific population and is characterized by an emphasis on narrow objectives, integrated communication channels, and a predetermined time period (16). The primary

Table 1. Program and theoretical models matrix

Program-organizing model	Theoretical model					
	Social (norms)	Cognitive (knowledge/belief)	Community-level structural (access)	Individual-level structural (income, etc.)	Drive or trait (personality)	Behaviorist (consequences)
Public information campaigns (example: U.K. AIDS Campaign): cognitive emphasis	Influence public opinion	**Facts about AIDS**	Involve community groups		Refer to counseling services	Appeal to public benefits
Structural interventions (example: family planning counseling): structural emphasis	Use peer influence	Facts about methods	**Distribute contraceptives**	**Target women**	**Counsel on family planning methods**	Give praise and support
Behavioral analysis interventions (example: Blue Cross/Blue Shield safety belt program): consequence emphasis	Make contest public	Facts about contest		Target people with cars		**Contest/prizes**

assumption of campaigns is that knowledge and attitude lead to behavior. Campaigns often focus on a specific call to action, such as "Call for further information . . . ," "See your local doctor . . . ," "Get a mammogram . . . ," or "Just say no to drugs." They are used to influence social norms that in turn influence individual behavior. The "Just Say No to Drugs" program in the United States, for example, was both an appeal to individual behavior and an effort to create a new social norm relating to drug abuse.

Like military campaigns, public communication campaigns are neither single battles (a series of television announcements) nor the entire war (urging everyone at risk of HIV infection to use a condom). Public communication campaigns are integrated programs aimed at a specific tactical objective—the Smokey the Bear campaign was designed to raise awareness about forest fires. The tactical objective of most public communication campaigns is to create greater awareness or knowledge. This objective falls into the cognitive model category; that is, the audience has a deficit of specific knowledge (information) or attitudes (motivation), which therefore explains the absence of a desired behavior. Program objectives frequently change over time, as the audience matures or as new risk factors are targeted. Therefore, the war is often composed of several sequential campaigns, e.g., "AIDS kills," "You could be at risk of AIDS," and "Don't discriminate against persons living with AIDS."

One of the largest, best-funded, and most systematic recent public communication campaigns has been the United Kingdom's Public Education Campaigns on AIDS (U.K. AIDS Campaigns). The U.K. experience illustrates the main elements of the campaign approach.

Narrow cognitive objectives

Campaign one (March to November 1986) was designed to inform the general public about specific facts and myths (knowledge deficit) and influence public opinion to permit a higher-profile approach to AIDS prevention (attitude change). Campaign two (November 1986 to March 1987) focused on who is at risk and what they should do through messages such as "The more partners, the greater the risk" and "Protect yourself, use a condom" (11).

Integrated channels

Campaign one relied heavily on print and press media as a means to influence public opinion. Campaign two, at a cost of about $15 million, integrated press announcements, street posters, radio and television, and a mass mailing to all 23 million U.K. households and included special programs for the armed forces, police, prisons, colleges, youth organizations, and medical organizations (14). One distinguishing characteristic of a campaign is that the same or very similar messages are diffused through coordinated channels during a specific time frame.

Large scale

The large scale of the U.K. effort is obvious, but it is useful to point out the value of scale in such a program. A rigorous nationwide evaluation showed that 82% of the U.K. population could accurately describe one of the campaign materials. In this case, television spots were the most-remembered element, accounting for 91% of the people who recalled at least one component of the campaign (14). The U.K. campaign targeted all adult citizens. If a smaller subset of a population was targeted, scale would be related to the size of that intended audience. It is less important to reach 10 million versus 1 million than it is to saturate 50 to 80% of a target audience.

Predetermined time period

Because a campaign is a tactical element designed to achieve a set of objectives, it should neither go on forever nor just fade away. Campaigns are carefully planned to accomplish their objectives in a predetermined time period. The U.K. campaign one lasted from March to November 1986, and campaign two lasted from November 1986 to March 1987 (18). The presence of a specific time line distinguishes campaigns from other approaches by giving organizational discipline to them—adding urgency, emphasizing timely integration, and allowing for objectives to be clearly measured when each campaign ends.

Few campaigns are as large or as costly as the U.K. effort, but all campaigns are distinguished from other organizational models by this combination of (i) narrow objectives, (ii) integrated channels, (iii) proportionally large scale, (iv) predetermined time period, and (v) a focus on cognitive (knowledge and/or attitude) deficits.

Structural Interventions

Structural interventions focus on removing obstacles to successful behavior change. They are distinct from campaigns in several respects, particularly in their commitment to more interactive, more intensive face-to-face, and much longer interventions. These interventions often take on characteristics related to the obstacles being addressed. For example, external obstacles such as personality trait or drive barriers (low self-esteem or the need for emotional support) are often addressed in counseling interventions. External policies or structures that discriminate against or inhibit behavior, such as laws against condom advertising, norms favoring multiple partners, or discrimination against men who have sex with men, typically call for empowerment or organizational change interventions. Inadequate access to resources needed to adopt specific behaviors, for example, condoms or STD treatment services, is often solved through service delivery interventions. In the real world of program implementation, various combinations of counseling, empowerment, and service delivery are often woven together into more complex structural interventions.

The most common identifying characteristic of structural interventions is an emphasis on active participation and interactive responsiveness among users and providers. All three subsystems (counseling, organizational empowerment, and service delivery) devote much effort to the quality of interpersonal systems. The intent of structural interventions is not so much to alter how people see the world (as cognitive programs do) or to provide new reward systems for behavior (as behaviorist programs attempt to do), but rather to identify and then remove internal obstacles, such as poor problem-solving skills, or external obstacles, such as ineffective services, social norms, discrimination, or poverty.

Counseling, for example, focuses on internal psychological obstacles. Such one-on-one encounters between a trained provider and a potentially high-risk individual are among the best known and most accepted intervention strategies. Counseling's primary role is to help an individual deal with internal obstacles such as low self-esteem, problem solving, or a sense of isolation and abandonment. In addition, counseling also transmits facts and often teaches skills. STD counseling has often been limited to the periods immediately preceding and following sessions when individuals were most accessible, but experience suggests that longer-term follow-up counseling may be necessary to maintain behavior change over time.

Other behavior change programs also have extensive and well-documented experience with counseling. The family planning community, for example, has relied successfully on counseling interventions. Data from studies in Tunisia show that home counseling led to greater increase in contraceptive use than adding a new service center. Three groups were compared—a community with a new service center, a community with trained counselors, and a community with both. The area with counseling only had a 125% increase in new contraceptive users versus a 65% increase in the area with a new service center only (6). Counseling also helps sustain new behavioral practices over time. In Jakarta, Indonesia, 90 and 79% of intrauterine device users who received counseling were still users after 1 and 2 years, respectively, while only 52 and 29% of noncounseled new users continued after the same respective periods (3).

Empowerment has an equally long and distinguished place in the history of behavior change. Here, the salient obstacle is an oppressive or inhibiting social norm, policy, or law that prevents people from adopting behaviors they understand and are individually motivated to try. Individual action is insufficient to remove the obstacle (18). Community organization brings people together to plan interventions that empower the community to remove the obstacle (change the law or policy) or establish a new norm (make stable sexual relationships more fashionable among homosexual couples).

Service delivery programs to improve access to needed services also play a fundamental role in structural interventions. These include government and private efforts to improve the availability of STD treatment, distribute sterile needles to intravenous drug users, provide drug treatment to drug users, and increase contraceptive services. Data from international immunization programs, for example, suggest that under some circumstances, significant improvement in service delivery of vaccines alone, even without serious educational efforts, increases immunization coverage rates dramatically (6).

Again, examples of combined approaches are common. The community response in the United States, Europe, and Australia to provide counseling and service delivery and to influence public policy on AIDS has operated through programs like those sponsored by the Shanti Project, San Francisco, the Gay Men's Health Crisis, New York City, and the Whitman-Walker Clinic, Washington, D.C., just a few examples of programs that have combined elements of all three structural approaches.

Applied Behavioral Analysis

The applied behavioral analysis paradigm emerges from the fields of empirical psychology, the psychology of learning, social psychology, and, to some degree, physiological psychology. It emphasizes observable events as opposed to feelings and knowledge and is closely tied to the field of experimental analysis of behavior. Since 1973, much of this work has been referred to as behavioral medicine. Blanchard (3) defines the concept as the "systematic application of the principles and technology of behavioral psychology to the field of medicine, health, and illness." He goes on to define the elements he feels are central to this field, including (i) detailed analysis of observable behavior and objective assessment of what people do; (ii) understanding the cues that trigger behavior (antecedents), the behavior itself, and what happens to the person after performing the behavior (consequences); and (iii) shaping behavior through discrimination (learning to recognize what we do) and generalization (the transfer of what works in therapy to the real world).

For the purpose of this chapter, the consequence approach to organizing behavior change interventions is most important. Managing positive consequences, such as prizes, verbal praise, group achievement, and public recognition, and disincentives, such as fines, peer pressure, loss of privileges, and reprimands, to reward or punish compliance with the targeted behaviors may be particularly important in constructing more comprehensive STD prevention efforts.

Blue Cross and Blue Shield of North Carolina, for example, organized a carefully controlled experiment to determine whether an applied behavioral analysis program could significantly increase the use of automobile seat belts among its 1,013 employees. The program's antecedents consisted of a 20-min awareness session for all employees conducted by the senior staff. The session included a lecture and a film and distribution of a printed flyer, a brochure describing the value of safety belts, and a flyer describing a company-wide reward program for using safety belts. In many ways, these antecedents parallel the activities of a mini-public communication campaign.

The Blue Cross program went further to add a consequence strategy that provided specific rewards for correct performance. For example, \$5 coupons were distributed randomly for 1 month to occupants of vehicles who were wearing seat belts when they passed through the company's parking lot entrance. The coupons were also tickets for a \$100 gift-certificate drawing. Unobtrusive observations of shoulder-belt use during the 1-month intervention period and for 1 month afterward showed that shoulder-belt use increased from 10% before the program to 54% during the program to 24% during the month after the program. The program cost about \$1,945, or about \$1.75 per employee (19).

Behavioral management need not be community-wide. An example of these same principles applied to an individual, self-managed program is illustrated below

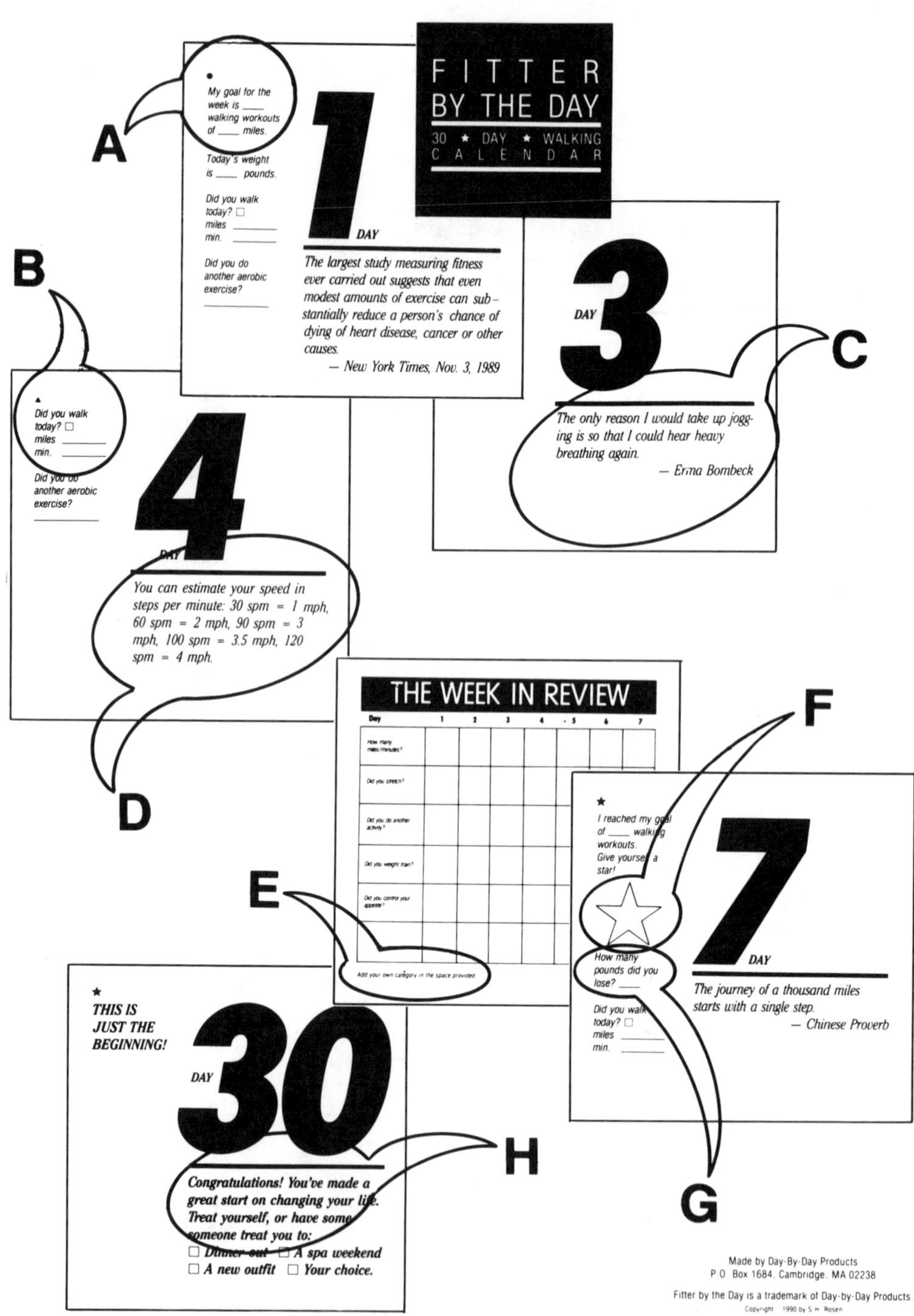

FITTER BY THE DAY
30 ★ DAY ★ WALKING CALENDAR
A
My goal for the week is ____ walking workouts of ____ miles.
Today's weight is ____ pounds.
Did you walk today? ☐ miles ______ min. ______
Did you do another aerobic exercise? ______
1 DAY
The largest study measuring fitness ever carried out suggests that even modest amounts of exercise can substantially reduce a person's chance of dying of heart disease, cancer or other causes.
— New York Times, Nov. 3, 1989
B
Did you walk today? ☐ miles ______ min. ______
Did you do another aerobic exercise? ______
4 DAY
You can estimate your speed in steps per minute: 30 spm = 1 mph, 60 spm = 2 mph, 90 spm = 3 mph, 100 spm = 3.5 mph, 120 spm = 4 mph.
D
3 DAY
C
The only reason I would take up jogging is so that I could hear heavy breathing again.
— Erma Bombeck
THE WEEK IN REVIEW
Day 1 2 3 4 5 6 7
How many miles/minutes?
Did you stretch?
Did you do another activity?
Did you weight train?
Did you control your appetite?
Add your own category in the space provided
E
F
I reached my goal of ____ walking workouts. Give yourself a star!
How many pounds did you lose? ____
Did you walk today? ☐ miles ______ min. ______
7 DAY
The journey of a thousand miles starts with a single step.
— Chinese Proverb
G
THIS IS JUST THE BEGINNING!
30 DAY
Congratulations! You've made a great start on changing your life. Treat yourself, or have someone treat you to:
☐ Dinner out ☐ A spa weekend
☐ A new outfit ☐ Your choice.
H
Made by Day-By-Day Products
P.O. Box 1684, Cambridge, MA 02238
Fitter by the Day is a trademark of Day-by-Day Products
Copyright 1990 by S.H. Rosen

in a weight-loss program packaged commercially as a 30-day Walking Calendar (17). Figure 1 illustrates selected pages from the calendar and shows how specific behavioral analysis principles are built into this clever behavior modification program.

Behavioral analysis interventions are also eclectic. They often integrate various theoretical explanations to create comprehensive action programs to promote large-scale behavior change. The antecedent elements of these models resemble many aspects of information campaigns. For example, campaignlike activities are often used to cue and model specific behaviors. A television spot illustrating how a young man can ask to buy a condom without embarrassment, a poster showing a woman demanding that her boyfriend use a condom, and the Gay Men's Health Crisis program's use of a safety pin as a nonverbal cue for safe sex all constitute classic behavioral cues or antecedents and overlap conceptually with many of the activities identified with public communication campaigns.

It is, however, the systematic and large-scale use of consequence strategies that represents the unique operational contribution that behavior analysis can make. From a Happy Baby Lottery in The Gambia, West Africa, that taught 11,000 illiterate women in 5 weeks to correctly prepare a complex diarrheal remedy (15) to thousands of contests and lotteries operated to motivate sales staff throughout industry (19), consequence strategies provide concrete ways to stimulate the first trial of difficult new behavior and new ways to shape and sustain behavior change over time.

I have described three broad organizational approaches that emerge from a review of real-world programs. (i) Public communication campaigns emphasize cognitive explanations for absent behavior and use multiple channels to saturate a particular audience with messages to correct a knowledge or attitudinal deficit and to influence the perception of social norms. (ii) Structural interventions are heavily influenced by counseling, community empowerment, and increased access to services and are designed to overcome structural obstacles, either personal or organizational, that hinder compliance with selected behavior. (iii) Behavioral analysis interventions manipulate antecedents and, especially, consequences of a specific behavior to shape new behaviors over time.

In all the examples cited, it is clear that eclectic combinations of theoretical models are common. While the U.K. AIDS Campaign's primary focus was to provide effective information about AIDS, referral counseling services and analysis of the benefits or rewards people would find salient were built into the program as well. While projects like the Shanti Project in San Francisco focus on increasing access to counseling for HIV-positive individuals, they also use mass media

---

Figure 1. (A) A behavioral goal is clearly established, and (B) the individual is told to measure success at regular intervals. (C) The task is made fun by adding humor. (D) Truly new and useful information is given—information people do not already have. (E) People are allowed to individualize their response. (F) A successive self-reward system is built in, with (G) markers that allow people to document and thereby notice success. Finally, (H) a larger reward is built in for final success.

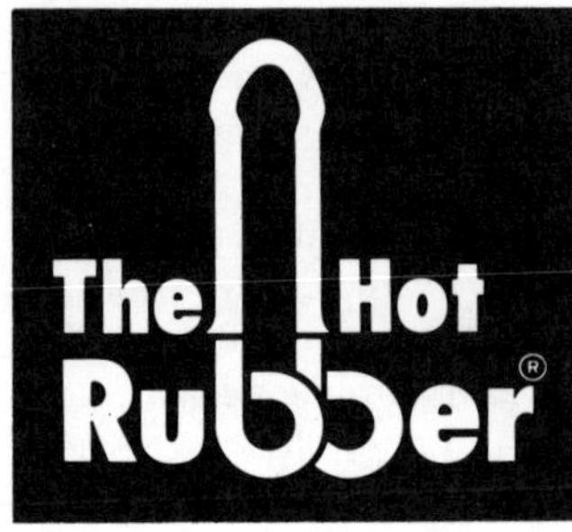

Figure 2. Swiss Hot Rubber campaign logo.

messages and positive rewards to influence attitudes and social norms about sexuality in a broader audience. And while the Blue Cross and Blue Shield program was distinguished by its emphasis on prizes as rewards for specific behavioral compliance, it also used posters and pamphlets (cognitive intervention) to improve knowledge and attitudes, and it changed company policy (structural intervention) to support, rather than hinder, seat belt use.

The primary dilemma facing program planners today is in choosing what combination of possible interventions is best suited to the particular behaviors they wish to promote and the audience they wish to reach and is acceptable to the program directors they propose to support. In the real world, all three of these elements interact to produce interventions. The next part of the chapter describes social marketing, one of the most comprehensive and practical systems we have for helping program planners consider, select, sequence, and integrate various program activities into practical and effective behavioral interventions.

SOCIAL MARKETING

Social marketing has been defined as the application of commercial marketing to the exchange of ideas, goods, or services that have a social purpose. This section begins with an illustration of a social marketing program in action, the Swiss (Hot Rubber) Campaign (20). The Swiss AIDS Foundation recognized early in the AIDS epidemic that homosexual men in Switzerland were at the epidemiological epicenter of HIV infection but that condoms were virtually unused among this high-risk population. An aggressive program to introduce condoms and increase their regular use among homosexual men was initiated. Audience research revealed that commercially available condoms had little or no appeal to the target audience and were difficult to find. Fear appeals were identified as counterproductive for the population. Therefore, the campaign adopted the notion of eroticizing safe sex.

The first marketing decision was to select a special condom for the homosexual man as the central product and to create a clever name and package that positioned the condom with "attractiveness and sexiness." The condom was called "The Hot Rubber," and a humorous trademark reinforced the upbeat pleasurable tone (Fig. 2).

Using price to add value to products is a common marketing tactic. The pricing decision for this condom was not limited to commercial considerations of profitability but also reflected a careful analysis of attitudes toward price and quality among the target population. As a result, the monetary price told users that these condoms were a quality product.

The distribution strategy went far beyond commercial systems and targeted areas most likely to increase timely and easy access to condoms. Informal meeting places, along with bars and saunas frequented by homosexual patrons, were selected as the primary distribution points, rather than drugstores and other commercial outlets used by existing condom distributors. This distribution strategy was so effective after the first 2 years of the program that in several bars a customer could order "a beer with . . ." and receive a free condom.

Promotion was particularly aggressive. A monthly poster, for example, adapted to seasonal changes and using images attractive to the homosexual audience, rapidly increased name recognition of the Hot Rubber brand and carried out the positioning strategy of "Hot Rubber equals fun, eroticism, and pleasure."

Sales figures of the Hot Rubber condom increased from 2,000 condoms in 1985 to around 300,000 in 1987. The decision of homosexual men in Switzerland to use condoms was potentially influenced by factors other than the Hot Rubber campaign. During the same period, the press frequently carried news stories about AIDS and homosexual men. The high infection rates among homosexual men in Switzerland (the highest per capita rate in Europe in 1985 to 1987) also meant that many of them knew friends or had lovers who were ill or who had died of AIDS. Sales increases of other condoms, however, never approached the sales increases recorded by the Hot Rubber brand (20).

Social marketing has become increasingly popular as a way to organize behavioral interventions, particularly in public health. The Stanford Heart Disease Prevention Program is a good example of a social marketing program (7). The National Cancer Institute used social marketing as one operating paradigm in its recent guide to health communication (1). The international public health community, particularly the U.S. Agency for International Development, has pioneered the application of social marketing to family planning, child survival, and, more recently, HIV disease and drug-abuse prevention (1). Several texts on social marketing are now available (5, 9, 10, 15). These books document dozens of applications ranging from political campaigns to teenage pregnancy. Indeed, social marketing has become something of a public health fad.

Social marketing is sometimes confused with public communication campaigns because of its frequent use of mass media as a promotional technique. Social marketing has been unfairly criticized as inherently manipulative and characterized incorrectly as "selling," because the popular notion of advertising and marketing is one of manipulation and sales. But, as we learn more about behavior change on a large scale, social marketing (as defined in recent texts and manuals and shaped by almost 20 years of experimentation) comes to represent a comprehensive, practical, and unique process for designing and implementing behavioral interventions that

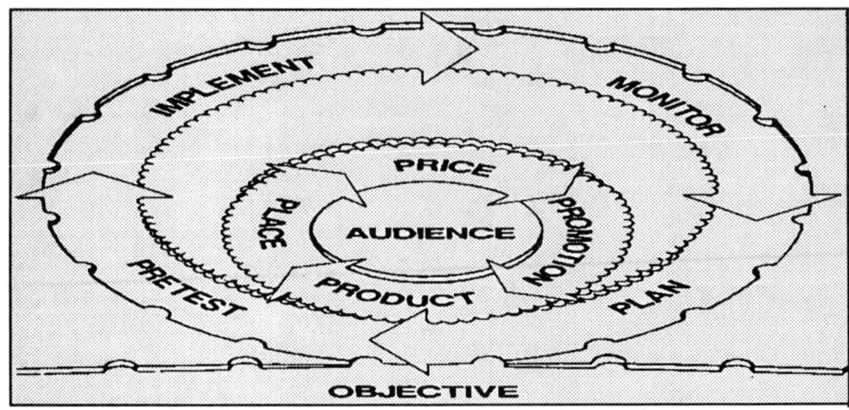

Figure 3. Social marketing process wheel.

integrate lessons learned from all three theoretical and organizing models discussed above.

What makes social marketing uniquely valuable is the completeness of its planning structure combined with the simplicity of its planning process. Its completeness is best expressed through the four Ps of the marketing mix (product, place, price, and promotion) (22). Its simplicity is reflected clearly in its program-planning process (assess, plan, pretest, implement). As illustrated in Fig. 3, the marketing mix and the program-planning process interact to create a practical and comprehensive system that helps program planners to understand and address cognitive, structural, and behaviorist explanations for absent or unhealthful behavior.

The four Ps of the marketing mix form the framework that ensures that planners will consider all the elements discussed above that might influence behavior in a particular audience.

The product in marketing represents the decisions associated with selecting and shaping the idea, commodity, behavior, or service to be promoted to meet the consumer's needs. Social marketing products can be much more than commodities. For example, a hotline service, safe-sex practice, genital self-examination—these are all legitimate social marketing products, although they cannot be physically packaged or priced. Central to social marketing is the conviction that products must have benefits or rewards that consumers perceive as valuable. The analysis of products from this perspective of rewards is heavily influenced by formal behaviorist models.

Our ability to control the product (commodity, service, or behavior) in public health is often severely hampered by the limits of our science. For example, we have yet to develop a condom that adds pleasure rather than decreases sensation or a measles vaccine that doesn't require refrigeration. These products present much more difficult problems to solve than making a cereal more crunchy or a soft drink more sweet. Often, in public health, we are forced to select rather than shape products, choosing from a range of difficult and unrewarding alternatives those behaviors that we believe will be most acceptable to the user, given all the constraints. Clearly, for example, most public health officials recognize that sexual abstinence is the best clinical prevention for STDs, but abstinence, for most populations, is not an acceptable or reasonable behavioral alternative. Consequently, condoms, fewer partners, and better partner selection are the compromise behaviors or products from which we can make strategic selections for given populations.

Price in social marketing refers to more than monetary expenditure. It includes opportunity cost, status loss, and consumer time. That a young woman pays no money for an STD treatment does not mean that the treatment costs her nothing. Indeed, her time and inconvenience or the risk of social stigma may constitute perceived costs that far outweigh her perceived benefits, particularly if she doesn't adequately understand or give importance to the possible long-term consequences of delayed treatment. These considerations lead to strategic decisions for given populations about which costs are most important and which set of benefits best offset those costs for that population. Pricing strategies relate to that aspect of structural tactics that deals with internal obstacles such as self-esteem or status. Social marketing has adopted research techniques from anthropology, sociology, and psychology to understand and address these costs.

The concept of place refers to the channels through which products (commodities, messages, health services) flow to users and the points at which these products are offered. Place focuses largely on access obstacles commonly identified in structural interventions, such as access and policy. Product availability and distribution, for example, may involve not only retail and wholesale supply systems but also the efforts of health providers, volunteer workers, friends, and neighbors. Place may be a store, a health center, or even a person, such as a community volunteer who distributes condoms and services. Place considerations also encompass the activities that go into making these outlets effective, including staff training, physical organization, scheduling, and interpersonal counseling skills. Place strategies in marketing resolve the access barriers identified in structural interventions and help ensure that those barriers are understood and addressed.

Promotion includes the functions of advertising, public relations, user education, and interpersonal support. Promotion includes decisions on messages, or what's communicated about the product, and decisions on channels (mass media, print, and interpersonal), or how that message gets to the right people. Promotion is concerned with a wide range of interpersonal systems—including counseling, patient education, and nonformal, community-based support systems—as well as broadcast and print media. Promotion's role is to organize the cognitive (knowledge and attitude) prerequisites that help people decide to use and continue to use healthful products, practices, and services. Public communication campaigns are a common promotional strategy, but public relations and face-to-face persuasion/consequences are also important promotional technologies.

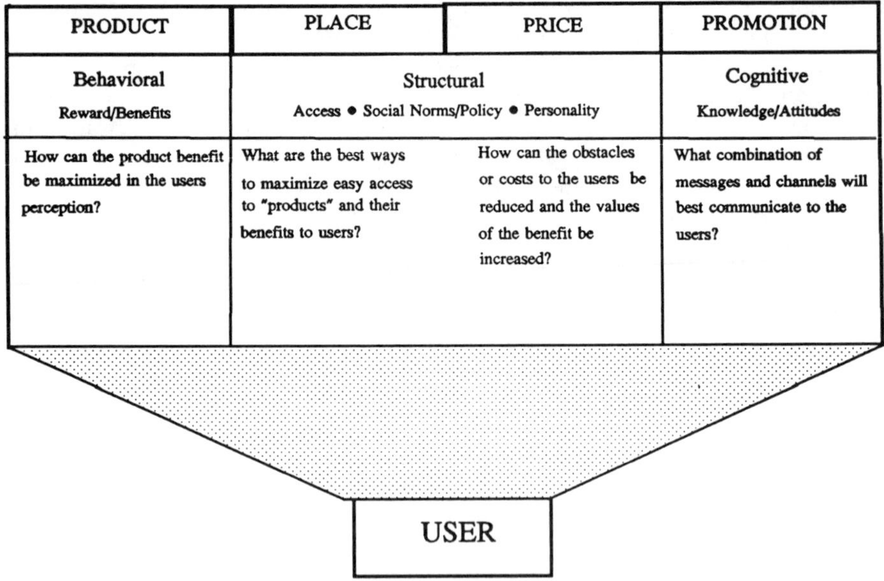

Figure 4. Marketing mix and behavior change.

As illustrated in Fig. 4 and described briefly above, the four Ps of marketing address each of the three major organizing paradigms described above. Product strategies deal primarily with behavioral explanations, price and place strategies deal primarily with structural explanations, and promotion deals primarily with cognitive explanations. In the real world, these domains often overlap and interact. For example, a social norm such as "Real men don't use condoms" represents a cost or price issue that program managers must understand and reduce if a safe-sex program is to be successful. This social norm is best reshaped in the promotion activity of the program. It is common in the social marketing of practices that carry no monetary value for price analysis to identify the obstacles and promotion to be the means to overcome them.

As we saw in the Swiss example, the unique contribution of social marketing is to focus all program planning on the user—on what benefits users will perceive, how to reduce obstacles users might experience, and how to reach users in their cognitive world, using their language, linking with their belief system, and communicating through channels they find credible and persuasive. Few other organizing systems have such a determined, comprehensive, and single-minded focus on user satisfaction as the key to success.

Three important social marketing concepts emphasize the central role of user satisfaction: audience segmentation, product positioning, and integrated marketing communication.

Audience segmentation rests on the conviction that important differences exist among even seemingly homogeneous groups of users. For example, segmentation studies in Tijuana, Mexico, showed that female sex workers were divided into very different segments by the benefits they saw to condom use—one group was motivated by the appeal to protect their unborn children from HIV infection, and the other by its fear of clients' refusal to use a condom (1). A single appeal would have missed one-half of this important population.

While the notion that people are different is hardly revolutionary, social marketing has given us a set of sophisticated research tools—integrating qualitative and quantitative research techniques—to identify audience segments and allow us to better understand, target, and address users' needs as they perceive them.

Product positioning is a process for understanding the way the user thinks about a problem or behavior and then placing or positioning that product, service, or behavior in a way that makes it attractive and appealing and enhances its perceived benefits to the user in relation to competing choices. Positioning is particularly powerful in public health because it leads planners to focus on the behaviors that compete for attention to the public health solution. It forces planners to recognize what they are asking people to give up as well as what they are offering them in exchange.

For Tijuana's sex workers, for example, for one group of women, condoms competed against the loss of money from dissatisfied clients. Therefore, condoms were positioned as a new negotiating tool to use with clients, giving women a way to improve their service to clients. For the women concerned about childbearing, however, condoms were competing against old beliefs that condoms were just annoying and that any STD could be easily cured (1). The program addressed this traditional criticism of condoms by positioning condoms as a way to preserve their capacity to have healthy children.

Finally, integrated marketing communication has taken health planners out of the world of mass media selling to a much more sophisticated and comprehensive focus on how to reach and influence people. It is a systematic process for assessing consumers' views and adjusting service channels and appeals to meet their needs. In traditional marketing, like much of traditional health education, the responsibility of the promotion or the education office was limited to little more than transmitting these messages about products or a service.

Today, integrated marketing communication has demonstrated that every aspect of a product or service communicates a message to the user about that service (A. De Moya and E. Guerrero, Int. Conf. AIDS, Stockholm, Sweden, abstr. 6514, 1988). It is not only what we tell people about STD clinics that matters, it is what they experience at that clinic that shapes their image of STD treatment. Long waiting periods, dirty environments, callous or hurried staff, lack of medical supplies, and incomplete information all communicate messages more powerfully than television spots, posters, or even counseling interviews. Social marketing helps us focus, through the practice of integrated marketing communication, on all the aspects that influence consumers' perceptions of the service we are offering.

The four Ps and these few marketing concepts are at the heart of marketing's unique organizing principle. Equally important, however, is marketing dedication

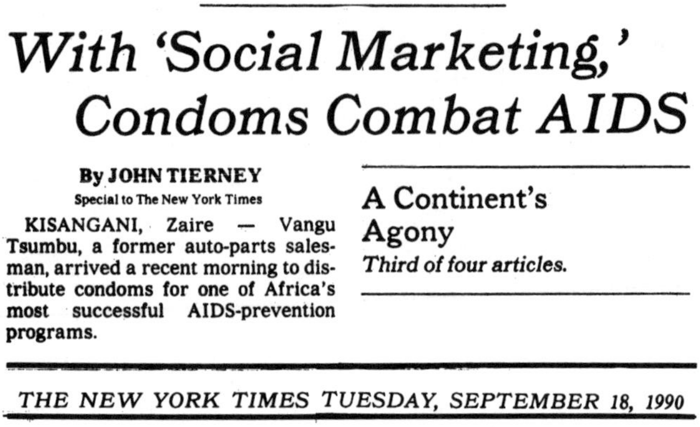

With 'Social Marketing,' Condoms Combat AIDS

By JOHN TIERNEY
Special to The New York Times

KISANGANI, Zaire — Vangu Tsumbu, a former auto-parts salesman, arrived a recent morning to distribute condoms for one of Africa's most successful AIDS-prevention programs.

A Continent's Agony
Third of four articles.

THE NEW YORK TIMES TUESDAY, SEPTEMBER 18, 1990

Figure 5. *New York Times* headline.

to a systematic planning process heavily committed to consumer and market research. In Fig. 3, the marketing mix rotates rapidly within the larger wheel of the program-planning process, in which each of the four Ps is planned for, pretested, implemented, and monitored. This process reflects the social marketer's deep conviction that user satisfaction must be assessed scientifically and constantly through consumer and product research.

Social marketing planning relies on a series of social science research tools that include observation trials; focus group, in-depth, and individual interviews; and surveys to help understand user behavior, the conditions under which that behavior occurs, the life-style setting of the user population, and the obstacles that inhibit the user's adoption of the new practice. Planners use these data to determine the relative importance of the marketing mix for a given behavioral problem and a given population. Implementation and monitoring follow sequentially, again each having addressed all four Ps at every stage. One of social marketing's most important contributions has been the ability to integrate comprehensive planning with systematic audience research.

The headline in Fig. 5 appeared on page 1 of the *New York Times*, 18 September 1990 (21). The article deals with several successful applications of social marketing to the sale of condoms in Africa. The headline is important not only because it highlights the growing visibility of social marketing and demonstrates its successful application in several developing countries but also because it exemplifies one of the most common misconceptions about the field—that marketing (social or not) is dominated by the sale of physical products.

A concluding example will illustrate how social marketing can be used to shape behavior rather than product sales. Condoms are still the issue, but the objective is correct condom use, not condom sales; i.e., condoms are being distributed free but are not widely used. The setting is the STD program in the Dominican Republic. The goal is to increase correct condom use among high-risk women (commercial sex workers) to help protect them and their clients from STDs, particularly HIV infection. The example illustrates not only how all four Ps of the marketing mix are assessed and addressed but also how social marketing functions as an ongoing decision-making framework for program managers to detect and then correct errors as they appear.

AIDS was first identified in the Dominican Republic in 1983. In 1989, the number of cases had grown to more than 800, with an estimated seroprevalence rate between 0.7 and 1%, or approximately 45,000 to 60,000 HIV-positive individuals. The ratio of male to female cases of AIDS, roughly 65:1 from 1983 to 1985, changed to 2:1 by 1987, with heterosexual transmission representing about half of all the cases. By late 1987, the Ministry of Health had a dual-track strategy in place to reduce HIV transmission on the island. Track 1 was a national education campaign to teach the basic facts about AIDS to the general public. Track 2 was an innovative, community-based strategy to reach specific high-risk groups, defined as homosexual men and female sex workers. The Program for the Control of Sexually Transmitted Diseases and AIDS, or PROCETS, was the coordinating agency for both tracks (13).

Condoms were already well known on the island and were available commercially and through a family planning program that was importing tens of thousands of condoms annually for free distribution through its centers (De Moya and Guerrero, Int. Conf. AIDS, 1988). Among female sex workers, however, anecdotal information and early qualitative research suggested that condoms were not popular for two reasons: condoms were believed to break easily, and they were considered too expensive to use regularly.

To address the issues, an aggressive, peer-based, street outreach program called Messengers of Health was begun. It included free condom distribution and informational talks at street contact points. By 1988, it was clear that the program was increasing condom availability among female sex workers (female sex workers were often found to be carrying many condoms on their persons), but condom use was still feared to be low (4). For example, one imaginative tracking study of motels (a favorite site for casual sex in the Dominican Republic) placed condoms in every room and then checked the room after each couple left. Results showed most condoms were left unused (E. Guerrero, personal communication). Also, complaints about condom breakage seemed to grow, particularly among the women who received free condoms.

Therefore, the program managers decided to take a comprehensive look at the program from a social marketing perspective, that is, a systematic analysis of each of the four marketing mix Ps. Their first step was to organize a program of consumer research that relied heavily on rapid assessment and qualitative techniques, particularly focus groups. In addition, existing surveys were reviewed, and a new knowledge, attitude, and practice survey directed at female sex workers was organized. Perhaps the most innovative research technique was a series of carefully controlled observation trials of 91 female sex workers that tested their skill in putting on and taking off condoms. This extraordinary research used a dildo as a surrogate model and included individual in-depth interviews about sexual practices, AIDS attitudes, and condom use. For the first time, with this survey, the program managers had a quantitative measure of condom skill deficits.

The research was designed to explore all four marketing variables. (i) Product: What about condoms might be improved? (ii) Place: Where could condoms be distributed to increase use and how could they be placed to improve use? (Emphasis was placed on use, not just access. Answers to questions such as "When did you get your condom?" and "Do you always carry a condom?" were assessed to identify relationships between immediate access and use.) (iii) Price: What are the obstacles (skills, embarrassment, partner referral, fears, etc.) to condom use? (iv) Promotion: What communication channels reach female sex workers, who do they listen to, and what convinces them that something is right or wrong for them?

An analysis of the condoms that were being distributed showed that many had passed the expiration date and were prone to breakage. The solution was to replace those condoms immediately with a new and more reliable product. Focus groups showed that no particular condom characteristic (lubrication, nonoxynol-9, color, etc.) was important.

The analysis of the distribution and location situation did not reveal much that was not already known. The program had already determined that street distribution dramatically increased availability and that distribution in motels and brothels reduced access as a major obstacle. The real dilemma was how to sustain free distribution over time. Given a small target population such as sex workers and its potential for extremely high risk behavior, the costs of free condom distribution seemed justifiable and affordable for several years until long-range commercial alternatives could be developed.

The analysis of price issues (obstacles to use) provided the most valuable new insights for this audience. The condom skill exercise, for example, uncovered important skill deficits. Of 91 women in the observation trials, 78% unrolled the condom completely before placing it on the model or removed the condom with excessive pulling using their long fingernails. Both behaviors contributed to the high breakage rate. These deficits were easy to correct. After only one observation of correct placement, all the women were able to correctly place and remove the condoms. The real problem was not the missing skill but that the lack of skill led women to be embarrassed about condoms and to avoid touching the packet or using them regularly, even though many of these women did carry condoms with them in their purses.

Perhaps most important, the interviews revealed that the women seldom put condoms on their male partners and even more rarely took off the condoms after intercourse. They considered condom management to be the men's responsibility.

These findings led to a major reshaping of the program strategy. Emphasis was shifted away from women alone to an emphasis on the relationship of the female sex worker to male clients. What could be done to lower the cost (price) of introducing a condom into this relationship? A three-part strategy was settled upon.

(i) Train female sex workers to desensitize condom use, increase skills, and reduce inhibiting attitudes about safe sex (negotiation skills with clients, condoms always break, I'm not really at risk, etc.). Female sex workers who were trained would then act as counselors to other women who might trust peers more than authorities.

(ii) Develop materials to cue condom use behavior at the moment it was needed and remind clients and women of how to put the condom on correctly. The prevalence of motels and brothels made the distribution of some print materials to the point and time of intercourse a practical option in the Dominican Republic.

(iii) Create television campaigns with a subtle but effective message: Don't stray from your steady partner—but if you do, always use protection. This was one of the first explicit mass media campaigns addressed to clients of female sex workers.

To develop the training exercises, recruiting procedures, materials, and television campaign, the program manager sought consumer (female sex workers and clients) input for materials development and testing. Again, small groups of women met to help design materials and test concepts. The resulting training design relied heavily on participatory exercises that helped women confront their own myths and assess more accurately their own risks and gave them the skills needed to put new pro-condom attitudes in action.

The material to cue condom use was originally to be a poster, but after working with the women, a sticker was selected as a better approach as it was much easier to apply above their beds and in motels. A dual positioning emerged as illustrated in Fig. 6.

Figure 6A shows the first and last panels in the condom instruction sticker addressed at women who used motels as points of sexual intercourse. Note how they differ in setting, dress, and interaction from Fig. 6B, which shows panels directed at women who worked at brothels. These differences emerged as important visual cues needed by each group to make the images salient to their own situation.

The successful development of this material also illustrates the critical role of program monitoring. Even after careful development of these visuals, site checks made after the initial distribution to motels showed that almost all the stickers had been removed. No confirmed explanation was ever found, but interviews with motel owners revealed that several clients had not liked to "think about AIDS" every time they had intercourse and had "probably" removed the stickers. This led to producing a smaller version of the sticker that was placed in the bathroom of the motel room rather than over the bed.

The television advertisement for men was developed by a local advertising agency (Young, Rubicam, & Damaris) working with the national program manager. As shown in Fig. 7, a trapeze analogy was used to illustrate the beauty of fidelity, the risks of multiple partners, and the need for a safety net (condom) if one strays from a permanent relationship.

The Dominican Republic case illustrates three important lessons. (i) Consumer research is fundamental to identifying obstacles to effective condom use. (ii) A comprehensive planning framework such as social marketing allowed program managers to review all the potential obstacles (product, price, place, promotion) and target the most important deficits. (In the Dominican Republic, planners

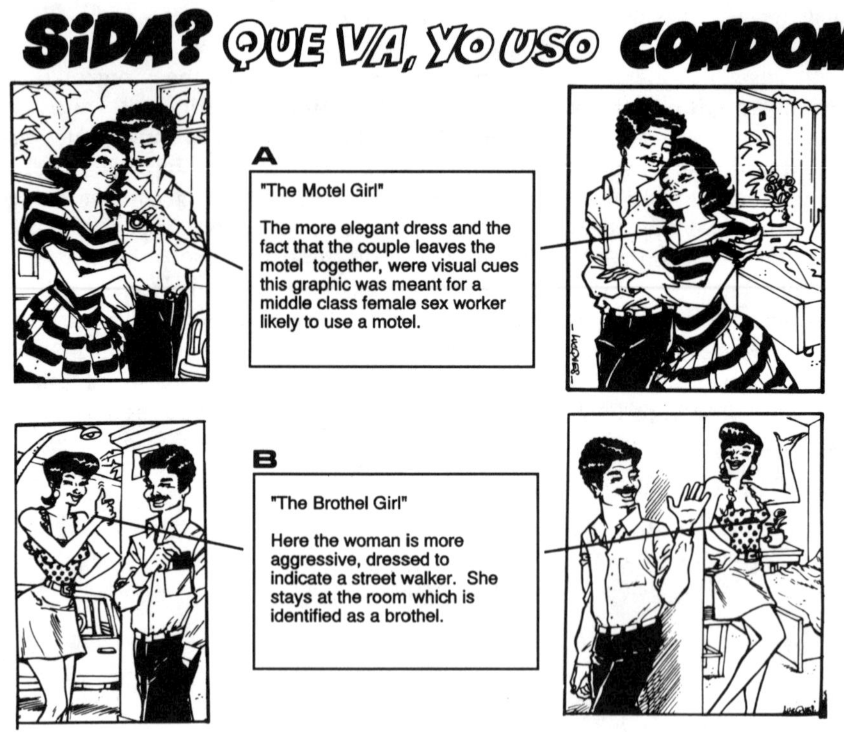

Figure 6. Dominican Republic condom instructions.

uncovered important surprises such as the expired condoms and the condom skills deficits that led to the women's unanticipated embarrassment in condom use.) (iii) Social marketing need not sell a product for money in order to be a useful organizing tool. As illustrated in Fig. 8, the conceptual framework of product, place, price, and promotion, driven by the technology of consumer research, was just as useful in addressing complex behavioral problems such as condom use as it was in addressing the somewhat less complex problem of condom sales.

SUMMARY

This chapter described three common organizing models for large-scale behavior change interventions appropriate for STD prevention. Public communication campaigns are highly organized systems for delivering messages through multiple channels designed to influence how people think or feel about a behavior. The focus is cognitive obstacles. Community-level intervention represents a quite different approach to behavior change, focused less on knowledge and attitude and more on noncognitive obstacles (internal or external) that inhibit people from

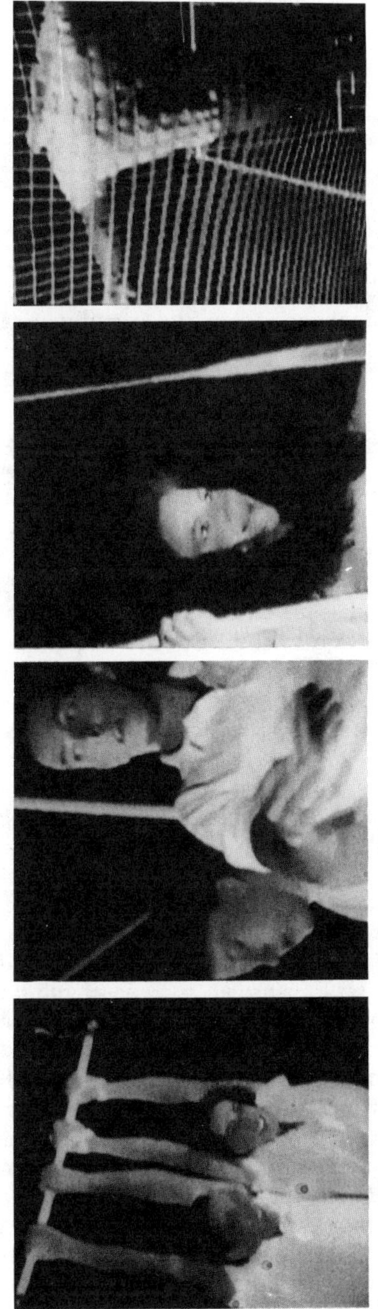

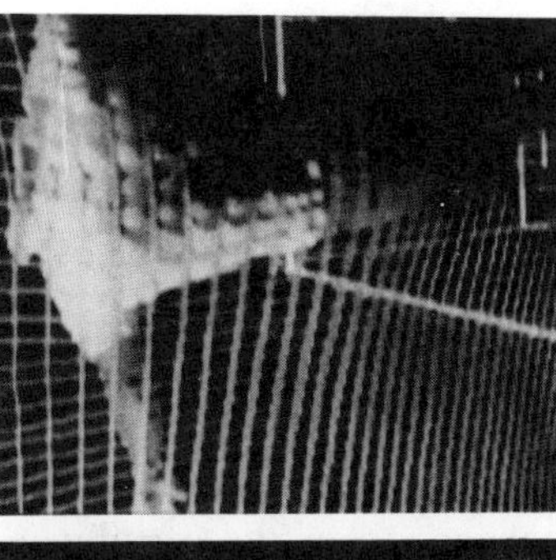

Figure 7. Dominican Republic TV spot.

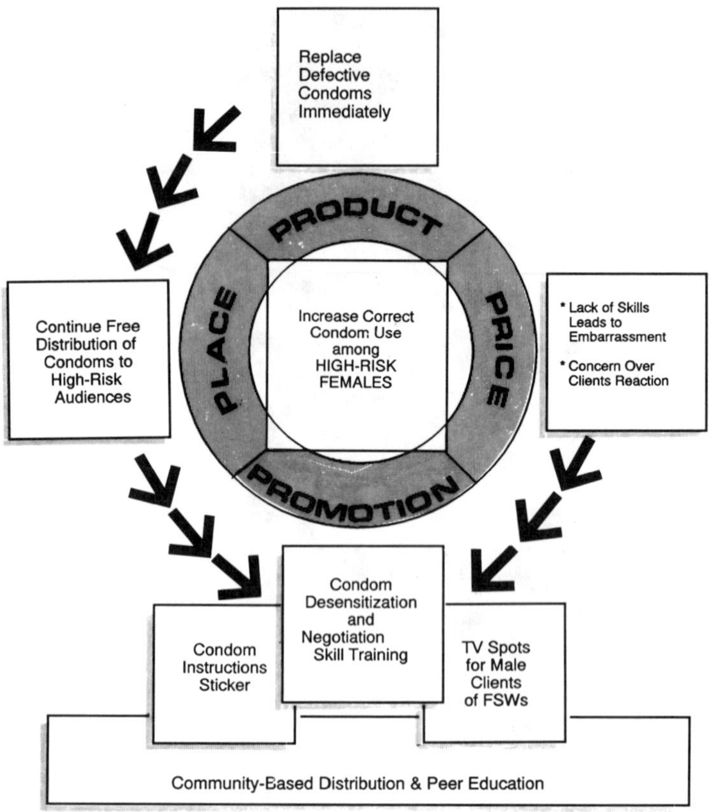

Figure 8. Social marketing and program decision-making in the Dominican Republic. FSWs, female sex workers.

adopting new behaviors. Particularly important here are improved access to services, empowerment, and policy and psychological or personality barriers such as self-esteem and problem-solving skills. Behavioral interventions are a third model and focus on the identification and delivery of positive consequences as a primary means to influence human behavior. In the real world, each model tends to be eclectic, borrowing from the tactics and technologies of the other two, but usually maintains a dominant paradigm related to cognitive, structural, or behaviorist explanations for absent behavior.

Social marketing is defined as a program-planning system that an STD program manager can use to select, organize, and monitor activities and approaches from various theoretical models. While social marketing is certainly not the only planning model available, it is unique in its determined focus on user satisfaction; its comprehensive yet straightforward planning paradigm of product, place, price, and promotion; and its eclectic integration of various social science research techniques to understand the user and the health problem and their interrelatedness. Perhaps most importantly, social marketing has already proved useful, in industrial and developing countries, for influencing a wide range of behaviors including product promotion, increased demand for services such as counseling and immunization, and individual life-style behaviors such as decisions to plan family size, treat infant diarrhea more effectively, and reduce the risk of cardiovascular disease.

Acknowledgments. I am deeply indebted to AIDSCOM, a project of the U.S. Agency for International Development and the Academy for Educational Development, for support in the preparation of this chapter.

LITERATURE CITED

1. **AIDSCOM Project.** 1988. *Psychographic Research for Condom Promotion among Female Sex Workers in Tijuana,* p. 4–6. Academy for Educational Development, Washington, D.C.
2. **AIDSCOM Project.** 1990. *Dominican Republic Implementation Plan,* p. 2–7. Academy for Educational Development, Washington, D.C.
3. **Blanchard, E. B.** 1977. Behavioral medicine: a perspective, p. 2. *In* R. B. Williams, Jr., and W. D. Gentry (ed.), *Behavioral Approaches to Medical Treatment.* Ballinger Publishing Co., Cambridge, Mass.
4. **De Moya, A. E.** 1988. *Toward an Epidemiology of Sexually Transmitted Diseases in Latin American Sex Workers and Their Clients: Early Responses to the AIDS Threat,* p. 13. World Health Organization on Prevention and Control of Sexually Transmitted Disease in Population Groups at Risk, Geneva.
5. **Fine, S.** 1989. *Social Marketing: Promoting the Causes of Public and Nonprofit Agencies.* Allyn and Bacon, Needham Heights, Mass.
6. **Foster, S. O.** 1984. Immunizable and respiratory diseases and child mortality, p. 12. *In* L. C. Chen and H. Mosely (ed.), *Child Survival: Strategies for Research—Population and Development Review,* supplement to vol. 10. The Population Council, New York.
7. **Frederiksen, L. W., L. J. Solomon, and K. A. Brehony.** 1984. *Marketing Health Behavior: Principles, Techniques, and Applications,* p. 15–17. Plenum Press, New York.
8. **Geller, E. S.** 1987. *Corporate Safety Belt Programs,* p. 79–80. Virginia Polytechnic Institute and State University, Blacksburg.
9. **Kotler, P., and E. Roberto.** 1989. *Social Marketing: Strategies for Changing Public Behavior.* The Free Press, New York.
10. **Manoff, R. K.** 1985. *Social Marketing: New Imperative for Public Health.* Praeger Publishers, New York.
11. **Mukesh, K., and K. Wellings.** 1989. The U.K. public education campaign evaluation and evolution, p. 108–110. *In AIDS Prevention through Health Promotion Monograph Series—Case Studies in Monitoring and Evaluation.* World Health Organization Global Programme on AIDS, Royal Tropical Institute, Geneva.
12. **National Institutes of Health.** 1989. *Making Health Communication Programs Work: a Planners Guide,* p. 1. NIH publication no. 89-1493. U.S. Department of Health and Human Services, Washington, D.C.
13. **Pareja, R., S. Rosario, W. A. Smith, M. Butler, and E. Guerrero.** 1989. Santo Domingo female sex workers' use and handling of condoms: research guiding the development of instructional material, p. 43–64. *In AIDS Prevention through Health Promotion Monograph Series—Case Studies in Monitoring and Evaluation.* World Health Organization Global Programme on AIDS, Royal Tropical Institute, Geneva.
14. **Population Information Program.** 1987. Counseling makes a difference. *Pop. Rep.* **15:**5.
15. **Rasmuson, M. R., R. E. Seidel, W. A. Smith, and E. M. Booth.** 1988. *Communication for Child Survival,* p. 9–79. HEALTHCOM Project, Academy for Educational Development, Washington, D.C.

16. **Rice, R. E., and C. K. Atkin.** 1989. *Public Communication Campaigns,* 2nd ed., p. 7–8, 87–104. Sage Publications, Newbury Park, Calif.
17. **Rosen, S. H.** 1989. *Fitter by the Day: 30 Day Walking Calendar,* p. 1–12. Day-by-Day Products, Cambridge, Mass.
18. **Ross, M. G.** 1955. *Community Organization: Theory, Principles, and Practice,* 2nd ed., p. 8. Harper & Row, Publishers, Inc., New York.
19. **Seltz, D. D.** 1979. *How to Conduct Successful Sales Contests and Incentive Programs,* p. 103. Dartnell Corp., Chicago.
20. **Staub, R.** 1989. The Swiss Hot Rubber Campaign: self-proclaimed gays taking the responsibility to inform their community, p. 37–39. *In AIDS Prevention through Health Promotion Monograph Series—Facing Sensitive Issues.* World Health Organization Global Programme on AIDS, Royal Tropical Institute, Geneva.
21. **Tierney, J.** 1990. With 'social marketing,' condoms combat AIDS. *The New York Times,* 18 September 1990, p. 1.
22. **Wells, W., J. Burnett, and S. Moriarty.** 1989. *Advertising Principles and Practice,* p. 85–87. Prentice-Hall, Inc., Englewood Cliffs, N.J.

Using Information To Change Sexually Transmitted Disease-Related Behaviors: an Analysis Based on the Theory of Reasoned Action

Martin Fishbein, Susan E. Middlestadt, and Penelope J. Hitchcock

Given that sexually transmitted diseases (STDs) are transmitted by individuals engaging in definable physical behaviors and that many STDs are not curable, it is clear that an effective STD prevention program must include a component that focuses on changing high-risk or maintaining low-risk behaviors. Furthermore, a behavior change program is also necessary to encourage people to determine whether or not they have been exposed to a particular STD, as well as to get them to seek and use available treatments. Elsewhere in this volume, Hornik and Smith provide general overviews of behavior change theories and behavior change strategies. In this chapter, we illustrate how one of the theories, the theory of reasoned action (1, 7, 8, 10), can be used to empirically identify the determinants of (i.e., the factors underlying) any given behavior. Perhaps more important, we also try to show how, once identified, information about these determinants can be used to develop interventions that can successfully influence behaviors involved in the control and spread of STDs, including AIDS.

The theory of reasoned action is particularly useful if one is attempting to develop an intervention that includes an informational, educational, or communication component. This type of intervention has often been criticized as ineffective in producing behavior change. From the perspective of the theory of reasoned action, the problem of changing behavior is not, as Hornik (this volume) suggests, one of converting knowledge to behavior, but instead, it is one of identifying the appropriate kinds of knowledge (or information) that must be provided and/or the structural changes that must be made if one wishes to influence the performance of a given behavior. To change or maintain a given behavior in a given population, one must first understand the determinants of that behavior in that population. The more one knows about the precise underlying factors influencing the decision to perform (or not to perform) a given behavior, the greater the probability that one can develop successful interventions to modify that behavior. Indeed, the key to successful behavioral interventions is the identification of the determinants of the specific behaviors that one wants to maintain or change.

Martin Fishbein – Department of Psychology, University of Illinois, Champaign, Illinois 61820. ***Susan E. Middlestadt*** – The Academy for Educational Development, Washington, D.C. 20037. ***Penelope J. Hitchcock*** – Sexually Transmitted Diseases Branch, National Institute of Allergy and Infectious Diseases, Bethesda, Maryland 20892.

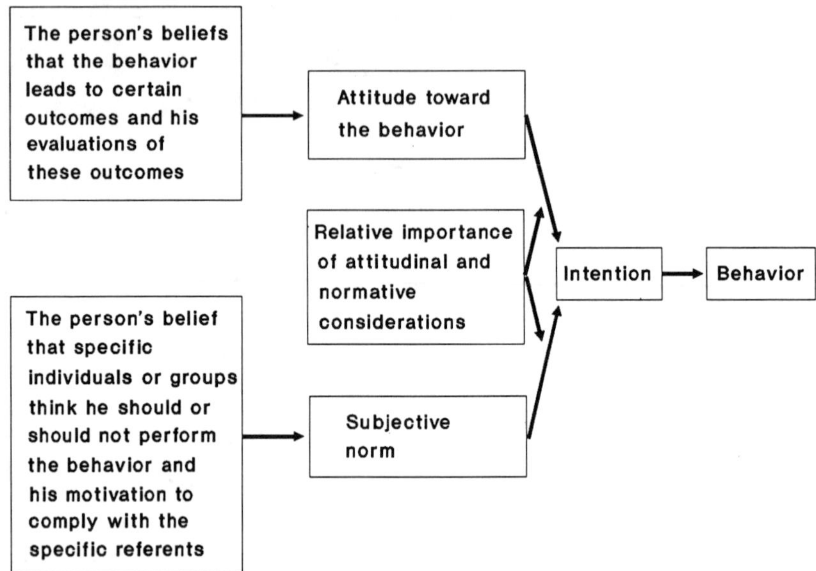

Figure 1. A theory of reasoned action: factors determining a person's behavior. Arrows indicate the direction of influence within hypothesized relationships. (From reference 1.)

A THEORY OF REASONED ACTION

First introduced in 1967, the theory of reasoned action (1, 7, 8, 10) is a general theory of human behavior that deals with the relations among beliefs, attitudes, intentions, and behavior. Each variable in the theory has been operationally defined, and standardized procedures for assessing each of these variables have been developed. Thus, it is possible to conduct empirical tests of the hypothesized relationships among variables.

The theory of reasoned action has been used successfully to predict and explain why people have (or have not) engaged in a wide variety of behaviors including smoking (6, 8), drinking (5, 21), signing up for a treatment program (12), using contraceptives (14, 17), dieting (20, 22), wearing seat belts or safety helmets (2, 4, 13), exercising regularly (15), voting (3, 23), breast-feeding (18), buying various goods and services (19), donating money to a university library (18a), and choosing a career (16).

Briefly, the theory assumes a causal chain that links beliefs to behavior. As can be seen in Fig. 1, behavior is viewed as a function of the intention to perform that behavior; intention is seen as a joint function of one's overall positive or negative feeling toward performing the behavior (i.e., one's attitude toward performing the behavior) and one's overall perception of social pressure to perform or not to perform the behavior (i.e., one's subjective norm with respect to performing the behavior); and attitude and subjective norm are, in turn, viewed as a function of underlying cognitive (i.e., belief) structures. More specifically, attitudes are viewed as a function of behavioral beliefs that performing the behavior will lead to certain outcomes and one's evaluation of those outcomes. Subjective norms are viewed as a function of normative beliefs that specific referents (i.e., certain individuals or groups) think one should or should not perform the behavior and one's motivation to comply with those referents. Thus, according to the theory, behavior is ultimately determined by a cognitive structure composed of underlying behavioral and normative beliefs. In the final analysis then, changing behavior is primarily a matter of changing this cognitive structure (i.e., of changing the underlying beliefs).

The Behavioral Criterion

The first step in applying the theory of reasoned action is to select and identify the behavior(s) of interest. A full identification of any behavior requires consideration of the four elements of action, target, context, and time. That is, every action occurs with respect to some target, in a given context, and at a given point in time. Although one may arrive at more general behavioral criteria by generalizing across one or more of these elements, a change in any one of the four elements redefines the behavior of interest. For example, using a condom is a different behavior from carrying or buying a condom (a change in action); going to an STD clinic is a different behavior from going to a family doctor or going to a human immunodeficiency virus counseling and testing site (a change in target); using a condom with a spouse or long-term partner is a different behavior from using a condom with a casual partner or with a commercial sex worker (a change in context); and going to an STD clinic on a Tuesday morning is a different behavior from going to the same STD clinic on a Saturday afternoon (a change in time). It is worth noting that using a condom *the next time* I have vaginal sex with my main partner is a different behavior from using a condom *every time* I have vaginal sex with my main partner (a different type of change in time).

Since each behavior is likely to be based on its own unique set of determinants (i.e., on a cognitive structure specific to that behavior), each behavior may require a different intervention strategy. For example, the information necessary to increase condom use with one's spouse or long-term partner may be very different from that required to increase condom use with a casual date or with a commercial sex worker. Similarly, the information necessary to increase condom use for oral sex may be very different from that required to increase condom use for vaginal or anal sex. To be effective, interventions must influence the beliefs that underlie the decision to perform (or not to perform) the targeted behavior.

Predicting Behavior from Intentions

The theory assumes that most socially relevant behaviors are under volitional control. Therefore, the most immediate determinant of any given behavior is the intention to perform or not to perform that behavior. This intention, however, must correspond exactly to the behavior in question (i.e., the intention must be defined in terms of the same four elements of action, target, context, and time that serve to define the behavior). There is now considerable evidence that such correspondent intentions provide very accurate predictions of most social behaviors. Thus, to change a specific behavior, one must change the intention to perform that behavior. For example, if the goal of an intervention is to increase homosexual mens' use of condoms for oral sex with their long-term partners, the intervention should be designed to increase homosexual men's intentions to "always use condoms for oral sex with my long-term partner" and not to increase their intentions to "avoid AIDS," to "practice safe sex," or even their general intentions to "always use condoms when I have sex." Indeed, as we shall see below, changing intentions to reach goals (e.g., to avoid AIDs) and/or to engage in a class of behaviors (e.g., to practice safe sex) are seldom effective strategies for producing change in specific behaviors.

Predicting Intentions from Attitudes and Subjective Norms

Given that correspondent intentions are viewed as the immediate determinants of behavior, the theory is primarily concerned with identifying the factors underlying the formation and change of these correspondent intentions. According to the theory of reasoned action, a person's intention to perform (or not to perform) a given behavior is a function of two basic determinants, one personal in nature and the other reflecting social influence. The personal factor is the individual's positive or negative feelings with respect to performing the behavior in question; this factor is termed *attitude toward the behavior*. The second determinant of intention is the person's perception of the social pressure put upon him or her to perform or not to perform the behavior. Since it deals with perceptions of what others think one "should" or "ought" to do, this factor is termed *subjective norm*. Generally speaking, individuals will intend to perform a behavior when they have a positive attitude toward performing it and/or when they believe that their important others think they should perform it. Note that the attitude (and the subjective norm) specified by the theory is the individual's attitude toward (or subjective norm with respect to) his or her own performance of the behavior in question. That is, like the intention, the attitude (and the norm) must be defined in terms of the same four elements of action, target, context, and time that define the targeted behavior.

Although attitudes and subjective norms may both influence the formation of a given intention, the relative importance of these two factors is expected to vary depending on the behavior and the individual. For some behaviors (and intentions), attitudinal considerations may be more influential than normative ones, while for other behaviors, normative considerations may predominate. Similarly, the intention to perform a given behavior may be primarily under attitudinal control for some individuals (or segments of the population) and predominantly under normative control for other individuals or groups. For example, in a recent study of undergraduate males' intentions to always use a condom, it was found that, in forming this intention, those who were sexually inexperienced tended to place more weight on attitudinal considerations, while those who were sexually experienced (i.e., who had had intercourse at least once) tended to place more weight on normative considerations (M. Fishbein and S. E. Middlestadt, unpublished data).

The discussion to this point can thus be summarized by equation 1,

$$B \sim I = f[w_1\text{Ab} + w_2\text{SN}] \tag{1}$$

where B is the behavior of interest (e.g., a dichotomous response to the question, "Do you always use a condom when you have vaginal intercourse with your wife?"), I is the intention to perform that behavior (e.g., the likelihood that "I intend to always use a condom when I have vaginal intercourse with my wife," measured sometime before the behavioral observation), Ab is the attitude toward performing that behavior (e.g., positive or negative feeling toward "my always using a condom for vaginal intercourse with my wife"), SN is the subjective norm concerning this behavior (e.g., the belief that "most of my important others think I should/should not always use a condom for vaginal intercourse with my wife"), and w_1 and w_2 are the weights (or relative importance) of the attitudinal and normative components, respectively.

Although this level of explanation provides some initial insight into why people behave the way they do, a more complete understanding of intentions requires an explanation of why people hold given attitudes or subjective norms. The theory of reasoned action also attempts to answer these questions.

The Cognitive Structure Underlying Attitude and Subjective Norm

As indicated above, the theory of reasoned action views behavior change as ultimately being a matter of changing the cognitive structure underlying that behavior. That is, one must change the evaluative implication of the behavioral beliefs underlying attitudes and/or the normative implication of the normative beliefs underlying subjective norms. Thus, to develop a successful intervention, one must first identify and examine the behavioral beliefs and outcome evaluations underlying the attitude as well as the normative beliefs and motivations to comply that determine the subjective norm.

Attitude and behavioral beliefs

A person's attitude toward performing a given behavior is a function of the person's salient (i.e., "top of the mind") beliefs that performing the behavior will lead to certain outcomes and the person's evaluation of these outcomes. The more one believes that performing the behavior will lead to positive outcomes (or prevent negative outcomes), the more favorable the person's attitude. Conversely, the more one believes that performing the behavior will lead to negative consequences (or prevent positive outcomes), the more negative the attitude.

This expectancy-value relationship between attitude and behavioral beliefs is expressed mathematically in equation 2

$$\mathrm{Ab} = f\left[\sum_{i=1}^{n} b_i e_i\right] \tag{2}$$

where Ab is the attitude toward one's own performance of the behavior in question (e.g., positive or negative attitude toward "my always using a condom for vaginal intercourse with my wife"); b_i is the belief that one's performance of the behavior will lead to a given outcome i (e.g., the likelihood that "my always using a condom for vaginal intercourse with my wife will reduce my sexual pleasure"); e_i is the person's evaluation of outcome i (e.g., how good or bad is "reducing my sexual pleasure"); and a behavioral crossproduct is formed for each of the n salient outcomes by multiplying the belief times the evaluation. Finally, the n crossproducts are summed. Note that not all of the possible outcomes of performing a behavior are seen as determinants of the attitude toward the behavior. The determinants of a given attitude in a given population are only those behavioral beliefs that are salient in the population under examination. Furthermore, one's attitude toward a behavior is determined by the evaluative implications of the total set of salient beliefs one holds; attitudes are not determined by any single belief.

Subjective norm and normative beliefs

A person's subjective norm with respect to a given behavior is a function of the person's normative beliefs that specific salient referents (either individuals or groups) think that he or she should or should not perform the behavior and the person's motivation to comply with those individuals or groups. Generally speaking, a person who believes that most referents with whom he or she is motivated to comply think he or she should perform the behavior will perceive social pressure to do so. Conversely, a person who believes that most referents with whom he or she is motivated to comply think he or she should not perform the behavior will have a subjective norm that puts perceived pressure on the person to avoid performing the behavior.

The relation between subjective norm and normative beliefs is expressed mathematically in equation 3

$$\mathrm{SN} = f\left[\sum_{j=1}^{n} b_j m_j\right] \tag{3}$$

where SN is the subjective norm (e.g., the person's belief that "most people who are important to me think I should/should not always use a condom when I have vaginal intercourse with my wife"); b_j is a normative belief that referent j thinks the person should/should not perform the behavior (e.g., the person's belief that "my parents think I should always use a condom when I have vaginal intercourse with my wife"); m_j is the person's motivation to comply with referent j (e.g., the belief that "generally speaking, I want to do what my parents think I should do"); and a normative belief times motivation to comply crossproduct is formed for each of n

salient referents. These n normative crossproducts are then summed. Again, note that only salient referents influence one's subjective norm. And, here too, the theory designates that subjective norms are determined by the normative implications of a set of salient normative beliefs rather than by the perceived normative pressure being exerted by any one referent.

Salient outcomes and referents

Just as one must determine whether a given behavior in a given population is under attitudinal or normative control, one must also identify the behavioral and normative beliefs that underlie the attitude or subjective norm. Salient outcomes and referents vary from behavior to behavior and population to population. The top-of-the-mind consequences one thinks about when one considers using a condom with a spouse or long-term partner may be very different from those that are salient when one considers using a condom with a casual or one-time partner. For example, one may think about loss of trust when one considers using a condom with a spouse but not with a casual or one-time partner. In addition, the outcomes and referents that are salient vis-à-vis either of these behaviors are quite likely to differ depending on the gender, culture, and socioeconomic status of the population of interest. Thus, in applying the theory to a new behavior or with a different population, it is imperative to conduct pilot research in a sample of the population of interest to identify salient outcomes and referents for that behavior in that population.

DESIGNING SUCCESSFUL BEHAVIORAL INTERVENTIONS

In this half of the chapter, we consider more directly the issues and questions involved in designing successful interventions aimed at interrupting transmission of STD pathogens or interrupting disease progression. Although one's ultimate goal may be to have an impact on a disease (e.g., reduce STD rates), and although one may believe that this can be accomplished by increasing the likelihood that a person will engage in a category of behaviors (e.g., engage in safe-sex practices), the target of an intervention should be one or more specific behaviors rather than a behavioral category or a behavioral outcome.

According to the theory of reasoned action, to be effective, an intervention must have an impact on a person's beliefs. As has been pointed out elsewhere (11), any given communication can be viewed as one or more belief statements. A receiver can accept or reject the information contained in (i.e., the belief statements composing) the communication. If the information is accepted, this reinforces or changes the receiver's beliefs. In other words, communications essentially provide information that may lead to belief change. According to the theory of reasoned action (Fig. 1), by changing behavioral or normative beliefs, one can change corresponding attitudes and/or subjective norms, and by changing attitudes and/or subjective norms, one can change corresponding intentions. Moreover, if one changes a behavioral intention, this should influence the performance of the correspondent behavior.

Since intentions are the immediate determinants of behavior, a change in a behavioral intention should lead to a change in the correspondent behavior. In marked contrast, if one changes an intention to reach a goal, to achieve an outcome, and/or to engage in a class of behaviors, there is no guarantee that this will result in goal attainment or produce change in specific behaviors. Goal attainment often involves a number of nonbehavioral factors, many of which are beyond an individual's control. In addition, there is usually no single behavior whose performance ensures goal attainment. Instead, there are typically several behaviors, each of which increases the likelihood of reaching the goal in question. For these reasons, intentions to reach goals are often very poor determinants of actual goal attainment or of the particular behavior(s) one might perform in attempting to attain that goal.

Similarly, knowing that a person intends to engage in a category of behaviors does not mean that the person intends to perform a specific behavior within that category. Different people may define a behavioral category in different ways, and hence a person may not include a specific behavior within his or her definition of the category. In addition, a person may not know or may be incorrectly informed about the behaviors that another person would define as composing the behavioral category. For example, a commercial sex worker may have a different definition of safe sex than a doctor or a public health worker. And, even if the person knows or is told the definition of the behavioral category, there is no guarantee that an intervention that is successful in changing intentions to engage in that behavioral category will also change intentions to perform (or the actual performance of) a specific behavior within that category. Thus, if one's objective is to decrease anal sex or to increase condom use, one should focus on changing people's intentions to abstain from anal sex or their intentions to always use condoms and not on their intentions to "avoid STDs" or to "practice safe sex." To design successful behavioral interventions, it is necessary to (i) select and clearly specify an appropriate behavior to change and (ii) empirically identify the beliefs underlying (i.e., the cognitive determinants of) the targeted behavior.

Which Behavior(s) Should Be Changed?

From the biomedical perspective, the behavior to be changed must be one that, if altered, will result in a reduction of the spread or progression of STDs. That is, one must identify risk factors rather than risk markers (see Padian et al., this volume). Obviously, if a valid behavioral risk factor is not identified, an intervention that is successful at modifying the behavior will not reduce or eliminate the health problem. Unfortunately, choosing and defining the behavior (or behaviors) one wishes to maintain or change is not a simple process. We often focus on outcomes (avoiding STDs, staying healthy) and behavioral categories (seeking health care, practicing safe sex) rather than specific behaviors. Moreover, a behavior for one person may be a goal for another. For example, although condom use is a behavior for men, it is a goal for women. Women do not use condoms; only their partners do. At best, women can put a condom on their partner or they can attempt to influence the likelihood that their partners will use condoms. Thus, rather than trying to increase women's intentions to "use condoms" (a goal), a more appropriate intervention would address their intentions to engage in behaviors such as "putting a condom on my partner," "telling (or asking) my partner to use a condom," or "refusing to have sex if my partner does not use a condom."

To complicate matters even further, it is becoming increasingly clear that differences in context and target are quite important in the identification of sexual behaviors. Recall that behaviors are defined by the four elements of action, target, context, and time. Not surprisingly, our research is revealing that using a condom for oral sex is a different behavior from using a condom for vaginal or anal sex. Similarly, telling one's long-term partner to use a condom is a very different behavior from telling a casual or one-time partner to use a condom. Since "using a condom" and "telling my partner to use a condom" each refer to a number of different behaviors, they may best be viewed as behavioral categories rather than single behaviors.

Strictly speaking, variations in any one of the four elements define different behaviors. Thus, for example, "telling my *long-term* partner to always use a condom for oral sex" is a different behavior from "telling my *casual* partner to always use a condom for oral sex" or "telling my *long-term* partner to always use a condom for vaginal sex." Given practical considerations, however, it is often necessary to generalize over one or more of these elements in choosing an intervention objective. For example, one may wish to increase the likelihood of "telling *all* my partners to always use a condom for *vaginal* sex." For successful interventions, these decisions about which elements to generalize across should be based on research (both epidemiological and behavioral). That is, research is necessary to determine which generalizations are acceptable and to determine which types of specification are crucial.

This initial step of selecting and identifying the behavior(s) to be influenced by an intervention is a crucial one that requires substantial collaboration among behavioral scientists, medical researchers, and epidemiologists familiar with the prevention and treatment of STDs.

What Are the Determinants of the Selected Behavior(s)?

Once a behavior has been selected and properly specified, it is necessary to identify the determinants of that behavior. As described above, the immediate determinant of any behavior is the intention to perform the behavior. Intentions are, in turn, determined by attitudes and subjective norms, which are themselves determined by underlying cognitive structures. It is important to recognize that every behavior will have its own unique set of determinants, and thus each behavior may require a different type of intervention. For example, it is quite likely that one may have to design different interventions if the objective is to increase the frequency with which someone uses a condom for vaginal intercourse for all partners than if the goal is primarily to increase condom use for vaginal sex with casual partners. Indeed, it is conceivable that the intention to use a condom for vaginal sex with all partners is under normative control, while the intention to use a condom for vaginal sex with casual partners is under attitudinal control. Similarly, it is possible that even if these behaviors were both under attitudinal control, a key factor that might negatively influence a person's intention to use a condom for vaginal sex with all partners could be the belief that this behavior "will lead to a loss of trust between me and my partner." Yet this belief may be unimportant and/or nonsalient when one considers using a condom for vaginal sex with a casual or one-time partner.

Relative importance of attitudinal and normative factors

In designing a behavioral intervention, it is necessary to determine whether the intention is primarily under attitudinal control or normative control or whether it is influenced by both types of considerations. According to the theory of reasoned action, if one wants to change or reinforce a given intention, one must change or strengthen the attitude toward performing that behavior and/or the subjective norm with respect to that behavior. Whether one should change the attitude or subjective norm, however, depends on the relative importance of these two components as determinants of that intention. If a behavior is primarily under attitudinal control, attempts to change that behavior through the use of normative pressure will not be very successful. Similarly, if the members of some group perform a given behavior because they believe that their significant others think they should perform the behavior, little will be accomplished by trying to change their attitudes toward performing that behavior.

Recall, however, that the relative weights of the two components may vary from population to population. For example, while sexually experienced male U.S. college students' intentions to "always use a condom" appear to be primarily under normative control, this same intention appears to be predominantly under attitudinal control in a sample of sexually experienced male Mexican college students (9). Thus, this step, as in all steps of the application of the theory of reasoned action, must be based on research conducted in the population that is the focus of the intervention.

Salient outcomes and referents

Once one has determined whether a given behavior (or intention) is attitudinally or normatively controlled, one must identify salient outcomes (e.g., costs and benefits of performing the behavior) and/or salient referents vis-à-vis the behavior. This can be done by asking a representative sample of the population of interest to report what they see as advantages and disadvantages of performing the behavior (to identify salient outcomes of performing the behavior) and to indicate people or groups who would approve or disapprove of their performing that behavior (to identify salient referents).

It is again important to recognize that salient outcomes and referents will vary as one moves from behavior to behavior and population to population. This can perhaps best be illustrated by considering some of the salient outcomes obtained in a study of condom use among commercial sex workers. More specifically, in the key participant interviews conducted as part of the Centers for Disease Control's AIDS intervention demonstration projects, commercial sex workers were asked to separately indicate what they saw as the advantages and disadvantages of using condoms for oral, anal, and vaginal sex. Not surprisingly, most of these women felt that using a condom for vaginal or anal sex would protect them from AIDS and other STDs. It is interesting that protection from AIDS was not frequently reported as an advantage of using a condom for oral sex. However, a unique perceived advantage of using a condom for oral sex was that it meant that one did not have to get semen in one's mouth. And, not surprisingly, a unique advantage of using a condom for vaginal sex was that it would prevent pregnancy.

With respect to negative consequences, many of the professional sex workers reported that using a condom would reduce their clients' satisfaction. Breakage was seen as a major disadvantage of condom use vis-à-vis anal sex, while "it tastes bad" was frequently cited as a disadvantage of using a condom for oral sex. Even more important, the key disadvantages of using a condom differed across ethnic groups. While Hispanic sex workers were worried that using a condom could be painful and lead to injuries (e.g., it would increase friction; it would lead to urinary tract diseases; it would get stuck inside and get infected), black sex workers felt that using condoms would decrease their own sexual pleasure (e.g., it's not natural; it doesn't feel right; it's not skin-to-skin), and white sex workers worried about the mechanics of condom use (e.g., they're difficult to buy and/or to put on; they're expensive; they make the client last longer). These findings should make it clear that different populations may have very different concerns about the same behavior. More important, they provide clear evidence that different beliefs may have to be addressed and therefore that very different interventions may be necessary to change the same behavior in different populations.

Which aspects of the underlying cognitive structure to address

Once one has identified outcomes and referents that are salient in the population of interest for the behavior of interest, one must then decide which of these behavioral or normative beliefs to target in an intervention. As described above, data must be gathered assessing two aspects for each salient outcome and two aspects for each salient referent. More specifically, with respect to each outcome, one must assess (i) the strength of the behavioral belief that performing the behavior will lead to the outcome and (ii) the evaluation of that outcome. Similarly, with respect to each salient referent, one must assess (i) the strength of the normative belief that the referent thinks the person should or should not perform the behavior and (ii) the motivation to comply with that referent. If the relative weight of the attitudinal component is high, further analyses need to be conducted on the behavioral beliefs and evaluations underlying the attitude component. If the relative weight of the normative component is high, further analyses need to be conducted on the normative beliefs and motivations to comply.

These analyses should be used to identify those beliefs, outcome evaluations, and motivations to comply that discriminate between people who do and do not intend to perform the behavior in question. Once identified, these differentiating items are good aspects to address with interventions.

Consider the behavior of "telling my partner to use a condom every time I have sexual intercourse" that we examined in two groups of college women (S. E. Middlestadt and M. Fishbein, VIth Int. Conf. AIDS, abstr., vol. 3, p. 265, 1990). One of the salient outcomes of performing this behavior was that it would "protect me from STDs." Given that protection from STDs is a salient concern of these women, it would seem reasonable to develop a message directed at increasing the women's beliefs that telling their partners to use a condom would protect them from STDs. However, our analyses of the underlying cognitive structure indicated that while this message would be expected to be effective among sexually inexperienced college women, it is unlikely to be effective among college women who have had sexual intercourse at least once.

Among the inexperienced women, a comparison between those who do and do not intend to tell their partners to use condoms revealed a statistically significant difference in the degree to which their beliefs about STD protection contributed to their attitudes (i.e., in the behavioral belief times outcome evaluation crossproduct). Further analysis showed that this difference was due to a difference in belief strength rather than in outcome evaluation. That is, in comparison with inexperienced women who do not intend to tell their partners to use condoms, inexperienced women who intend to perform this behavior are significantly more likely to believe that telling their partners will protect them from STDs. Thus, a communication increasing the perceived likelihood of this salient outcome would make an inexperienced woman more positive toward performing the behavior, more likely to form a positive intention, and more likely to actually perform the behavior. In contrast, among the experienced women, intenders were similar to nonintenders with respect to the behavioral belief, the outcome evaluation, and the behavioral crossproduct of the two. Both intenders and nonintenders believed that it was quite likely that telling their partners to use condoms would protect them from STDs. The experienced women were thus homogeneous with respect to this belief. They all already believed the outcome would occur. There was little room for change, and addressing this belief would not be expected to successfully increase the targeted behavior.

In sum, given a targeted behavior, one can construct instruments to measure the correspondent intention, attitude, and subjective norm and then use these measures to empirically determine whether the behavior in question is under attitudinal or normative control. In contrast, one cannot simply construct instruments to measure the underlying cognitive structure. One must first empirically determine the outcomes and referents that are salient for the targeted behavior in the population of interest. Once a set of salient outcomes and referents has been identified, one can construct instruments to measure the strength of behavioral and normative beliefs as well as to measure evaluations of the salient outcomes and motivations to comply with salient referents. These measures can then be used to empirically determine those aspects of the underlying cognitive structure that would be effective ones to address in an intervention.

CONCLUSION

In this chapter, we tried to show how research based on the theory of reasoned action can be used to develop behavioral interventions. In the commercial world, interventions such as promotions and advertising campaigns are often based on extensive market research that attempts to identify the needs of consumers and/or the strategies that might be expected to influence consumer behavior. In contrast, within the health and other nonprofit domains, much less research is done. Assumptions are made about the kinds of information that should be provided to the public to achieve various goals (e.g., to reduce the spread of an STD) or to produce behavior change (e.g., to decrease the performance of behaviors that put one at risk for an STD). Educational programs, mass media communication campaigns, and other forms of health interventions are often based on intuition as to what needs to be changed and how to accomplish these changes. Rarely are the kinds of empirical and theoretical considerations discussed in this chapter taken into account. Most messages and interventions are constructed somewhat arbitrarily on the basis of what all too often turn out to be false assumptions about the determinants of the behavior one wishes to change. Indeed, more often than not, it has been assumed that providing people with information about a disease and how it is spread will lead to behavior change. However, as Hornick (this volume) and others have pointed out, this type of information is rarely converted into action.

One of the main reasons communications and other forms of interventions fail is that they often do not address appropriate beliefs. Messages are rarely directed at behavioral or normative beliefs about performing the behavior one is attempting to change. Instead, all too often, messages provide people with information they already have or try to convince them of something they already believe. If most members of a group already believe that performing some behavior will lead to a certain consequence or outcome (e.g., that "using a condom for anal sex will protect me from AIDS"), little will be accomplished by a persuasive communication that focuses on that information. Similarly, if most members of a group or some segment of the population are aware that their parents are strongly in favor of their telling casual partners to use condoms for vaginal intercourse, little will be accomplished by basing one's intervention on parental pressure.

It is our contention that information and education interventions can be highly effective behavior change devices. Communication of information (or knowledge) through educational or mass media channels can produce significant changes in behavior. However, the information must address the behavioral or normative beliefs underlying the behavior that one wishes to change. Given that epidemiological research has identified a behavioral risk factor, the goal of the intervention should be to change that behavior. To do this, the intervention should attempt to increase intentions to perform (or not perform) the targeted behavior. If this intention is primarily under attitudinal control, the intervention should try to change behavioral beliefs about the advantages and disadvantages of performing the behavior. If the intention is primarily under normative control, the intervention should try to change normative beliefs that specific referents think one should or should not perform the behavior. For the intervention to be successful, decisions about the specific behavioral or normative beliefs to address should not be based on intuition but must be determined empirically. We hope that medical and public health personnel concerned with STDs including AIDS will work closely with behavioral scientists to select and clearly define appropriate high-risk behaviors, to conduct the research necessary to identify the determinants of those behaviors, and to develop effective communications and other interventions that can influence these determinants.

LITERATURE CITED

1. **Ajzen, I., and M. Fishbein (ed.).** 1980. *Understanding Attitudes and Predicting Social Behavior*. Prentice Hall, Inc., Englewood Cliffs, N.J.
2. **Allegrante, J. P., R. G. Mortimer, and T. W. O'Rourke.** 1980. Social-psychological factors in motorcycle safety helmet use: implications for public policy. *J. Saf. Res.* **12:**115–126.
3. **Bowman, C. H., and M. Fishbein.** 1978. Understanding public reactions to energy proposals: an application of the Fishbein model. *J. Appl. Soc. Psychol.* **8:**319–340.
4. **Budd, R. J., D. North, and C. P. Spencer.** 1984. Understanding seat-belt use: a test of Bentler and Speckart's extension of the theory of reasoned action. *Eur. J. Soc. Psychol.* **14:**69–78.
5. **Budd, R. J., and C. P. Spencer.** 1985. Exploring the role of personal normative beliefs in the theory of reasoned action: the problem of discriminating between alternative path models. *Eur. J. Soc. Psychol.* **15:**299–313.
6. **Chassin, L., C. C. Presson, M. Bensenburg, E. Corty, R. W. Olshavsky, and S. J. Sherman.** 1981. Predicting adolescents' intentions to smoke cigarettes. *J. Health Soc. Behav.* **22:**445–455.
7. **Fishbein, M.** 1967. Attitude and the prediction of behavior, p. 477–492. *In* M. Fishbein (ed.), *Readings in Attitude Theory and Measurement*. John Wiley & Sons, Inc., New York.
8. **Fishbein, M.** 1980. A theory of reasoned action: some applications and implications, p. 65–116. *In* H. E. Howe and M. M. Page (ed.), *Nebraska Symposium on Motivation, 1979*. University of Nebraska Press, Lincoln.
9. **Fishbein, M.** 1990. AIDS and behavior change: an analysis based on the theory of reasoned action. *Interam. J. Psychol.* **24:**37–56.
10. **Fishbein, M., and I. Ajzen.** 1975. *Belief, Attitude, Intention and Behavior: an Introduction to Theory and Research*. Addison-Wesley Publishing Co., Reading, Mass.
11. **Fishbein, M., and I. Ajzen.** 1981. Acceptance, yielding and impact: cognitive processes in persuasion, p. 339–359. *In* R. E. Petty, T. M. Ostrom, and T. C. Brock (ed.), *Cognitive Processes in Persuasion*. Lawrence Erlbaum Associates, Inc., Hillsdale, N.J.
12. **Fishbein, M., I. Ajzen, and J. McArdle.** 1980. Changing the behavior of alcoholics: effects of persuasive communication, p. 217–242. *In* I. Ajzen and M. Fishbein (ed.), *Understanding Attitudes and Predicting Social Behavior*. Prentice Hall, Inc., Englewood Cliffs, N.J.
13. **Fishbein, M., J. M. Salazar, P. R. Rodriguez, S. E. Middlestadt, and T. Himelfarb.** 1988. Predicting Venezuelan students' use of seat belts: an application of the theory of reasoned action in Latin America. *Rev. Psicol. Soc. Pers.* **4:**19–41.
14. **Fisher, W. A.** 1984. Predicting contraceptive behavior among university men: the role of emotions and behavioral intentions. *J. Appl. Soc. Psychol.* **14:**104–123.
15. **Godin, G., and R. J. Shephard.** 1986. Psychosocial factors influencing intentions to exercise of young students from grades 7 to 9. *Res. Q. Exercise Sport* **57:**41–52.

16. **Greenstein, M., R. N. Miller, and D. E. Weldon.** 1979. Attitudinal and normative beliefs as antecedents of female occupational choice. *Pers. Soc. Psychol. Bull.* **5:**356–362.
17. **Jaccard, J. J., and A. R. Davidson.** 1972. Toward an understanding of family planning behaviors: an initial investigation. *J. Appl. Soc. Psychol.* **2:**228–235.
18. **Manstead, A. S. R., C. Proffitt, and J. L. Smart.** 1983. Predicting and understanding mothers' infant-feeding intentions and behaviors: testing the theory of reasoned action. *J. Pers. Soc. Psychol.* **44:**657–671.
18a. **Middlestadt, S. E.** 1990. Developing a research-based communication campaign to increase financial contributions to a University library: an application of the theory of reasoned action, p. 51–81. *In* R. W. Belk (ed.), *Advances in Nonprofit Marketing,* vol. 3. JAI Press, Greenwich, Conn.
19. **Ryan, M. J.** 1982. Behavioral intention formation: the interdependency of attitudinal and social influence variables. *J. Consumer Res.* **9:**263–278.
20. **Saltzer, E. B.** 1978. Locus of control and the intention to lose weight. *Health Educ. Monogr.* **6:**118–128.
21. **Schlegel, R. P., C. A. Crawford, and M. D. Sanborn.** 1977. Correspondence and mediation properties of the Fishbein model: an application to adolescent alcohol use. *J. Exp. Soc. Psychol.* **13:**421–430.
22. **Sejwacz, R., I. Ajzen, and M. Fishbein.** 1980. Predicting and understanding weight loss: intentions, behaviors and outcomes, p. 101–112. *In* I. Ajzen and M. Fishbein (ed.), *Understanding Attitudes and Predicting Social Behavior.* Prentice Hall, Inc., Englewood Cliffs, N.J.
23. **Shepherd, G. J.** 1987. Individual differences in the relationship between attitudinal and normative determinants of behavioral intent. *Commun. Monogr.* **54:**221–231.

Epidemiological and Ethnographic Methods for Research in High-Risk Behavior: Integrated Approaches to Acceptability and Intervention

Lucile F. Newman, Sally Zierler, and Donna Cheung

The epidemic of AIDS has challenged researchers to comprehend the persistence of risky behavior in potentially life-threatening circumstances and to favor interventions that can reduce risk for particular populations. The collaboration of multidisciplinary research teams enables project design that includes individual, group, and sociocultural aspects of behavior change. To change behavior in relation to sexually transmitted diseases (STDs) including human immunodeficiency virus (HIV), it is necessary first to understand the nature of behavior and its motivations, to describe the areas of human action, and to focus on those activities promoting contact and transmission of disease. With no preventive action against viral STDs or HIV immediately available, the first line of defense against these infections is still education. It is still necessary to convince people to change risky behavior. To do that, it is necessary to know what the behavior is that must be changed. What are the forms of risky behavior? What populations are most at risk? What are the contexts in which it takes place? By what authority is such change acceptable? Medical? Local leaders? Church? Schools? Peers?

Human behavior is circumscribed by customs, rules for interpersonal behavior, and symbolic meanings. Therefore, to understand how choices are made between perceived alternatives, one must understand both societal expectations and common experiences regarding particular areas of behavior. Behavioral interventions are most effective when aimed to change the normative context, to create an environment in which an innovation can become expected behavior.

Ethnographic research refers to a qualitative approach to research on cultural values, motives, and behavior (1, 5, 12). Rather than construct instruments embodying the conceptual categories and interests of the researcher, the researcher becomes a learner, with the subjects of study as experts on their own behavior. Language then becomes an essential part of what is learned. "Language is the public storehouse of tradition, the signal of just what it is in the world that is significant. . . ." (2). Thus, the goal of qualitative research is to investigate the language and cultural context of behavior to improve the validity of information collected for an epidemiological study. The goal of an epidemiological study is to provide a valid estimate of disease occurrence in relation to a potential determinant

---

Lucile F. Newman and Sally Zierler – Department of Community Health, Brown University, Providence, Rhode Island 02912. ***Donna Cheung*** – Department of Anthropology, Brown University, Providence, Rhode Island 02912.

of disease. The contributions of the qualitative methods of ethnographic research in integration with quantitative methods are described in this chapter. It begins with a discussion of integration of qualitative and quantitative methods, description of ethnographic methods, then acceptability research, the analytic concept of "context variables," and finally, acceptability of interventions.

INTEGRATION OF QUALITATIVE AND QUANTITATIVE RESEARCH METHODS

Epidemiology provides descriptions of the occurrence of disease in human populations. From these descriptions, investigators are able to discern patterns of occurrence, and these patterns lead to thoughts of causal connections between characteristics of populations and their frequency of disease. Ultimately, the goal of such thinking is to prevent disease. But the path from description of disease occurrence to the removal of a disease cause often leads to dead ends, or circuitous routes that may yield little new knowledge about risk factors for disease. Sometimes, identification of causes follows a relatively simple path, such as the discovery that most lung cancers can be attributed to cigarette smoke. Often, intensive searching comes up with little evidence that can explain disease frequency, as witnessed by nearly 50 years of research on the etiology of birth defects.

There are inherent limitations to epidemiological studies because there are inherent limitations to what is knowable. Furthermore, errors in conceptualization, design, data collection, and analysis reduce the ability to identify causes of disease (6, 19). Ethnographic studies, as precursors to epidemiological studies, define an epistemology that can shape the nature and language of a study and enhance its potential to identify risk factors that may explain some of the disease frequency in a particular population. For example, much epidemiological evidence comes from self-reported information on exposure histories. The validity of these self-reports is improved by ethnographic study of context communities in conjunction with interviews that are sensitive to the domain of inquiry and phrased in a language that is familiar to the respondents.

Much of the research on identification of risk factors for transmission of HIV infection has depended on self-reported sexual activities. These behaviors are difficult to describe not only because of the variability of their occurrence but also because of the personal, cultural, and moral sensitivities that affect acknowledgment of their experience. In the context of a study of modes of sexual transmission of HIV infection, the goal of data collection may be to classify individual sexual behaviors according to the dose, duration, and route of entry of possibly infected body fluids. In reality, epidemiologists resort to a crude proxy for this conceptual determinant by classifying people according to their lifetime number of sexual partners, or whether they use a condom or other latex barrier during genital sex. The acceptability of the questions designed to identify sexual modalities for HIV transmission will affect the validity of the response, which in turn will affect the ability to identify a preventable cause of disease. Even if a preventive strategy has been identified (such as use of latex barriers for genital sex), subsequent interventions to increase use of barrier methods or to empower partners to negotiate sexual activities would necessitate an appreciation of the social, religious, and cultural mores to gain acceptability. In this way, the epidemiological intervention is not designed in a cultural vacuum.

Ethnographic methods are essential to enable a view of the context community separate from the immediate problem of infection, enhance the reliability of self-reports, and enlarge the view of action to include the meaning of interventions to the actors. The limitation of these studies is in establishing representatives of in-depth interviews with a small number of people. The combination of qualitative with quantitative methods helps to mitigate this problem. They promote working simultaneously on normative and attitudinal forces (see Fishbein et al., this volume), on cultural context, and on individual change. In essence, they provide a qualitative base for a quantitative study.

QUALITATIVE METHODS: FROM THE PARTICULAR TO THE GENERAL

There are many forms of ethnographic investigation. Ethnographic study may be a long-term full-scale ethnography of context, behavior, and interaction in a particular community. It may be a short-term observation of particular limited domains of behavior, such as sexual behavior or risk taking or institutionalized bisexuality. It often includes in-depth interviewing to ascertain individual and collective attitudes and perceptions, such as the effects of legal restrictions on behavior. Group interviews enable exploration of norms of expectable behavior. Taken together, these methods of investigation provide an understanding of the values of a community, the chain of events that can lead to infection, and description and interpretation contributory to the objectives of quantitative studies.

Ethnography is a method of in-depth observation and description of social structure and human behavior based on the concept of culture. Hammel (12) defines culture as "an evaluative conversation constructed by actors out of the raw materials afforded by tradition and ongoing experience." It is constantly negotiated. Ethnography is sometimes termed "participant observation" because of its emphasis on open-ended interviews, cultural context, and an attempt to gain individual as well as collective views. Of importance is identification of significant coactors in a social network (12). Observation of the experience of everyday life enables an interpretation of human experience, the social determinants of cultural meanings, and processes of change for both individuals and societies. Ethnographic approaches to understanding contact, transmission, acceptable intervention, and the social impact of STDs and HIV include observation and description of cultural and subcultural belief systems, patterns of interaction, and practices that support or inhibit contact and spread of disease. Objectives of ethnographic study of a subset of larger epidemiological studies are to provide an in-depth analysis of risky behavior and to identify points of intervention that are culturally sensitive and that take advantage of the strengths of a community (3, 11, 12, 14, 16, 17).

ETHNOGRAPHIC FIELD METHODS

Preliminary methods for investigation of a community at risk for HIV infection include a variety of approaches. Methods include several phases of interviewing with different groups. The first interviews are case histories, which are individual extensive interviews. Individual in-depth life history interviews enable an orientation to the community. Then ethnographic interviews are done. These are open-ended interviews with knowledgeable individuals in the community of study. Phase one, language elicitation, is done with a range of knowledgeable individuals who may be active community members or medical, psychological, or health counselors familiar with the community. Objectives of phase one interviews are to define domains of interaction, patterns of partnership, and language to prepare questionnaires. Language elicitation provides class, location, and ethnic group-appropriate terminology, including slang or simplified terms to avoid imposition of professional language and categories on the research situation. Phase two, group interviews, may be focus group interviews with small groups who have some commonality, i.e., age, language, ethnic identity, or residence. The objective of these interviews is to determine cultural norms for particular groups in relation to values, sexual aesthetics and behavior, and risk taking. Group interviews also identify language and domains of interaction. Focus groups, because they are a public performance, enable identification of collective values and publicly held points of view. Phase three includes individual interviews with respondents sampled, for example, by geographical area or block, or attendees at a clinic. Objectives of individual interviews are to, in this instance, identify sexual behavior and aesthetics, use of STD-preventive actions, use of health services, self-protective knowledge and practices, and acceptability of interventions. This provides a continuing presence in the community.

All these activities assist in research design ("What are the key questions to be answered?"), language elicitation for question formation, and categories for coding responses that are sensitive to the characteristics and values of the group to be studied. They provide preliminary and cost-effective feasibility and hypothesis-generating phases of problem identification.

Continuing study would, in addition to the above, include ethnographic interviews with a subsample of the target population. These methods answer questions of what people are doing ("What kind of behaviors are occurring?") rather than "How many are doing it?" How does environment affect behavior? What interventions could change risky behavior?

Analysis of narrative material includes coding for categories of response, ranking of various behaviors in terms of risk, and eliciting explanatory models of disease. The ethnographer also keeps notes on personal or idiosyncratic points of view, a general view of how the interview went, and an estimate of reliability on the part of each respondent.

The benefits of an ethnographic subset study then include feasibility and hypothesis-generating studies preliminary to a larger study; ability to elicit appropriate language and concepts for questionnaire development; a continuing presence in the community to monitor the larger studies; and a built-in opportunity for achievement of target group participation in intervention design and effective intervention evaluation.

ACCEPTABILITY RESEARCH

Acceptability research objectives are designed to study those attributes of behavioral interventions that could affect their acceptance in various sociocultural settings, with a focus on risk-taking behavior and risk factors for STDs and HIV. Acceptability refers to the degree to which an intervention or any of its attributes is perceived by people to be consonant with their well-being (13). Acceptability varies among individuals by age, gender, stage of life cycle, and social class and among cultural and ethnic groups. It includes perceptions of advantage and disadvantage, perceived side effects, perceived effectiveness, social implications of use, and risks and hazards of changing behavior.

The need for comparable data in acceptability research requires a standard format, but one that is at the same time flexible enough to accommodate the variations required by the field conditions of each research setting. Emphasis is placed on analysis of qualitative material to identify localized influential context variables, as well as quantitative material to understand existing consistencies in behavior. Recently, plans to develop an intervention to prevent transmission of HIV among prostitute women prompted use of ethnographic methods. The goals of the project are to provide women with safe sex and intravenous drug use information, to provide a safe space for prostitutes to discuss their concerns about HIV and about changing behaviors, and to assist sex workers who want to change careers or change their life-style. To begin thinking about the nature of this intervention, prostitute women were interviewed for their perspective on the usefulness of this kind of program. In addition, they provided specific information on the nature and language of sex work and needs not directly HIV related, such as housing, child care, and educational, personal, and professional goals. The information provided by these women will be used to develop an intervention, including measurement instruments for evaluation of the effect of the intervention on changing behaviors associated with HIV risk.

ANALYSIS OF QUALITATIVE MATERIAL: CONTEXT VARIABLES

For such a study, the questions are as follows. Where in the causal chain can intervention take place? How can we block the sufficient cause of inevitable HIV infections? The recommendation is to expand the scope of epidemiological research to contextual areas and experiences further from (more distal to) the disease itself. Identification of the normative context of particular groups and subgroups has been undertaken through the conceptual framework of "context variables" or context descriptive factors (15). Ethnographic approaches focus on the relations of social and cultural factors to behavior. In a certain sense, context variables attempt to identify sociocultural *determinants* of determinants of behavior.

Context variables were originally derived from research on the acceptability of contraceptive methods (15). Their framework is based on a demographic model that begins with the definition of proximate variables, i.e., those closest to the index behavior and potentially predictive of outcome (4), for example, number of partners; and of intermediate variables, or conditions that are required for the index outcome (7), for example, hazardous life-style. Context variables refer to cultural, ideational, and normative factors through which variations in behavior are influenced and potential changes in behavior are anticipated. They are qualitative rather than predictive but are essential to understanding the context community and meanings of actions to those who engage in them and locating possible areas of resistance and intervention points as well as unacceptable interventions. Some examples follow, including ideological variables, relational variables, sexual aesthetics, variables of the marketplace, and perceived risks and hazards of changing behavior.

Ideological variables in reference to STDs and HIV infection may include religious prohibitions of any interference with intercourse, repression of women's interests, national rejection of drugs or AIDS as a problem (with concomitant refusal to test blood), political controls of information, prevailing values of bravery and risk taking, and situations of tourism in which denial of disease promotes economic advantage.

Relational variables include patterns of partnership, separation of values of sex and reproduction, expectation of both formal and informal unions, flexibility in gender identity and gender role, acceptance or rejection of partner communication, and dominance patterns and forms of negotiation in sexual relationships. (Patterns of partnership refer to marriage, nonmarital persisting relationships, and informal, casual, and random contacts between same- or opposite-sex individuals.)

Sexual aesthetics and values of underground behavior include that which is considered good and right in sexual relationships, romantic concepts of honor or taboos against certain forms of sexual behavior, symbolic representations of risk-taking behavior, barriers to acceptance of interventions, and known unacceptable interventions. In some societies, there may be periods of uncontrolled behavior, "seasons of abandon," when everything is permitted—masked identity, abandonment of mind and daily life, rule breaking, acting out of sexual contradictions, institutionalized transvestism, ambiguous sexuality, stylized male-to-male dominance activities of casual and anonymous penetration—which go unremarked as aspects of bisexual behavior.

Variables of the marketplace include sex as currency, as a means to other ends, as a trade for drugs, economic advantages of drug trade, official secrecy to protect tourism, and the power of the marketplace as a motivating factor in people's lives.

Perceived risks and hazards of changing behavior include participating in research or intervention programs, being seen as an informer, and trying new ideas and technologies with attendant risks to relationship, honor, status, or fear of exposure to ridicule.

BARRIER METHODS STUDY

A pilot study, now in its second phase, involved interviews on acceptability of barrier methods among women, with one group of university women and another older clinic population in a small city (D. Cheung, M.A. thesis, Brown University, Providence, R.I., 1991). This total population is a low-risk group but not a no-risk group. The domain of behavior investigated was how women felt about negotiating with a partner, whether they had a sense of ability to negotiate. All the sexually active women had had unprotected intercourse at some time. However, the consistent risky behavior in this population was identified as ambivalence and not asserting themselves in interpersonal interactions. It was clear in the interviews that women were confused about having control of pregnancy prevention through use of the pill, yet feeling loss of control over HIV prevention, and at the same time learning that STDs are more prevalent than they had thought and, as cofactors in HIV, more dangerous. The sense of loss of control just when coitus-independent birth control made sex seem safe is especially difficult in sexual decision-making (8, 10, 19).

Context variables in the barrier methods studies are described briefly. Ideological descriptive factors included a sense of lack of control, a habit of not discussing sex with potential partners, and a sense of pregnancy as immediate and visible as a problem and solved by the pill, while viral STDs and HIV were yet another interference with sexual activity while appearing remote and invisible.

Sexual aesthetics in this population included a romantic notion of the woman as unprepared and open only to spontaneous sexual union, a position that is enhanced by coitus-independent fertility-regulating methods but which increases risk of STDs and HIV.

Relational descriptive factors were the center of the responses in that the interview focused on negotiation and locus of control. Attitudes toward negotiation were expressed as ambivalence by the older clinic population, while the student group was characterized more by confusion and denial. The lack of congruence in responses between perceived control and actual preventive behavior indicated an ideal of anticipation attenuated by the actual relationship and suggested interventions in the area of self-respect, relationship, negotiation, and intensive health education.

INTERVENTION

Intervention programs were suggested by the barrier methods project specific to these populations. Intervention programs were the subject of focus group discussions for both groups. Of particular concern were difficulties of consistent condom use and problems of a sense of equity in relationships. The women's concerns were about trust and a lack of control in the negotiation of sexual relationships and a lack of effective prevention other than barrier methods. The purpose of the studies was to expand on these issues and to suggest culturally sensitive interventions in behavior.

Reliance on the condom or abstinence characterizes the approach of official American programs of intervention. While the condom may be useful as a barrier to STDs and HIV, it requires consistent use and partner cooperation (18). An important part of negotiation is couple communication—the more casual the interaction, the less likely is effective use of a condom. This suggests interventions focused on the point of sexual negotiation and enhanced with female-usable methods.

If a cause of risky behavior in this population (e.g., unprotected intercourse, multiple partners) is seen as ambivalence and denial of risk, then an intervention would be to create a normative climate that promotes taking responsibility for one's own actions and emphasizing personal control and participation in interactive decision-making. This could take the form, for the university group, a closed and accessible community, of assertiveness-training programs, role-playing interactive scenarios in dormitories or through peer counselors, and print material on female-usable methods (9). The university population is especially open to new methods, both the female condom and those of their own devising, and would find new method trials acceptable.

Interventions for the clinic population would be quite different but could include support group discussions regarding discontinuity between expressed views and actual behavior. Another intervention could include health education materials which recognize that the model of the pill (coitus independent, a private sense of control of fertility regulation) is not yet available for prevention of viral STDs including HIV. Both interventions should include discussion of STDs as cofactors increasing susceptibility to HIV, as well as precursors to other life-threatening diseases. Other interventions would be to promote discussion of these issues in clinic environments through focus groups or other means of enabling group discussions.

Epidemiological measures of the effect of these interventions would reflect, then, not only the acceptability of the program but also the efficacy of the intervention in reducing disease occurrence. Without the ethnographic studies, an inability to detect an effective intervention could be due to the underlying unacceptability of a truly useful strategy that had been applied to the wrong population.

CONCLUSION

The integration of qualitative with quantitative studies enables a more cost-effective identification of research directions. The focus in ethnographic study is on specific sexual and risk-taking behaviors, as well as on normative and attitudinal factors in the experience of particular populations. A preliminary ethnographic study provides a feasibility study, a hypothesis-generating capability, and language elicitation for instrument design and for defining important dimensions of behavior. Continuing presence in the community enables identification of cultural acceptability of interventions as well as what interventions would be unacceptable, and finally, ensures involvement of target group members in the development of educational materials and interventions. The larger objective of the study is to use the methods in identifying risky behaviors, language, and domains of concern to improve the validity of methods of an epidemiological study.

LITERATURE CITED

1. **Agar, M. A.** 1985. *Speaking of Ethnography. Sage University Paper Series on Quantitative Research Methods,* vol. 2. Sage Publications, Beverly Hills, Calif.
2. **Agar, M. A.** 1986. *The Professional Stranger: an Informal Introduction to Ethnography.* Academic Press, Inc., New York.
3. **Amaro, H.** 1990. Women's reproductive rights in the age of AIDS: new threats to informed choice. *Genet. Resource* **5:**39–44.
4. **Bongaarts, J.** 1978. A framework for analyzing the proximate determinants of fertility. *Popul. Dev. Rev.* **4:**105–132.
5. **Catania, J. A.** 1990. The AIDS epidemic: quantitative assessment. *In* A. Chouinard and J. Albert (ed.), *Human Sexuality: Research Perspectives in a World Facing AIDS.* The International Development Research Centre 1DRC-MR269e, Ottowa, Ontario, Canada.
6. **Catania, J. A., D. R. Gibson, D. D. Chitwood, and T. J. Coates.** 1990. Methodological problems in AIDS behavioral research: influences on measurement error and participation bias in studies of sexual behavior. *Psychol. Bull.* **108:**339–362.
7. **Davis, K., and J. Blake.** 1956. Social structure and fertility: an analytic framework. *Econ. Dev. Cultural Change* **4:**211–235.
8. **DeBuono, B. A., S. H. Zinner, M. Daamen, and W. M. McCormack.** 1990. Sexual behavior of college women in 1975, 1986 and 1989. *N. Engl. J. Med.* **322:**821–825.
9. **Drew, W. L., M. Blair, R. C. Miner, and M. Conant.** 1990. Evaluation of the virus permeability of a new condom for women. *Sex. Transm. Dis.* **17:**110–112.
10. **Ehrhardt, A. A.** 1988. Preventing and treating AIDS: the expertise of the behavioral sciences. *Bull. N.Y. Acad. Med.* **64:**513–519.
11. **Fullilove, M. T., R. E. Fullilove, K. Haynes, and S. Gross.** 1990. Black women and AIDS prevention: a view towards understanding the gender rules. *J. Sex Res.* **27:**47–64.
12. **Hammel, E. A.** 1990. A theory of culture for demography. *Popul. Dev. Rev.* **16:**455–485.
13. **Marshall, J. F.** 1977. Acceptability of fertility regulating methods: designing technology to fit people. *Prev. Med.* **6:**65–73.
14. **Newman, L. F.** 1990. Ethnographic approaches to AIDS: understanding contact, transmission, and prevention. *In* S. J. Blumenthal, A. Eichler, and G. Weissman (ed.), *Women and AIDS: Promoting Healthy Behavior.* National Institute of Mental Health, Washington, D.C.
15. **Newman, L. F. (ed.) with J. Nyce.** 1985. *Women's Medicine: a Study of Indigenous Fertility Regulating Methods.* Rutgers University Press, New Brunswick, N.J.
16. **Page, J. B., D. L. Chitwood, P. C. Smith, N. Kane, and D. C. McBride.** 1990. Intravenous drug use and HIV infection in Miami. *Med. Anthropol. Q.* **4:**56–71.
17. **Singer, M., C. Flones, L. Davison, G. Burke, Z. Castillo, K. Scanlon, and M. Rivera.** 1990. SIDA: the economic, social, and cultural context of AIDS among Latinos. *Med. Anthropol. Q.* **4:**72–79.
18. **Stein, Z. A.** 1990. HIV prevention: the need for methods women can use. *Am. J. Public Health* **80:**460–462.
19. **Zierler, S., D. Laufer, L. Feingold, I. Kantrowitz, C. Carpenter, and K. Mayer.** 1990. Heterosexual behavior and HIV infection: the New England Behavioral Health Study. *Rhode Island Med. J.* **73:**285–292.

Behavioral Interventions for Prevention and Control of Sexually Transmitted Diseases Including HIV Infection

Approaches to Sexually Transmitted Disease Control in North America and Western Europe

Edward W. Hook III

As discussed earlier in this monograph, efforts to control sexually transmitted diseases (STDs) may be divided into those that attempt to prevent acquisition of infection (primary prevention) and those that attempt to prevent development of complications and interrupt transmission from already-infected individuals to sexual partners (secondary prevention) (4) (Table 1). In practice, there is often overlap between these two types of prevention, and successful primary or secondary prevention efforts may also accomplish the goal of tertiary prevention—attempting to minimize the effects of STD complications and their sequelae. While primary prevention efforts may originate from a wide variety of sources, secondary prevention, which relies heavily on diagnosis and therapy to accomplish its goals, is largely the responsibility of health care providers and public health programs.

Despite the obvious potential benefits to be derived from STD control efforts, there are few if any examples of nations that have successfully eliminated STDs or kept their populations free of STDs for sustained periods. A number of different strategies for STD control have been developed and, in some instances, implemented with partial success; however, important questions regarding approaches to STD control and their applicability from pathogen to pathogen remain. This chapter reviews the various approaches currently utilized or suggested as part of efforts to control STDs, discusses how different biological characteristics of STD pathogens have an impact on their susceptibility to control strategies, and describes and comments on the role of dedicated STD clinics in efforts to control STDs in North America and Western Europe.

Approaches to STD control, as well as prioritization of which STDs to emphasize for control, vary from nation to nation and are influenced by variables such as the distribution and perceived importance of the diseases, the prevailing systems of health care, and health care resources (6). In developing countries, as pointed out by Piot and Laga (this volume), until recently other health care issues such as diseases of children and malnutrition have received primary emphasis by public health specialists. Only since recognition and appreciation of the significance of the ongoing epidemic of human immunodeficiency virus (HIV) infection and its sequela, AIDS, has STD prevention become a public health priority for developing nations. In North America and Western Europe, however, where resources have been greater, organized STD control efforts have been carried out since early in the

Edward W. Hook III – Johns Hopkins University School of Medicine and Clinical STD Services, Baltimore City Health Department, Baltimore, Maryland 21205.

Table 1. Potential STD control measures for North America and Western Europe

Primary prevention
Health education and counseling
General population
Targeted risk groups
Health care professionals
Vaccines
Secondary prevention
Screening programs
Provision of care (diagnosis and therapy)
Assurance of treatment efficacy (susceptibility monitoring)
Partner notification
Mass treatment

20th century, when campaigns to prevent the spread of infectious syphilis were begun. Currently, in some Western European nations and some parts of rural America, responsibility for STD diagnosis and treatment is distributed among all medical care providers, while in other European nations and urban North America, specialized STD clinics are available to provide STD diagnostic and treatment services (6).

The quality of STD diagnosis and therapy, whether practiced by health care providers working in dedicated STD clinics or in the context of other settings (e.g., general practice, family planning or obstetrics and gynecology clinics, etc.), may vary greatly. Barriers to optimal STD diagnosis and prevention efforts in non-STD clinic settings include the problems that providers may not be versed in current standards of STD care; that they may be uncomfortable taking an STD history; or that they may erroneously assume that their patients are not at risk for STD. Even in some STD clinics, because of the belief that care of STD patients is an undesirable task, some providers may be working in those locations because of their need for employment, rather than by desire. In addition, because STD clinics are often judged by the numbers of patients seen rather than the quality of care provided, providers working in such settings are sometimes pressured to see patients quickly, possibly at the expense of time spent in counseling and explanations regarding their patients' problems. In some countries, specialized STD clinics devote a large proportion of their efforts to care of potential high-frequency transmitters such as prostitutes or (more so in the past than presently) homosexually active men, while others serve a broader mix of patients (6).

Temporal trends in national STD morbidity are often used to guide decisions regarding the allocation of funding for STD control and prioritization of individual STDs for resource utilization. In the United Kingdom and Sweden, where most STDs and STD syndromes are reportable and where reporting is relatively complete, public health strategists are able to use these data to direct STD control efforts. In most other nations, however, reporting is not required or, if required, is often incomplete. In the United States, reporting of gonorrhea, syphilis, chancroid, and AIDS is sought by the U.S. Public Health Service, while information on patients with chlamydia, HIV infection, and most other STDs and STD syndromes is not. In addition, U.S. STD clinic attendees tend to be disproportionately lower socioeconomic status minority residents of urban areas. It is estimated that only about one-half of all diagnosed cases of reportable STDs (primarily gonorrhea and syphilis) are actually reported to the U.S. Public Health Service. Reporting from public facilities is usually more complete than reporting from private sources. About one-half of reported STD cases originate from publically funded facilities such as STD clinics, while the remainder (but a smaller proportion of the total cases seen in these settings) are from other sources of health care (e.g., hospitals, private medical offices and clinics). As a result, national figures reporting U.S. STD morbidity disproportionately reflect epidemiological trends among the lower socioeconomic class patients served by public facilities. The lack of accurate population-based data on STD prevalence relegates public health officials to basing their control strategies on estimates of the burden of STDs and their distribution within the population.

STD control efforts are also influenced by the origins of the funds that pay for them. Although in some locations patients are expected to pay for STD treatment, the funds collected support only a small part of the measures needed for comprehensive efforts to control STDs. The costs of educational efforts, partner notification programs, STD screening programs, and diagnostic and therapeutic quality assurance programs cannot be readily paid for by individual patients. Further complicating the issue, STDs tend to be concentrated among hard-to-reach members of communities who may not have the resources or appreciate the need to pay for STD-related care, i.e., individuals who are asymptomatically infected and members of core groups of high-frequency transmitters such as prostitutes or persons with limited access to health care (12, 13, 18). Irrespective of the organization of the medical care system, because of the importance of these hard-to-reach core group members for STD endemicity, as well as the tendency for STDs to concentrate in lower socioeconomic groups, governmental public health agencies tend to bear a disproportionate burden for organizing and implementing secondary STD prevention and control efforts in most industrialized countries.

Few nations have sufficient resources to allow them to spend an equal effort to control all STDs. In addition, only in recent years has there been sufficient knowledge beyond simple reports of incidence to begin to prioritize control efforts for the expanding spectrum of STD pathogens based on their vulnerability to intervention efforts and their relative public health importance. Early in the 20th century, syphilis was the first disease in the United States to be systematically approached from the perspective of public health disease control efforts. In the late 1960s and early 1970s, a national gonorrhea control program was embarked on, using the methods that had been previously applied to syphilis. More recently, there has been discussion of development of a national chlamydia control initiative; however, a number of factors, including limited financial resources, have hindered nationwide implementation. Since the mid-1980s, following recognition of HIV as the causative agent of AIDS, control of this lethal STD has become the highest STD control priority for U.S. public health officials, with at least a portion of the funding for these efforts being derived from funds previously utilized for control of other STDs. The effect of the reallocation of funds from gonorrhea and syphilis control efforts to HIV prevention has been a subject of debate. Some experts attribute at least a portion of recent declines in gonorrhea rates observed in North America (2) and Western Europe to behavioral changes resulting from increased knowledge about HIV and the desire not to acquire it, while others have taken an opposing view, attributing the dramatic increases in U.S. syphilis rates since 1985 to the effects of decreased funding for syphilis control. Given the nonhomogeneous distribution and epidemiological differences between these two diseases, it is possible that both perspectives are, at least in part, correct.

BIOLOGICAL CONSIDERATIONS REGARDING STD PATHOGENS

As discussed elsewhere in this volume (Anderson; Brunham and Ronald), for sexually transmitted infectious diseases to be sustained within communities, each case must generate at least one new case; i.e., the disease must have a reproductive rate exceeding 1.0, otherwise the disease will "burn itself out." The amount by which a disease's reproductive rate exceeds (or is below) 1.0 determines how rapidly the disease will spread within (or be eliminated from) the community. The success of STD control efforts in turn could be assessed by the magnitude of their effect on STD reproductive rates, with the magnitude of such changes in turn being reflected by temporal STD trends.

Theoretically, prioritization of STD control efforts should incorporate careful consideration of the different biological characteristics of the various STD pathogens since those characteristics influence each disease's relative vulnerability to different intervention strategies. A number of biological characteristics of STD pathogens influence their reproductive rate and thus the potential utility of different control efforts (Table 2). These biological parameters include transmission efficiency, incubation time between acquisition of infection and transmissibility, the clinical manifestations of infection (e.g., the presence and severity of symptoms, owing to their impact on an individual's impetus to seek diagnosis and therapy), and other characteristics of the natural history of an infection (7). More efficiently transmitted infections can contribute to rapid increases in disease incidence through the activities of potential high-frequency transmitters such as prostitutes. In these instances, control efforts that reduce transmission by core group members may rapidly affect STD incidence. On the other hand, diseases with lower efficiencies of transmission, requiring multiple exposures for transmission, are likely to spread more slowly and be less concentrated within communities; once established, these diseases may also be more difficult to control. The infectivity of different STD pathogens may vary in terms of likelihood of transmission following a single exposure. Emerging data suggest that despite similarities in their modes of transmission and the clinical spectrum caused by the two infections, transmission of gonorrhea is more efficient than transmission of chlamydia (11). Infectivity may also vary from pathogen to pathogen over the natural history of untreated

Table 2. Biological factors affecting the utility of STD control efforts

STD	Incubation period (days)	Prominence of symptoms	Susceptible to curative or preventive therapy
Syphilis (*T. pallidum*)	10–90	+ +	Yes
Gonorrhea (*N. gonorrhoeae*)	2–5	+ + + (males) + + (females)	Yes
Chlamydia (*C. trachomatis*)	7–14	+ + (males) + (females)	Yes Yes
Herpes simplex virus	4–21	+ + to + + + (50–70% of first episodes are asymptomatic)	No
HIV	14–49	Acquisition usually asymptomatic	No
Human papillomavirus	60–90	+ (80–90% of patients are asymptomatic)	No
Hepatitis B virus	30–60 (following mucosal route of infection, shorter for parenterally acquired disease)	+	No (other than passive immunotherapy for exposed individuals)

infection. The infectivity of syphilis is greatest early in the disease, when infectious cutaneous and mucosal lesions are most often present, and declines to nearly zero in individuals infected for more than 2 years, who rarely have potentially infectious cutaneous manifestations of disease. In contrast, for HIV infection, following a relatively brief period of high infectivity soon after acquisition of infection, infectivity is thought to decline, only to gradually increase over the course of the disease.

Several additional biological parameters also influence STD incidence rates and the vulnerability of those STDs to intervention efforts. STDs vary with respect to the time between disease acquisition and the time at which an individual is infectious to sex partners (incubation periods). Short incubation times translate to a need for more rapid identification and treatment of exposed individuals if such efforts are to be employed to help prevent these individuals from, in turn, transmitting infection to other sex partners. Postexposure preventive therapy is more likely to be an effective control measure for individuals exposed to sex partners who have STDs with long incubation periods than for STDs with short incubation times. For example, the short (2- to 5-day) period between exposure and infectiousness of gonorrhea probably represents a far greater challenge to efforts to prevent transmission through interventions directed at recently exposed sex partners than the longer incubation times of more slowly dividing STD pathogens such as *Chlamydia trachomatis* or *Treponema pallidum* (syphilis).

The prevalence and severity of clinical manifestations of infection also influence STD epidemiology and control efforts in important ways. Most STDs begin with "presymptomatic" periods during which individuals have not yet become symptomatic and thus may transmit infection unknowingly. In addition, for most STDs, a proportion of infected individuals remain asymptomatic for prolonged periods. The greater the proportion of individuals with asymptomatic infection, the more readily the disease will be transmitted and spread within the community (12). Finally, there may be differences in the prevalence of disease symptoms and/or their specificity between men and women infected with the same pathogen. Again, gonorrhea and chlamydia illustrate these principles; symptoms are more prominent and asymptomatic infections are less common in patients with gonorrhea than in patients with chlamydia (7). In addition, women with either infection are more likely to be asymptomatic than men. Similarly, while some STDs are typically associated with prominent symptoms that may even make sexual activity painful (e.g., the genital ulcerations associated with classical initial outbreaks of genital herpes or chancroid), others more typically cause little or no discomfort (the ulcerations associated with syphilis or recurrent genital herpes). Diseases with less prominent symptoms or a higher proportion of asymptomatically infected individuals are better detected through screening of individuals at risk or by efforts to locate, evaluate, and treat sexual contacts of identified cases.

Finally, the success of STD control efforts is also shaped by the differential susceptibilities of STD agents to curative antimicrobial therapy or therapy to prevent development of infection (and transmissibility) in individuals who are exposed but still incubating those STDs. In general, bacterial STDs, such as those caused by *Neisseria gonorrhoeae*, *C. trachomatis*, *T. pallidum*, *Haemophilus ducreyi*, etc., are susceptible to antimicrobial agents that can modify subsequent infectivity. Clinically significant antimicrobial resistance leading to treatment failures has been described for *N. gonorrhoeae* and *H. ducreyi*. Although it has not yet clearly contributed to increased treatment failure rates, resistance of *C. trachomatis* and *T. pallidum* to antimicrobial agents commonly used for therapy of these pathogens has been described as well. In contrast, viral STDs (HIV, herpes simplex virus, human papillomavirus, etc.) are chronic infections that are not currently susceptible to curative antimicrobial therapy and thus are associated with prolonged, sometimes lifelong infectivity, thereby limiting the utility of medications as measures to help control the spread of the diseases.

APPROACHES TO STD CONTROL

Optimally, efforts to control STDs should be multifaceted. They should encourage individuals to avoid behaviors likely to result in disease acquisition and transmission, identify infected individuals by screening for education and therapy, and ensure that therapies utilized for STD treatment are optimally effective. Health education is also important to help individuals at risk identify themselves, to inform individuals of the variability of risk associated with specific sexual practices, and to facilitate making choices regarding behavioral changes to reduce the likelihood of STD acquisition. In addition, effective educational efforts may help individuals appreciate signs or symptoms of infection that might otherwise be overlooked. The explosion of information regarding HIV and AIDS and the rapidly increasing levels of knowledge about the disease among diverse population groups are ample testimony to the ability of programs to educate large portions of the population. A more important question is whether or not such increases in knowledge translate into altered behavior and therefore help to reduce rates of disease acquisition and transmission.

Identification of individuals with sexually transmitted infections also plays an important role in efforts to control these diseases. Infected individuals can be detected by a number of different approaches. These include screening of individuals at high risk for STD (10), utilization of syndromic diagnosis and treatment to increase the availability and rapidity of STD treatment, partner notification efforts to inform asymptomatic or mildly symptomatic infected individuals who might not otherwise seek care to do so, or occasionally even the utilization of mass treatment to try to eradicate a reservoir of infected individuals from groups identified to have a high prevalence of STD.

Role of Dedicated STD Clinics in STD Control

The role of STD clinics in efforts to control STDs goes beyond the obvious role of providing diagnosis and therapy for infected patients. The staffs of dedicated STD clinics often have specialized training and ready access to tests that enable them to arrive at accurate diagnoses for patients with genitourinary complaints at the time of clinic attendance, attributes that make them particularly efficient sites for timely, accurate STD diagnosis and therapy. Because STD clinics by and large serve the needs of patients at increased risk for STDs relative to the general population, they also provide access to a population in need of primary prevention efforts to reduce their risk for subsequent STD acquisition. Since many patients attending STD clinics have recently acquired the treatable STDs diagnosed at the time of clinic attendance, clinicians have the opportunity to emphasize to patients their vulnerability for future STD acquisition, pointing out that future risk for STD includes potential acquisition of untreatable as well as treatable STDs. In some STD clinics, nonclinician staff members are utilized to supplement STD counseling and risk reduction efforts, often at the time of efforts to promote partner referral or obtain information for partner notification efforts. Furthermore, STD clinic attendance may provide the opportunity to screen for otherwise inapparent STDs that may be present alone or concomitant with the other problems that brought the patient to the clinic. The practice of routine serological screening for infections such as latent syphilis or HIV results in identification of substantial numbers of these infections among patients attending STD clinics for other reasons. In addition, STD clinics provide systematically collected data on disease trends within communities. Finally, in nations in which partner notification is utilized as part of disease intervention efforts, patients attending STD clinics often serve as the point of initiation for such efforts (see below).

However, while STD clinics have the capacity to make important contributions to STD control efforts both for the individual and on a programmatic level, they have several shortcomings. Not the least of these is that they generally derive their funding from governmental or other public funding sources and, as a result, tend to be susceptible to funding shifts that in turn may lead to troublesome fluctuation in the availability of program resources. In addition, because of their acknowledged role as sites for STD diagnosis and care, attendance at dedicated STD clinics is sometimes considered embarrassing by persons who might benefit from utilization of available services. Consequently, some asymptomatic high-risk patients assiduously avoid visits to such facilities, missing the potential benefits of screening. Symptomatic patients likewise sometimes prefer to seek care at other sites, where there may be less expertise in STD diagnosis or where the results of diagnostic testing may not be as readily available, resulting in inaccurate diagnoses and/or delays in initiation of therapy. Still more troublesome is the fact that some individuals, rather than seeking care from health professionals, attempt self-treatment, a practice that may fail to cure their infection, that has been linked to development of antimicrobial resistance, and that fails to address the problem of possible infection in recent sex partners. Finally, there is little information as to whether STD clinics succeed in their roles as sites for efforts at primary prevention. The problem-oriented nature of most care provided in STD clinics results in the inability of STD control programs to document the success of their primary prevention efforts while providing a continuing and potentially demoralizing reminder of patients in whom such efforts fail.

The operation of STD clinics varies substantially, both from area to area within countries and from country to country. In the United States, STD control programs are funded and coordinated on a national level by the U.S. Public Health Service (the Centers for Disease Control), working through state and local health departments. National STD treatment guidelines and control priorities are periodically updated through cooperative efforts between Centers for Disease Control staff and national expert committees composed of representatives of local health departments and universities. Thus, while regional programs may vary with respect to prioritization of STD control efforts, they do so as part of a nationally coordinated effort. In contrast, in the United Kingdom, there is no nationally coordinated STD control program. Rather, each department of genitourinary medicine is autonomous, with its priorities and treatment protocols determined by the consultant physicians who direct the clinics.

STD Control Efforts in Non-STD Clinic Settings

STD diagnosis and therapy are also provided in a wide variety of settings other than dedicated STD clinics, including emergency rooms, walk-in clinics, private physicians' offices, and other specialty clinics (e.g., family planning, prenatal, urology, dermatology, etc). STD screening is likewise often practiced in a variety of non-STD clinic settings (3, 10). For example, screening for syphilis, gonorrhea, and sometimes chlamydia is often a component of routine family planning and prenatal care. While there has been considerable effort to assess the utility of and most efficient strategies for providing STD care in these settings, there has been relatively little formal assessment of the frequency with which this care is actually provided, the quality of the care provided, or its effectiveness. Likewise, there appears to be substantial variation among providers in these settings as to their investment in primary and secondary prevention efforts. Characterization and quantification of STD control efforts in non-STD clinic settings should be a priority for future research efforts.

Partner Notification for STD Control

Partner notification or contact tracing has been suggested to have a number of potential benefits as a method for STD control. For curable bacterial STDs, it provides opportunities to identify and treat asymptomatically infected individuals who would otherwise not be treated, thereby preventing further transmission to new sexual partners (3, 15). For gonorrhea or chlamydia, it leads to treatment of asymptomatic infected female partners of men with proven infection, preventing complications such as salpingitis or its sequelae, infertility and ectopic pregnancy. For exposed individuals who do not have microbiological evidence (culture or serological test data) of infection, partner notification may also permit administration of prophylactic treatment for incubating STDs. Even for diseases for which there is currently no curative therapy, such as herpesvirus or HIV infections, evaluation of exposed sexual partners may have several benefits. For exposed partners who have not yet acquired infection, identification provides the opportunity for risk reduction counseling to reduce the likelihood of subsequent acquisition of infection (e.g., abstinence, condom use, etc.). Asymptomatically infected partners of identified persons with incurable infections may benefit by permitting those individuals to avoid transmission of infection to others, as well as by permitting them to seek therapeutic options that, although not curative, may be beneficial. For instance, HIV-infected individuals identified through partner notification have the opportunity to avail themselves of therapies that have been shown to slow progression of disease (zidovudine) and to be prophylactic against development of complicating infections such as *Pneumocystis carinii* pneumonia.

Partner notification may be accomplished by direct referral of sex partners by infected individuals or through the mediation of public health professionals trained to accomplish this task while preserving the confidentiality of the index case (14, 17). (Although neither common nor a new problem, the desire to preserve the confidentiality of index cases is occasionally in conflict with the duty to warn individuals at risk for continued exposure and, in the AIDS era, requires public health officials to grapple with difficult choices.) In the United States, these individuals, who were previously called public health advisers but are now referred to as disease intervention specialists, are trained to interview infected individuals (the index cases) regarding the identity of or, if the identity is unknown, at least to obtain descriptive locating information about, recent sex partners (contacts). Disease intervention specialists then attempt to locate and inform contacts regarding their exposure and to explain to them the need for evaluation and/or treatment.

Disease intervention specialists work to provide both the index case and his or her contacts with information regarding the importance of STDs (and particularly the STD in question) to their reproductive health and measures that they might pursue to avoid future STD acquisition or exposure (16). Disease intervention specialists must carefully balance their efforts to educate and inform contacts of their risk against the need to preserve the confidentiality of the index case, since it is often the assurance of confidentiality that provides the disease intervention specialist with the ability to obtain pertinent locating information regarding recent sexual contacts.

The utility of partner notification as a method of STD control has been evaluated most completely for gonorrhea and syphilis. Partner notification has been shown to be a useful method for identification of men with asymptomatic gonorrhea (9), and preventive therapy for patients exposed to partners with syphilis has been demonstrated to significantly reduce the proportion of exposed individuals who develop infection (5). Recently, however, as use of illicit drugs has become increasingly linked to gonorrhea and syphilis, the utility of partner notification may have diminished, possibly owing to the increased frequency of transmission of infection to anonymous partners in the context of exchange of sex for drugs or money to purchase them (1, 15).

Vaccines and Mass Treatment for STD Control

Vaccination of individuals at risk for infection and mass treatment of populations with a high prevalence of disease but in whom other control strategies are not effective share the similar goal of trying to effect widespread changes in STD prevalence, thereby substantially diminishing transmission opportunities and leading to reduction in an STD's reproductive rate. Vaccines for the most part remain only theoretical means for reducing risk for STD acquisition. The only STD for which there is currently an effective vaccine is hepatitis B. Unfortunately, to date efforts to implement hepatitis B control programs based on vaccine administration to susceptible individuals have not been successful. Similarly, although theoretically useful, mass treatment programs are rarely employed for STD control. Nonetheless, such strategies might be useful in containing and controlling localized outbreaks within relatively closed communities in which repeated transmission between members of the community sustains the outbreak. Such an approach has been demonstrated to be effective for reducing STD prevalence in the prostitute population and may prove useful for STD control in hard-to-reach groups such as drug users (8).

STD CONTROL AT THE THRESHOLD OF THE 21ST CENTURY

In the nearly 50 years since the end of World War II, knowledge regarding STDs, the agents that cause them, and their sequelae has increased dramatically. In the early 1980s, a new, incurable, probably uniformly fatal STD, AIDS, was described, leading to reappraisal of methods for STD control and their utility.

Currently in North America and Western Europe, secondary STD control has been the responsibility of STD specialists, whose efforts are not uncommonly hampered by limited resources, and of private practitioners, who may be uncomfortable discussing STDs with their patients and who are sometimes not well versed in STD diagnosis and therapy. The design of most current STD control efforts is based on approaches developed to control syphilis, failing to utilize recently available biological and epidemiological data to adapt approaches for control of different STDs to the methods best suited for that purpose.

As described throughout this monograph, for the 1990s and beyond, STD control efforts need to incorporate strategies for primary prevention, to emphasize both behavioral and biological intervention efforts, and to appreciate that STD control is part of the larger effort to improve reproductive health. New strategies for STD control should make efforts to fully integrate other components of reproductive health care, such as contraceptive and family planning measures that may reduce STD risk, screening for genitourinary cancers and conditions that predispose individuals to them, and behavioral efforts to encourage safer sex, into coordinated reproductive health programs that might more efficiently and effectively lead to improved STD control. To accomplish this will require further evolution of current STD control strategies, moving away from the current number-driven, categorical programs that emphasize diagnosis and treatment of disease to efforts that utilize recognized STDs or STD risk as points for initiation of more comprehensive, complete reproductive health care and counseling.

Acknowledgments. I thank Koren Waters for her patience and assistance in manuscript preparation and John Gallwey for his comments and helpful perspective regarding STD control in the United Kingdom and Europe.

LITERATURE CITED

1. **Andrus, J. K., D. W. Fleming, D. R. Harger, Y. Chin, D. V. Bennett, J. H. Horan, G. Oxman, B. Olson, and L. R. Foster.** 1990. Partner notification: can it control epidemic syphilis? *Ann. Intern. Med.* **112:**539–543.
2. **Aral, S. O., and K. K. Holmes.** 1990. Epidemiology of sexual behavior and sexually transmitted diseases, p. 19–44. *In* K. K. Holmes, P.-A. Mardh, P. F. Sparling, P. J. Wiesner, W. Cates, Jr., S. M. Lemon, and W. E. Stamm (ed.), *Sexually Transmitted Diseases*. McGraw-Hill Book Co., New York.
3. **Curran, J. W., M. V. Schrader, J. K. Moyer, M. A. Kramer, J. G. Lossick, and W. E. Brown.** 1980. Gonorrhea in the emergency department: management, case follow-up, and contact tracing of cases in women. *Am. J. Obstet. Gynecol.* **138:**1105–1108.
4. **Ehrhardt, A. A., M. Fishbein, E. Washington, W. Smith, K. K. Holmes, and the NIAID Study Group.** 1990. Issues in designing interventions. *Sex. Transm. Dis.* **17:**204–207.
5. **Hart, G.** 1980. Epidemiologic treatment for syphilis and gonorrhea. *Sex. Transm. Dis.* **7:**149–162.
6. **Hart, G., M. W. Adler, A. Stapinski, T. F. Mroczkowski, and P. Weisner.** 1990. Evaluation of sexually transmitted disease control programs in industrialized countries, p. 1031–1040. *In* K. K. Holmes, P.-A. Mardh, P. F. Sparling, P. J. Wiesner, W. Cates, Jr., S. M. Lemon, and W. E. Stamm (ed.), *Sexually Transmitted Diseases*. McGraw-Hill Book Co., New York.
7. **Hook, E. W., III, C. A. Reichart, P. Ray, L. Bergman, D. D. Celentano, D. M. Upchurch, and T. C. Quinn.** 1990. Comparative epidemiology of gonococcal and chlamydial infections in Baltimore STD clinic patients, p. 580–583. *In* W. R. Bowie, H. D. Caldwell,

R. P. Jones, P.-A. Mardh, G. L. Ridgeway, J. Schachter, W. E. Stamm, and M. E. Ward (ed.), *Chlamydial Infections. Proceedings of the Seventh International Symposium on Human Chlamydial Infections.* Cambridge University Press, Cambridge.

8. **Jaffe, H. W., D. T. Rice, R. Voigt, J. Fowler, and R. K. St. John.** 1979. Selective mass treatment in a venereal disease control program. *Am. J. Public Health* **69:**1181–1182.
9. **Johnson, R. E.** 1979. Epidemiologic and prophylactic treatment of gonorrhea: a decision analysis review. *Sex. Transm. Dis.* **6:**159–167.
10. **Judson, F. N., K. G. Miller, and T. R. Schaffnit.** 1977. Screening for gonorrhea and syphilis in the gay baths—Denver, Colorado. *Am. J. Public Health* **67:**740–742.
11. **Katz, B. P., V. A. Caine, and R. B. Jones.** 1990. Estimation of transmission probabilities for chlamydial infection, p. 567–570. *In* W. R. Bowie, H. D. Caldwell, R. P. Jones, P.-A. Mardh, G. L. Ridgeway, J. Schachter, W. E. Stamm, and M. E. Ward (ed.), *Chlamydial Infections. Proceedings of the Seventh International Symposium on Human Chlamydial Infections.* Cambridge University Press, Cambridge.
12. **May, R. M.** 1981. The transmission and control of gonorrhea. *Nature* (London) **291:**376–377.
13. **Phillips, L., J. J. Potterat, R. B. Rothenberg, C. Pratts, and R. D. King.** 1980. Focused interviewing in gonorrhea control. *Am. J. Public Health* **70:**705–708.
14. **Potterat, J. J., and R. Rothenbert.** 1977. The case-finding effectiveness of a self-referral system for gonorrhea: a preliminary report. *Am. J. Public Health* **67:**174–176.
15. **Potterat, J. J., D. E. Woodhouse, C. I. Pratts, G. S. Markewich, and J. S. Fogle.** 1983. Women contacts of men with gonorrhea: case-finding yields. *Sex. Transm. Dis.* **10:**29–32.
16. **Thin, R. N.** 1984. Health advisers (contact tracers) in sexually transmitted disease. *Br. J. Vener. Dis.* **60:**269–272.
17. **Toomey, K. E., and W. Cates.** 1989. Partner notification for the prevention of HIV infection. *AIDS* **3:**S57–S62.
18. **Yorke, J. A., H. W. Heathcote, and A. Nold.** 1978. Dynamics and control of the transmission of gonorrhea. *Sex. Transm. Dis.* **5:**51–57.

Current Approaches to Sexually Transmitted Disease Control in Developing Countries

Peter Piot and Marie Laga

The health status of the population of the developing world provides a grim picture, as expressed by high infant, child, and maternal mortality rates, low life expectancy, acute and chronic malnutrition, and considerable morbidity from preventable and curable infectious diseases. Most efforts in disease control have focused on communicable diseases of children and on malnutrition. However, there is a growing concern that more attention should be paid to health concerns of adults in the Third World. This is a result of an increasing awareness of the considerable burden of diseases in adults in developing countries (R. G. Feachem, C. Murray, and M. A. Phillips, *The Health of Adults in the Developing World*, in press). Several populations are experiencing a transition from an epidemiological environment dominated by infectious diseases and malnutrition to a disease profile that increasingly involves noncommunicable diseases of adults in a population with a relatively larger proportion of sexually active individuals than in pretransition societies (16).

Until recently, sexually transmitted diseases (STDs) have received very little attention from the public health sector in developing countries. They are at best briefly discussed in papers on public health priorities in the developing world (21). The emergence of human immunodeficiency virus (HIV) infection and AIDS as a major public health problem in many parts of the Third World, better documentation of the economic and social impact of STDs, and the identification of several STDs as risk factors for the spread of HIV are all contributing to a global awareness of the importance of STDs (17, 19, 22; M. Over and P. Piot, *in* D. T. Jamison and W. H. Mosley, ed., *Evolving Health Priorities in Developing Countries*, in press) (see Brunham and Ronald, this monograph).

While the biomedical infrastructure for STD prevention and control is often weak in developing countries, the analogous infrastructure for HIV prevention and control is essentially nonexistent. Therefore, we are focusing on current infrastructure and approaches to STD control, because they are potentially important for behavioral interventions for both HIV infection and other STDs.

This chapter reviews current methods used for the prevention and control of STDs in developing countries, with emphasis on approaches other than behavioral interventions for the latter (see Holmes and Aral, this volume). It should be stressed that there is a wide variation in epidemiological content, health systems,

Peter Piot and Marie Laga – WHO Collaborating Centre on AIDS, Department of Microbiology, Institute of Tropical Medicine, 2000 Antwerp, Belgium.

and policy among the developing countries and that by necessity we have often generalized. Our experience is mostly in Africa, which is the environment discussed in most of this chapter.

THE EPIDEMIOLOGICAL ENVIRONMENT

The epidemiology of STDs in the developing world is reviewed in depth by Brunham and Ronald (this volume), and only some broad features will be mentioned here.

First, prevalence rates for the various STDs are often high, particularly in the cities but also in some rural populations. Because of increased child survival and continuing high population growth rates, the size of the population of adolescents and young adults will increase over the next decades (in contrast to the situation in the Western world). Thus, the sexually active population at risk for STDs will become even larger than at present.

Second, the incidence of severe complications and sequelae of STDs in women and neonates is significantly higher than in the industrialized world as a result of both high infection rates and inadequate management of STDs in women (22).

Third, in many populations of the Third World, particularly in sub-Saharan Africa, the Caribbean, Latin America, and some parts of Asia, HIV infection is a major problem as well. It is mainly spread through heterosexual contact in the very populations that already have high rates of STDs.

A fourth feature is the poor quality and low accessibility of the health system in general and the inadequate management of patients with STDs in particular. As for other health problems, epidemiological surveillance data are usually poorly developed.

Finally, STD control has not been a political priority for most countries and development agencies, and very few countries have a functioning STD control program. Lack of awareness of the problem of STDs and their sequelae, competition for resources to control other important health problems, and, in some cases, reluctance to deal with diseases transmitted by sex have all played a role. This situation now seems to be changing rapidly in many countries as a result of the launching of AIDS control programs, although the problem of resource allocation for STD and HIV control compared with other health problems has not been resolved.

GOALS AND OBJECTIVES OF STD CONTROL

The major goals of STD control are (i) the prevention of infection and (ii) the prevention of the development of complications of STDs through early detection and treatment.

Traditionally, STD control has put most emphasis on the latter (secondary prevention). However, primary prevention is receiving increased (and sometimes even exclusive) attention, because of the emergence of incurable viral STDs, particularly HIV infection. The importance of secondary prevention as a control strategy is one of the major current differences in approach between STD and AIDS control. But because of the recent identification of STDs as a risk factor for HIV transmission, lowering levels of STDs in some populations should become an important part of AIDS control programs.

The goals of STD control can be achieved through strategies such as (i) reducing exposure to infection by health education and promotion of condoms; (ii) providing adequate diagnostic and treatment facilities for STD patients; (iii) limiting complications by early detection (case finding and screening and adequate treatment); and (iv) limiting further transmission by counseling and partner referral (14). In practice, activities under these strategies are interdependent.

BEHAVIORAL INTERVENTIONS

Interventions to prevent the transmission of STDs through changes in sexual behavior should be an integral part of any STD control program. Unfortunately, such interventions have traditionally been neglected in favor of management of patients with STD. However, they currently receive much attention within AIDS prevention programs and will undoubtedly also have an impact on the incidence of STDs. Strategies and issues on this important topic are discussed by Smith (this volume).

In addition to health promotion as a strategy for the primary prevention of STDs and HIV infection, developing health care-seeking behavior to promote early diagnosis and treatment of STD is an important strategy in STD control (see Amaro and Gornemann, this volume). These activities are usually not part of HIV-oriented health promotion and are often a much-neglected part of STD control in the developing world.

A striking feature of behavioral interventions for STD control is the lack of coordination between STD and AIDS prevention efforts in many countries. As mentioned in a World Health Organization consensus statement, a combined health promotion strategy to prevent STD and HIV infection is more cost-effective and is synergistic for both programs (24).

There are other programs for which coordination is needed. For example, family planning programs reach sexually active individuals eligible for targeted health promotion for STD prevention. Maternal and child health (MCH) programs promote early presentation of pregnant women at antenatal clinics in a successful program to control neonatal syphilis.

SOME CHARACTERISTICS OF CLINICAL SERVICES FOR STDs

The confidence of the public in a program and the image of STD control depend to a great extent on the effectiveness of clinical services for STDs.

For many decades, adequate management of STD patients has been the cornerstone of STD control. The major public health aims are to reduce the duration of infectivity and the risk of development of complications.

The main objectives of clinical management are to provide diagnosis (ideally etiological diagnosis) and treatment, to offer counseling on STD prevention through behavior change and condom use, to encourage treatment of patients' sex partners, and to screen for other STDs, including HIV infection (3, 13, 14).

Types of Services

STD management may be provided at all levels of the health care system. In most developing countries, most patients with STDs are seen in primary health care settings, where they represent one of the commonest causes of medical consultations. The private medical sector as well as an informal sector (pharmacists, nurses and healers, vendors) plays a very important role in STD care in many countries.

Several countries have opted for some type of vertical system for STD management. In a fully vertical system (such as in Senegal), categorical STD clinics function in parallel with the primary health care system and are responsible for the care of patients with STDs at all levels of the health system.

Some countries (e.g., Zambia) are building a network of STD clinics at the district level for referral of patients who fail to respond to syndromic management at the primary health care level. In other countries, such as Kenya, public categorical clinics staffed by a specialist exist in the major cities. Such clinics function both as a primary care facility and as a referral center for STD patients. They may also be responsible for the first-line treatment of STDs detected in primary care facilities such as MCH and family planning clinics (e.g., neonates with ophthalmia neonatorum or congenital syphilis, pregnant women with a reactive syphilis serology, women with pelvic inflammatory disease).

Many countries have no specialized STD clinics, and STDs are treated throughout the regular health care system. Most care is delivered by paramedical personnel, using clinical algorithms for diagnosis and therapy.

Whatever the official system for STD control is in a country, the private sector (using either Western or traditional approaches) often bears a major share of STD management. For instance, among 1,200 female prostitutes participating in a survey in Kinshasa, Zaire, 87% had signs and symptoms suggestive of an STD during the last year, but only 32% had visited an official health care facility (M. Laga, N. Nzila, and A. Manoka, unpublished data). However, hardly any information is available on sources of health care for STD-related problems in the developing world and on the effectiveness of non-medically approved practices, such as self-medication and treatment by traditional healers. Reasons to prefer the more expensive private sector may include lack of confidence in the public health care sector in general, health providers' attitudes, poor quality of public clinics, and fear of lack of confidentiality. The common attitude of STD control programs has been to fight the private and certainly the traditional sector. It may be rewarding to explore the possibility of involving and training drug sellers and traditional healers in STD diagnosis, treatment, and counseling, following the model of traditional birth attendants.

Advantages and Disadvantages of Horizontal and Vertical Programs

From the point of view of STD control, categorical and fully integrated clinical services both have their disadvantages. An optimal approach will depend on a variety of local conditions, particularly the existing health system and the incidence of STDs. In general, clinical STD services should aim at maximum coverage and good accessibility and ensure the possibility of patient referral, either to a specialized service or to a competent outpatient clinic at the district level.

Vertical clinical services are usually preferred by STD specialists. Their major advantage is the ability to offer a comprehensive spectrum of STD clinical services by personnel with STD expertise. The services offered may include a diagnostic laboratory, prompt treatment with adequate antibiotics, and facilities for counseling and partner notification. In reality, such clinics lack funds, are often understaffed, have poorly trained personnel, lack appropriate drugs and diagnostic reagents, and spend minimal time on counseling.

A major disadvantage of categorical STD clinics is their inherent inability to reach a large, if not the major, proportion of women with an STD, since STDs in women are often asymptomatic and the clinical manifestations of most STDs in women are nonspecific. This implies that women with an STD have no particular reason to go to an STD clinic, although they may decide to go to a general primary health care facility because of urogenital and/or abdominal problems or because of the desire for family planning or antenatal services. Moreover, the laboratory tests required to diagnose the major treatable STDs in women (gonorrhea, chlamydial infection, and syphilis) are often as unavailable in STD clinics as in general primary health care facilities or in private practice. Added to all this, an often misogynistic or stigmatizing attitude in many STD clinics discourages women from returning a second time to such a clinic. STD clinics are probably cost-effective in very large cities where the incidence of STDs is usually higher, but it may be too expensive to organize special facilities in smaller cities and rural areas.

Major disadvantages of general primary health care services for STD care include the low level of technical expertise of the staff, the lack of diagnostic means and of appropriate drugs, and the unavailability of counseling. Some advantages are better accessibility, particularly to women, less stigma, and easier coordination and integration of primary and secondary prevention activities with other programs.

Constraints on Case Management

Counseling and health promotion activities

Because of financial, geographical, and sociocultural barriers, STD referral is a problem in many developing countries. Therefore, STD control programs should attempt to implement simplified and adequate approaches for case management at the primary health care level.

In general, management of patients in primary health care settings is guided by considerations such as the following (7). (i) The diagnosis should use a problem-oriented approach and be based on history, physical examination, and simple laboratory tests, if available. (ii) Investigations should be performed only if they influence the management of the health problem. (iii) The total time spent on one patient usually cannot exceed 5 min. (iv) Therapy should be rational, and treatment regimens should be standardized. (v) Patients should only be referred to a higher level of the health care system when initial management has failed.

It is obvious that it is very hard if not impossible to include health promotion and counseling activities in these 5 min. In addition, most clinics have no room for confidential, face-to-face counseling sessions. There is a need to develop innovative and appropriate approaches to counseling in the context of clinical services in the developing world.

Laboratory services

In general, laboratory services are among the weakest components of the health system in developing countries. A major problem is the availability of diagnostic reagents, which usually have to be bought abroad and paid for in often scarce foreign currency. As for STD diagnosis, even simple tests such as the rapid plasma reagin test for syphilis may not be available at the district level. In some countries, the isolation of *Neisseria gonorrhoeae* (still the standard method for diagnosis of gonorrhea in women) can be performed in only a few laboratories in the capital. Furthermore, most African countries are unable to assess the antibiotic susceptibility of local gonococcal isolates, making the formulation of rational treatment guidelines difficult. Inexpensive, simple, and rapid tests for the diagnosis of gonococcal and chlamydial infections in women are still not available (6a). In practice, all this means that diagnosis of gonorrhea and chlamydial infection in women is rarely possible. In the absence of better alternatives, tests with a very low predictive value, such as a Gram-stained smear for the diagnosis of gonorrhea in women, are still widely used, even at the referral level.

Syndromic approach

Several STD syndromes can be properly managed by using simplified clinical algorithms for diagnosis and treatment (18, 24). They are increasingly used in primary health care settings in the developing world, although they have not been properly evaluated in different clinical settings. An example of a decision tree for the management of genital ulcer disease is shown in Fig. 1. Basic assumptions in this case are that single-dose therapy is preferable, that chancroid is the major cause of genital ulceration and is rarely asymptomatic, that syphilis is the most severe cause in terms of systemic complications, and that most cases of chancroid respond well to the proposed antibiotic. This algorithm also considers the management of the patients' sexual contacts.

Unfortunately, this clinical approach for the diagnosis of gonococcal and chlamydial infections in women is insufficient because of the low sensitivity and specificity of clinical signs and symptoms associated with these infections (1; M. Laga, M. Gernier, I. Lebughe, K. Mahamba, N. Nzila, B. Edidi, F. Behets, R. Ryder, and P. Piot, submitted for publication). The development of simple and inexpensive bacterial antigen detection tests may offer the only solution with a reasonable sensitivity for these two major treatable STDs in women.

Availability of drugs

Drugs recommended for STD treatment should be available where patients are seen. Some of the antimicrobial agents included in the latest World Health

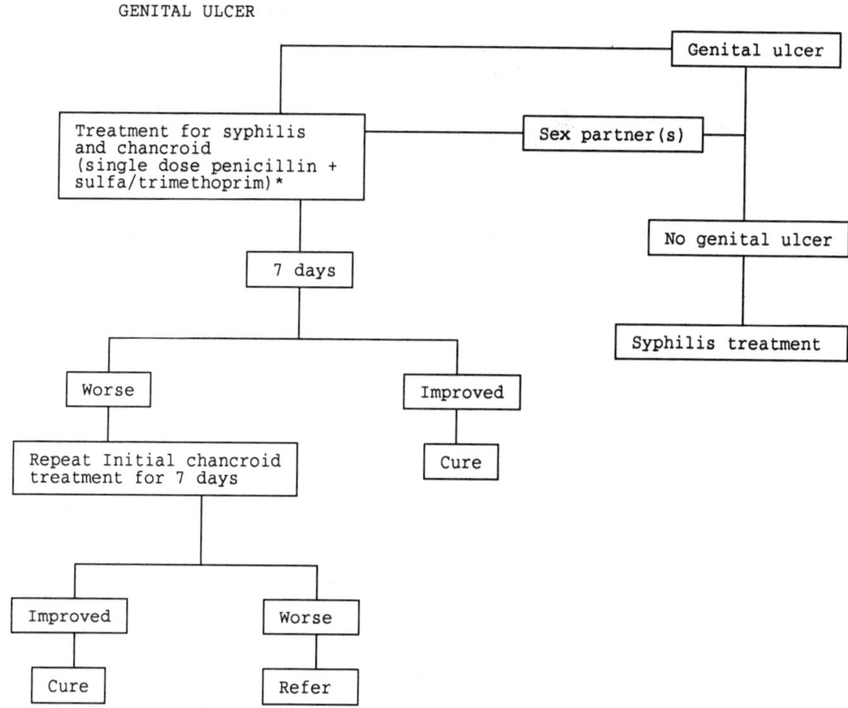

Figure 1. Management of genital ulcer disease in a population in which both syphilis and chancroid are endemic. *, choice depends on local resistance pattern of *H. ducreyi*.

Organization STD treatment guidelines are not part of the Essential Drug List and may not be available through the public system in several developing countries (e.g., the quinolones, which are now recommended as first-choice drugs for the treatment of gonorrhea) (23). Again, this illustrates the need for coordination with other programs. Another severe problem is the spiraling prevalence of antimicrobial resistance among STD pathogens, particularly the gonococcus and *Haemophilus ducreyi*, the causal agent of chancroid. This problem is much more severe in the developing world than in North America and Europe. It is probably related to strong antibiotic pressure and frequent self-medication with common antibiotics for STDs and other diseases. Despite restrictive laws on antibiotic prescription in most countries, antibiotics are easily available in pharmacies, markets, bars, etc. One of the consequences has been the loss of two of the least expensive antibiotics—penicillin and tetracycline—for effective treatment of gonorrhea in most of the developing world.

Partner notification

Some form of partner referral is being recommended by STD control programs for at least gonorrhea and syphilis. As mentioned earlier, this is rarely implemented because of lack of resources and because of sociocultural barriers concerning STDs and sex in general. Patient-initiated partner referral with contact slips has been used with reasonable success in some places, even through regular primary health care centers (12). The feasibility and effectiveness of using primary health care workers in partner notification activities is clearly an underexplored area.

INTERVENTIONS

Several types of interventions against STDs are routinely used in developing countries, but there is still room for increasing their effectiveness, and a critical review of their impact and cost-effectiveness should be performed in each country.

Ocular Prophylaxis at Birth

Eye prophylaxis at birth with silver nitrate was introduced by Credé in 1880 and has often been praised as one of the successes of preventive medicine. It resulted in a spectacular decline in the rate of blindness in young children in Europe, at a time when there was no effective treatment for gonorrhea. Today, this technique remains as valid as in the 19th century and is remarkable for its simplicity and low cost.

Because of high prevalence rates of gonorrhea among pregnant women, particularly in urban populations in much of the Third World, the incidence of gonococcal conjunctivitis in the newborn can be as high as 1 to 5% (8). In populations with a maternal prevalence of gonococcal infection as low as 0.5%, eye prophylaxis at birth with silver nitrate drops or tetracycline ointment is the most cost-effective strategy to prevent gonococcal (but not chlamydial) neonatal conjunctivitis (9) (Table 1). Such prophylaxis is a priority STD control activity in all countries where health care coverage is not optimal, because (i) gonococcal ophthalmia neonatorum is a sight-threatening disease, (ii) effective therapy of established eye infection is expensive and often not available at the primary health care level, and (iii) case finding for gonorrhea in pregnant women is usually not possible.

Despite its proven effectiveness and cost benefit, several developing countries with high rates of gonorrhea are not implementing or even recommending eye prophylaxis at birth. The reasons for this are that some West European countries have abandoned this policy, that silver nitrate often causes (benign) chemical conjunctivitis, and the belief that gonorrhea cases should be detected and treated in women before delivery. This is a tragic example of lack of understanding of the epidemiological reasons for changing a public health policy (the current very low prevalence rate of gonorrhea in pregnant women in Western Europe) and/or of an unrealistic recommendation (case finding for gonorrhea in women when such facilities are not available).

Other obstacles to the implementation of eye prophylaxis at birth include lack of training of midwives and traditional birth attendants in the proper instillation of the product and unavailability of the prophylactic agents. Once more, close

Table 1. Cost of interventions against congenital syphilis and gonococcal ophthalmia neonatorum per 1,000 pregnant women (in U.S. dollars) (from references 6 and 8)

Breakdown	Intervention cost	
	Screening pregnant women for syphilis	Eye prophylaxis at birth with tetracycline ointment
Tests	\$200	\$ 0
Treatment or prophylaxis	\$200	\$60
Training and educational material	\$100	\$ 5
Miscellaneous equipment	\$100	\$ 0
Cost per 1,000 women	\$600	\$65
Cost per woman	\$ 0.60	\$ 0.06
Cost of averting a case of adverse outcome	\$ 12[a]	\$ 1.40[b] \$11[c]

[a] Prevalence of maternal syphilis in the study was 8%; adverse outcomes: abortion (17 cases), perinatal deaths (19), congenital syphilis (14), low birth weight (16), premature delivery (5).
[b] Prevalence of maternal gonorrhea of 10%.
[c] Prevalence of maternal gonorrhea of 1%.

collaboration between the MCH and STD programs is a prerequisite for successful implementation.

Early Disease Detection

General population

Since many individuals with STDs, particularly women, may be asymptomatic for a long period, they will not seek early medical care. Yet they are infectious for their sex contacts. Women may transmit the infection to their fetus or newborn and are at risk for developing severe complications. Such persons can be identified through early detection efforts.

Early detection activities may consist of (i) promotion of health care-seeking behavior; (ii) availability of diagnostic tests for STDs at the primary health care level; (iii) case finding programs (i.e., disease detection by STD testing of patients who present for other health problems); and (iv) screening programs (i.e., active testing of populations).

Testing all pregnant women for syphilis and prompt treatment of seroreacters is a classic example of case finding and has been a successful strategy for the control of congenital syphilis. It is cost-effective, even in populations with prevalence rates as low as 0.01% (20), and it is officially recommended in virtually all developing countries. Unfortunately, this intervention is inconsistently implemented, even in countries with active syphilis prevalence rates as high as 15 to 25% among pregnant women. The major reasons for this include low awareness of the problem among public health officials and health care workers, unavailability of serological tests, poor organization of the intervention, and poor rates of antenatal clinic attendance in general or during early pregnancy.

Figure 2 shows how such a program is organized in one major city that has a categorical STD clinical service. Supposing that she follows the flow chart, and supposing that all steps are correctly performed, a seroreactive woman has to go at least three times to two different clinics, one of which (the STD clinic) will most likely be far away from her home. At least three different facilities of the health system are involved, but no particular health care worker is responsible for the process. It is no surprise that many women with syphilis are not detected or treated at delivery in such a system.

To be successful, a program to control congenital syphilis must be integrated into MCH care and should test and treat pregnant women during a single antenatal visit. Zambia is successfully implementing such a program, which in addition aims at increasing early (before 16 weeks of pregnancy) attendance at antenatal clinics through targeted health education (6). Although antenatal clinic attendance, screening, and treatment are still suboptimal, the intervention has reduced syphilitic adverse outcomes by two-thirds. The cost of each prenatal screening in this program is U.S. $0.60 (including training, equipment, and health education materials), with a cost of $12 for each case averted (Table 1).

In many populations with moderate to high prevalence rates, case finding for gonococcal and genital chlamydial infections in pregnant women is also a cost-effective intervention to prevent low birth weight, premature delivery, postpartum infections, and neonatal conjunctivitis and pneumonia. However, for fiscal and logistic reasons, and because of lack of appropriate diagnostic tests, such case finding is only rarely practiced.

High-risk groups

Regular STD screening of female prostitutes is performed in several countries and even legally required in some. This may be the only STD control activity in some countries and is usually politically popular. However, the impact on the incidence of STDs and the cost benefit of such programs have not been evaluated. The STD detection methods used are often questionable (i.e., Gram-stained blind cervicovaginal smear), and the approach may have a stigmatizing effect. There is often also a lack of primary prevention activities such as promotion and distribution of condoms.

Figure 3 shows the impact of monthly gonococcal culture followed by treatment with spectinomycin in infected women on the monthly incidence of gonorrhea in a large group of prostitutes in Kinshasa, Zaire (Laga et al., unpublished data). Although there seems to be over a 50% reduction in monthly incidence, the intervention appears insufficient for further decreases in the incidence of gonorrhea, despite intensive promotion of condom use. It may be that, to be effective, screening and treatment must be complemented by behavioral interventions and

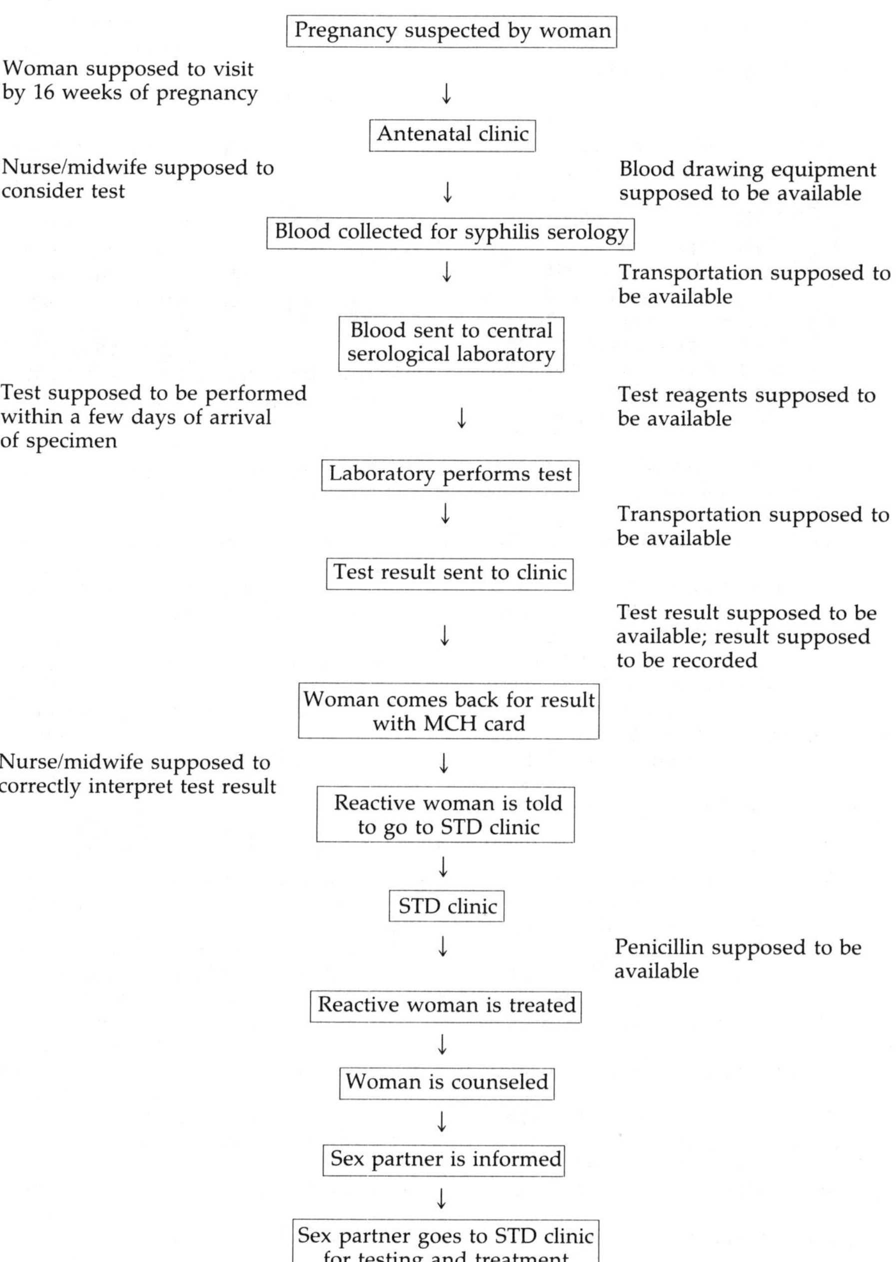

Figure 2. Steps involved in the control of congenital syphilis in city A: the "supposed to" syndrome at work.

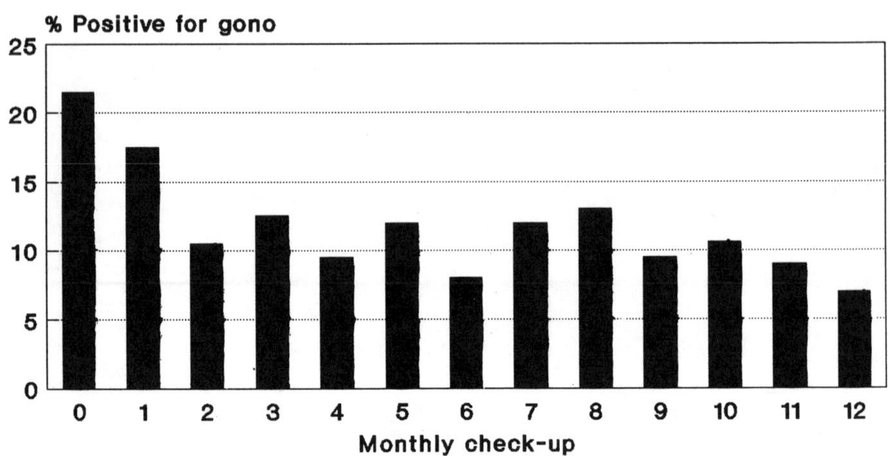

Figure 3. Effect of monthly case finding and treatment on the incidence of gonorrhea (gono) (solid bars) among 460 female prostitutes (from Laga et al., unpublished data). Month 0 represents prevalence of gonorrhea at entry to the study.

that services should be available to members of all high-risk groups in the community as well as to their partners.

There is a strong rationale for targeting STD prevention and control activities to core groups of high-frequency transmitters of STDs, since such interventions are potentially more cost beneficial and may have an amplifying effect (5, 10). For instance, Moses et al. (S. Moses, F. A. Plummer, P. Waiyaki, M. Bosire, N. J. D. Nagelkerke, J. O. Ndinya-Achola, A. R. Ronald, and E. N. Ngugi, Vth Int. Conf. AIDS Afr., abstr. T.RT.F.5, 1990) estimated that one female prostitute with HIV infection in Nairobi was the source of 12 cases of HIV infection in the general population of that city. With 50% condom use in this population of prostitutes, over 5,000 cases of HIV infection per 1,000 prostitutes per year would be prevented in the general population. These data are even more spectacular for STDs with a higher rate of transmission, such as gonorrhea (15).

The same may be true for targeted interventions in other core groups such as the military, long-distance truck drivers, and clients of prostitutes. Individuals belonging to these groups all have high rates of various STDs, including HIV infection in some countries (4, 10).

SOCIETAL INTERVENTIONS

Societal interventions for STD control may include regulation of prostitution, nightclubs, and alcohol and even of premarital and extramarital sex. They may be favored by cultural or religious beliefs and provide the public the feeling that the authorities are controlling the situation. However, history has shown that such measures do not control the spread of STDs and may even be counterproductive (2). The case of China suggests that draconian regulation of society may succeed in controlling STDs at least temporarily at the price of severe restrictions of human rights.

Some social and economic developments, which are usually not considered as part of STD control programs, may in the long run have a great impact on the STD epidemic in many countries. They include (i) targeting job training and employment opportunity programs for women, particularly economically deprived women, since this may prevent women from using prostitution as a survival strategy; (ii) creating inexpensive housing for families, resulting in a more equal sex ratio in cities of the Third World where there may be up to 50% more sexually active men than women, creating a demand for commercial sex (11); (iii) encouraging family planning, which will eventually result in a smaller proportion of people in their sexually active years and in a decrease of unemployment; and (iv) increasing access to health care by expanding affordable and effective primary health care. Unfortunately, current societal trends in the developing world (outside of parts of Asia) are actually favoring rather than slowing the spread of STDs.

SOME PRIORITIES FOR STD CONTROL IN THE DEVELOPING WORLD

This chapter has presented quite a sobering view of the current status of STD control in most of the developing world. As is often the case, the obstacles are highest where the needs are greatest and STD control programs are weak. This is largely due to competition for resources with other programs. In addition, however, it results from low awareness of the public health and economic importance of STDs, which in many cases is reinforced by political and cultural objections to dealing with STDs and the societal problems that foster them. Ironically, the AIDS epidemic and the associated interest of governments and donor agencies offer a historic momentum to change this defeatist picture.

A first priority is to change health provider and policymaker behavior to increase their interest in STD control and prevention, since this lack of interest and commitment is one of the reasons for the failure to implement biomedical interventions against STDs.

Some priorities for STD control in developing countries include (i) development of strategies and guidelines for STD control applicable to the different areas of the world; (ii) launching of a formal STD control program in each country; (iii) combination of STD and AIDS control programs and their implementation through primary health care and involvement of both the public and the private sectors; (iv) documentation and recognition of the differential impact of STDs on morbidity and mortality in women; (v) evaluation of clinical algorithms for case management and development of simple, inexpensive STD tests, particularly for the diagnosis of gonorrhea and chlamydial infections in women; (vi) integration of counseling and health promotion in clinical services seeing STD patients; (vii) evaluation of partner notification programs, especially through men with STDs, as a way of detecting and treating asymptomatically infected women; (viii) targeting of behavioral interventions to core transmitter groups; (ix) development of minimal standards for training of health care workers from the various sectors and for clinical services; (x) immediate implementation of case finding for syphilis in pregnant women and eye prophylaxis at birth; and (xi) assessment of prevention technologies controlled by women, such as spermicides and female condoms.

LITERATURE CITED

1. **Braddick, M. R., J. O. Ndinya-Achola, N. B. Mirza, F. A. Plummer, G. Irungu, S. K. A. Sinei, and P. Piot.** 1990. Towards developing a diagnostic algorithm for *Chlamydia trachomatis* and *Neisseria gonorrhoeae* cervicitis in pregnancy. *Genitourin. Med.* **66:**62–65.
2. **Brandt, A.** 1987. *No Magic Bullet.* Oxford University Press, New York.
3. **Cates, W., Jr., and A. Meheus.** 1990. Strategies for development of sexually transmitted disease control programs, p. 1023–1030. *In* K. K. Holmes, P.-A. Mardh, P. F. Sparling, P. J. Wiesner, W. Cates, Jr., S. M. Lemon, and W. E. Stamm (ed.), *Sexually Transmitted Diseases,* 2nd ed. McGraw-Hill Book Co., New York.
4. **D'Costa, L. J., F. A. Plummer, I. Bowner, L. Fransen, P. Piot, A. R. Ronald, and H. Nsanze.** 1985. Prostitutes are a major reservoir of sexually transmitted diseases in Nairobi, Kenya. *Sex. Transm. Dis.* **12:**64–67.
5. **Hethcote, H. W., and J. A. Yorke.** 1984. *Gonorrhea Transmission Dynamics and Control.* Springer-Verlag KG, Berlin.
6. **Hira, S. K., G. J. Bhat, D. M. Chikamata, B. Nkowane, G. Tembo, P. L. Perine, and A. Meheus.** 1990. Syphilis intervention in pregnancy: Zambian demonstration project. *Genitourin. Med.* **66:**159–164.

6a. **Hitchcock, P., J. N. Wasserheit, J. R. Harris, and K. K. Holmes.** 1991. Sexually transmitted diseases in the AIDS era: development of STD diagnostics for resource-limited settings is a global priority. *Sex. Transm. Dis.* **18:**133–135.

7. **Kasongo Project Team.** 1981. The Kasongo Project. *Ann. Soc. Belge Med. Trop.* **61**(Suppl.).
8. **Laga, M., A. Meheus, and P. Piot.** 1989. Epidemiology and control of gonococcal ophthalmia neonatorum. *Bull. W.H.O.* **67:**471–478.
9. **Laga, M., F. A. Plummer, P. Piot, P. Datta, W. Namaara, J. O. Ndinya-Achola, H. Nzanze, G. Maitha, A. R. Ronald, H. O. Pamba, and R. C. Brunham.** 1988. Prophylaxis of gonococcal and chlamydial ophthalmia neonatorum: silver nitrate versus tetracycline. *N. Engl. J. Med.* **318:**653–657.
10. **Lamptey, P., and M. Potts.** 1990. Targeting of prevention programs in Africa, p. 144–180. *In* P. Lamptey and P. Piot (ed.), *The Handbook for AIDS Prevention in Africa.* Family Health International, Durham, N.C.
11. **Larson, A.** 1989. The social context of HIV infection in Africa: a review of historical and cultural bases of East and Central African sexual relations. *Rev. Infect. Dis.* **11:**716–731.
12. **Latif, A. S., O. L. Mbengeranwa, E. Marowa, E. Paraiwa, and S. Gutu.** 1986. The decentralisation of the sexually transmitted diseases service and its integration into primary health care. *Afr. J. Sex. Transm. Dis.* **2:**85–88.
13. **Meheus, A., and P. Piot.** 1986. Provision of services for sexually transmitted diseases in developing countries, p. 261–272. *In* J. D. Oriel and J. R. W. Harris (ed.), *Recent Advances in Sexually Transmitted Diseases.* Churchill Livingstone, Ltd., Edinburgh.
14. **Meheus, A., K. F. Schultz, and W. Cates, Jr.** 1990. Development of prevention and control programs for sexually transmitted diseases in developing countries, p. 1041–1046. *In* K. K. Holmes, P.-A. Mardh, P. F. Sparling, P. J. Wiesner, W. Cates, Jr., S. M. Lemon, and W. E. Stamm (ed.), *Sexually Transmitted Diseases,* 2nd ed. McGraw-Hill Book Co., New York.
15. **Ministry of Health.** 1990. *National STD Control Programme (NASCOP). Two Year Plan for 1990–1991,* p. 77. Ministry of Health, Nairobi, Kenya.
16. **Omran, A. R.** 1971. The epidemiological transition: a theory of the epidemiology of population changes. *Milbank Mem. Fund Q.* **49:**509–538.

17. **Pepin, J., F. A. Plummer, R. C. Brunham, P. Piot, D. W. Cameron, and A. R. Ronald.** 1989. The interaction of HIV and other sexually transmitted diseases: an opportunity for intervention. *AIDS* **3:**3–9.
18. **Piot, P., and S. K. Hira.** 1990. Control and prevention of sexually transmitted diseases, p. 83–104. *In* P. Lamptey and P. Piot (ed.), *The Handbook for AIDS Prevention in Africa.* Family Health International, Durham, N.C.
19. **Piot, P., M. Laga, R. Ryder, J. Perriëns, M. Temmerman, W. Heyward, and J. M. Curran.** 1990. The global epidemiology of HIV infection: continuity, heterogeneity and change. *J. Acquired Immune Defic. Syndr.* **3:**403–412.
20. **Stray-Pedersen, B.** 1983. Economic evaluation of maternal screening to prevent congenital syphilis. *Sex. Transm. Dis.* **4:**167–172.
21. **Walsh, J. A.** 1988. *Establishing Health Priorities in the Developing World,* p. 151. United National Development Programme, New York.
22. **Wasserheit, J. N.** 1989. The significance and scope of reproductive tract infections among Third World women. *Int. J. Gynecol. Obstet. Suppl.* **3:**145–168.
23. **World Health Organization.** 1989. *STD Treatment Strategies.* WHO/VDT/89.447. World Health Organization, Geneva.
24. **World Health Organization.** 1990. *Consensus Statement from the Consultation on Global Strategies for Coordination of AIDS and STD Control Programmes.* WHO/GPA/INF/90.2, p. 5. World Health Organization, Geneva.

Behavioral Interventions in Industrialized Countries

Franklyn N. Judson and Maria E. M. Paalman

This chapter reviews behavioral interventions used to control sexually transmitted infections (STIs) in industrialized countries and discusses priorities for future research in this area. STI is a new acronym that combines an expanding list of sexually transmitted diseases (STDs) with human immunodeficiency virus (HIV) infections including AIDS. It is intended to unify a field in which AIDS, the most important and deadly STI, often has been viewed as separate from or different from other STDs and to emphasize that most STDs do not result from contact with clinically apparent diseases but rather with unnoticed and frequently subclinical infections. Thus, the most promising behavioral interventions are likely to focus on preventing infection or, at the very least, on detection and treatment before transmission or complications can occur.

We have made a number of pragmatic decisions about the content of this chapter and its relationship to other chapters. There is intentional overlap, some of which is needed for the chapter to stand on its own and some of which expresses the differing perspectives of the authors. We have elected to use a broad definition of behavioral interventions that encompasses any efforts that might be expected to alter one or more behaviorial determinants of STIs. This in turn required that citation of published and unpublished reports be highly selective. Selection criteria incorporated a desire to represent a variety of interventions, target groups, and countries as well as an element of referential incest (i.e., overreliance on publications related to the authors).

Several of the other chapters in this volume (e.g., those by Hornik, Smith, Fishbein et al., Newman et al., and Green and Washington) have introduced us to a sophisticated and disciplined approach to understanding, designing, and evaluating behavioral interventions. For analysis and discussion, we have accepted Hornik's descriptions of the better-established models for behavior change (see his chapter, this volume) and have grouped them into five major categories along with the salient implications for behavioral intervention control of STIs (Table 1). While we acknowledge that none of these models can currently be used to explain or prevent more than a minority of cases of STIs, we find them helpful in conceptualizing the issues.

This chapter is divided into two sections. The first reviews and comments on representative examples of prior behavioral intervention efforts to control STIs in industrialized countries. It takes into account a framework for organizing and

Franklyn N. Judson – World Health Organization, Geneva, Switzerland, and University of Colorado Health Sciences Center, Denver, Colorado 80204-4507. ***Maria E. M. Paalman*** – Dutch Foundation for STD Control, 3511 GE Utrecht, The Netherlands.

Table 1. Models of individual behavioral change and implications for behavioral interventions

Behavioral model	Implication(s) for behavioral interventions
Structural—community and/or individual	External factors determine which behavior options are available to an individual
Social expectations	Social or community norms determine individual behavior
Cognitive	Individual knowledge, attitudes, beliefs, values, and perceived self-efficacy determine individual behavior
Drive or trait	Enduring elements (i.e., heredity) of human personality influence individual behavior
Behaviorist	Individual behavior is shaped by the positive and negative outcomes of prior behavior

classifying the important determinants of sexual, health care-seeking, and health care provider behaviors (Table 2), as well as the objectives of specific behavioral interventions (Table 3). Behavioral interventions can be further categorized by the level of the intervention: (i) individual, (ii) defined groups or audiences, and (iii) the general population. Finally, some behavioral interventions clearly are aimed at more than one specific behavior and more than one level, and a few are best described as multiple-risk-factor interventions (6).

Utilizing the theoretical and conceptual framework established in the tables,

Table 2. Important determinants of sexual, health care-seeking and compliance, and health care provider behaviors

Type of behavior	Determinants
Sexual	Hereditary
	Knowledge, attitudes, and skills
	Social norms
	Behavior of sexual partners
	Use of addictive substances
	Public laws
Health care seeking and compliance	Knowledge, attitudes, and skills
	Social norms
	Availability of services
	Use of addictive substances
	Public laws
Health care provider	Knowledge, attitudes, and skills
	Community norms and priorities
	Community resources
	Public laws

Table 3. Objectives of specific behavioral interventions to control STIs

A. Reduce risk of exposure to and acquisition of STIs through changes in sexual behavior
  1. Postpone coital debut.
  2. Reduce numbers of sexual partners.
  3. Select sexual partners by infection status.
  4. Reduce use of substances that result in loss of control.
  5. Reduce sexual contact with individuals from high-STI-prevalence groups.
  6. Increase use of condoms and/or spermicides.
  7. Reduce frequency of sexual practices associated with higher rates of transmission.

B. Reduce risk of transmission and complications of STIs through improvements in health care-seeking and compliance behavior
  1. Increase early recognition of risk and/or symptoms of STI.
  2. Increase compliance with extended treatment regimens.
  3. Increase compliance with test-of-cure and other follow-up visits.
  4. Increase compliance with partner notification.

C. Increase accessibility and effectiveness of STI treatment and prevention services by improving health care provider behavior
  1. Improve STI training in professional schools.
  2. Provide STD and HIV prevention training centers.
  3. Establish STI specialty training and recognition.
  4. Improve private care providers' willingness and ability to detect and care for STIs.
  5. Improve and expand partner notification.
  6. Improve counseling on STI risk reduction.
  7. Improve promotion, distribution, and instructions for condoms.

D. Reduce transmission of STIs through the use of public laws
  1. Registration and/or periodic health examinations of prostitutes.
  2. Punitive fines and/or restrictive measures.
  3. Regulating and/or prohibiting certain establishments such as bathhouses for homosexual men and massage parlors.

the second section discusses future directions for behavioral intervention research and suggests priorities.

BEHAVIORAL INTERVENTIONS: A REVIEW OF PRIOR EFFORTS

In industrialized countries, the most extensive intervention efforts have been directed toward reducing an individual's risk of infection through modifying certain contributory aspects of sexual behavior. The common underlying assumption is that the targeted behaviors are under cognitive control. Thus, there is a preference for methods that emphasize information, education, and communications. Another explanation is that this approach simply is easier than modifying community norms and structural barriers, to say nothing of drive or trait influences (see Hornik, this volume).

Interventions directed at health care-seeking and compliance behaviors are intended to minimize the period of infectiousness for treatable STIs and to reduce secondary transmission rates for all STIs. More specific objectives have included earlier diagnosis; better compliance with treatment regimens, test-of-cure visits, and patient-initiated partner notification; and more recently, HIV testing and counseling. Objectives of interventions to improve health care provider behavior usually are less specific and are amenable mainly to process evaluation. They variably have consisted of establishment of STD and HIV training and prevention centers and networks of genitourinary medicine clinics staffed by STI specialists and provision of a more effective array of prevention services such as counseling, condom promotion, and partner notification (11).

Interventions to Reduce Risk of Infection

Most behavioral interventions have been designed to communicate information that will encourage individuals to change sexual behavior in ways that will reduce the risk of acquiring STIs. The first line of defense is to avoid exposure altogether. This may be accomplished by postponing coital debut, also a primary goal of successful behavioral intervention to prevent teenage pregnancies (33); by secondary celibacy, as adopted by significant numbers of homosexual men during the AIDS epidemic (6); and by selecting uninfected partners. In this regard, any type of sexual practice with an uninfected partner will be safer than safe sex with a partner known to be infected or whose infection status is unknown. Implications for privacy and established relationships as well as the dangers of stigmatization and discrimination have inhibited development of this type of intervention.

A second line of defense can be found in interventions that reduce but do not eliminate the risk of exposure. They stress having fewer sexual partners, particularly those who are anonymous and/or "one-night stands," and fewer involvements with persons likely to have high-risk life-styles. During the first half of this century, a very visible component of STI control programs in some industrialized countries consisted of warnings to the public, in general, and the military, in particular, about the dangers of consorting with prostitutes (7). These interventions could not be evaluated, and as effective treatments became available and the proportion of all STIs attributable to prostitutes was realized to be small, they all but disappeared.

There are a number of practical and human rights considerations that appropriately have deterred targeting homosexual men and inner city substance abusers for interventions aimed at preventing transmission of infections to individuals from low-prevalence populations. The principal challenge remains to prevent transmission within defined high-prevalence groups. Finally, given the adverse impact on STIs of alcohol and substances that cause loss of individual control over sexual behavior, it is discouraging that it took the HIV epidemic to draw resources to potentially important interventions in this area.

Some interventions represent a third line of defense and are designed to minimize the chances of infection when exposure to STIs occurs. They include reducing the frequency of high-risk sexual practices (e.g., receptive anal intercourse) and increasing the use of condoms and spermicides. Specific instructions on desired changes in sexual practices and on condom use are generally reserved for individual- and group-level interventions. Condom promotion has become a cornerstone of many HIV prevention programs. Although most studies can document some increase in condom use during active interventions as well as some relationship between regular use and lower rates of HIV transmission than in a comparison group, there are many methodological deficiencies, and measuring protective efficacy remains problematic (14).

The greatest recent experience with large-scale efforts, often involving multiple media, to modify sexual behavior in industrialized countries has been funded by and directed through HIV and AIDS control programs. Consequently, we have selected this area for extensive discussion according to the level of the interventions.

Interventions directed at the general public

There are several reasons to direct information, education, and communication about STIs to the general public (26). This level of intervention can raise personal and political awareness of the problem; favorably influence general attitudes toward STIs, safer sex, and health care-seeking behavior; counteract discrimination against and stigmatization of infected people and risk groups; and reach individuals who cannot be accessed through targeted programs. A mass media approach has the advantage of reaching large numbers of people at a low unit cost, generating free publicity and setting the stage for behavior change. The disadvantages are that the public nature of the communication often makes it necessary to compromise on the content of the messages, sometimes to the extent that many cannot identify with them. Also, after 1985, most of the AIDS information was going to individuals who were already well informed through nonintervention sources or who were not at risk.

Behavioral interventions for the general public commonly utilize a combination of information brochures, hotlines, mass media campaigns, and condom promotion and provision. In most countries, STD leaflets were available before the AIDS era but were limited in distribution to STD clinics, some family planning clinics, and an occasional general physician or specialist. They were rarely evaluated.

During the 1970s, the United States established the only free-access national STD hotline, while Sweden initiated mass media campaigns on STDs and condoms. Slogans such as "Ten Swedes are catching gonorrhea tonight" were used on posters in the streets. There followed a temporally associated long-term decline in gonorrhea incidence; however, the incidence of chlamydial infections continued to rise, bringing into question the causal relationship to the campaign (T. Ripa, personal communication). Some of the apparent disparity undoubtedly was owing to concurrent increases in testing for *Chlamydia trachomatis*.

With the arrival of AIDS, the number of interventions increased tremendously. All countries produced television spots, posters, brochures, and advertisements and distributed them widely. This generated the need for more information sources, which was met by AIDS hotlines in many countries. Hotlines can follow up on individual information requests, indicate areas that need extra attention in public campaigns, and identify groups that have not been adequately served with information (24).

Examples of interventions directed at the general public. Switzerland has the highest incidence of AIDS in Europe. In 1986, the first large-scale prevention operation was initiated, and an information booklet was distributed to every household. In 1987, the multimedia STOP-AIDS prevention campaign was launched (1, 10, 12). It focused on condom use with multiple or casual partners and on mutual faithfulness. Messages were simple, clear, and direct. Educational material for diverse target groups complemented the media campaign.

The University Institute of Social and Preventive Medicine has continually evaluated the prevention process by using social learning and communication theory. The evaluation was made up of 13 quantitative and qualitative measures of preventive knowledge, attitudes, beliefs, and practices. A telephone survey after the first campaign showed a decrease from 18 to 14% in those having occasional sexual relations and an increase from 25 to 45% in those using condoms some of the time and from 8 to 17% in those using condoms all the time. Self-reported behavior change was associated with an increase in the sale of condoms.

Since 1987, The Dutch Foundation for STD Control has conducted yearly mass media campaigns to prevent sexual transmission of HIV, especially among younger adults (8). The object of the first campaign was to make condom use socially acceptable and featured Dutch celebrities. The "Safe Sex on Holiday" campaign tapped into the fact that many adolescents engage in casual or new relationships during the summer holiday period. The "Excuses" campaign addressed inappropriate beliefs and rationalizations used to deny the risk of unsafe sex.

The campaigns were based on the Fishbein-Ajzen model of behavior change (see Fishbein et al., this volume). A variety of materials were produced and distributed through dedicated or mass media channels. Twice-yearly telephone surveys using the same random sampling procedures assessed knowledge, attitudes, intentions, and safer sexual behavior. Condom sales and the incidence of reported syphilis and gonorrhea were monitored.

After six surveys, 98% of respondents knew that condoms helped to prevent HIV transmission and the number who considered condom use a sign of distrust declined further. Over time, condoms were viewed more favorably. Among the 8% having casual partners, reported safer sex behavior rose steadily from 30% in April 1987 to nearly 70% in October 1988. Improvement was noted both for adolescents and for all respondents combined but not to the extent justified by their reported personal risk. The authors concluded that while many respondents still viewed their risk of HIV as small enough to disregard, this was not necessarily inappropriate given the very low HIV prevalence in the Netherlands outside of the main risk groups. Encouragingly, during the study period (1987 to 1989), respondents having casual partners and who used condoms sometimes or always increased respectively from 21 to 43% and from 9 to 40%. The remaining 17% still did not use condoms. Condom sales advanced 20%, and gonorrhea continued to decline, but in 1988, syphilis increased.

AIDS education in the United States has been directed at the general population (25). In October 1986, the *Surgeon General's Report on the Acquired Immune Deficiency Syndrome* was published. During 1987, Surgeon General Koop repeatedly advised using condoms to prevent HIV infection.

In the fall of 1987, the Centers for Disease Control initiated the U.S. National Information/Education Campaign to support local and state efforts to reduce the incidence of AIDS. The program consisted of public service announcements, a national mailing, minority outreach programs, a national AIDS hotline and associated clearinghouse for printed materials, outreach to private corporations, and research. In comparative surveys from 1986 and 1987, 7% of respondents reported changing sexual behavior, one-half of them by using condoms more frequently.

In the first 3 months of 1986, the United Kingdom conducted a newspaper AIDS information campaign for the general public. Knowledge about AIDS was assessed the following June and December with two mail surveys that used a 1-in-500 sample of Southampton citizens on the electoral roll. About two-thirds responded, and mean scores increased from 5.15 to 5.67 of 11 points (3). The results suggest that the free publicity on AIDS following the first campaign did increase the level of knowledge.

In early 1987, a nationwide distribution of leaflets was followed by intensive television, radio, press, and billboard advertising, known as the "Don't Die of Ignorance" campaign. During 1 week in March, 14 documentaries, talk shows, and other programs were aired by Britain's four television channels to inform the public and encourage changes in sexual behavior. Surveys of 1,000 adults taken immediately before and after the campaign indicated an increase in the general level of knowledge. A positive correlation between self-reported and tested knowledge was noted in both surveys, although the percentage who incorrectly considered themselves to be well informed rose from 3 to 15%. Independent of 17 other measures, viewing television programs was positively correlated with levels of knowledge, nonsupport for coercive measures, and possession of internal feelings of control. There were no reported changes in sexual behavior (35).

There are numerous difficulties in evaluating large public campaigns. Because there is a sense of urgency, interventions begin without good baseline data on STIs or on sexual knowledge, attitudes, beliefs, and practices. Clear-cut evaluable objectives are not developed, and relevant literature on health promotion to prevent other diseases may be overlooked.

Owing to concurrent targeted educational activities and many other uncontrolled or unrecognized influences on sexual behavior (Table 2), the opportunities for confounding are high. For example, to interpret what a doubling of condom sales means in terms of disease control, one needs to know how many sexual contacts took place, the prevalence rate of infection in the defined population, and whether the people exposed were the ones using the condoms. Usually, the bottom line of STIs prevented by the intervention is missing altogether.

Perhaps the Swiss approach of evaluating the total package of interventions is most realistic. It is not expensive (about $300,000 per year) and serves to reexamine the underlying assumptions of prevention policies in the country. Along with an extensive process evaluation in which choices are clarified, it can direct future actions.

Interventions directed at defined groups

Interventions directed at specific groups offer the opportunity to target information, education, and communication activities to meet the specific information needs of each group. Messages can be adapted to the social context and the specific language of the group. Successful projects so far have proved that it is essential to work through key group members who know the values and habits of other members, the channels to reach them, and the authorities they listen to.

Targeted groups or audiences can be defined by demographic indicators (age, sex, income, occupation, location [urban, rural, regional]); reference groups (race, language, sexual orientation); organizations through which they can be reached (health care facilities, factories, churches, cooperatives, schools, prisons, military institutions); and risk-prone behavior (multiple sexual partners, unsafe sexual practices, shared drug injection equipment).

From a disease control perspective, priorities should be set on the basis of firm epidemiological information. It is important to reach the people with the highest risk first, with the most convincing, intensive programs. Nevertheless, lower-risk groups cannot be ignored. To use a metaphor, when there is a fire, it must be fought where it is burning, but at the same time the fire brigade must keep the adjoining premises wet to prevent the fire from spreading. Thus, a justifiable fear of infection in health care workers has necessitated specific information and prevention programs. To prevent infections in a future generation, adolescents are an important target group. It is generally easier to develop safer sex behavior from the start than to change established unsafe habits.

The best group-specific behavioral interventions accommodate the different moral and communication standards pertaining to sexuality as well as different social contexts. What is only candid to one group can be offensive to another. Different target audiences need different behavioral strategies.

A large number of specific educational materials have been produced and distributed to different target groups, such as homosexual men, female prostitutes and their clients, ethnic minorities, women, tourists, young people, health workers, students, and military personnel. Because of its wide coverage in the industrialized world, school education is an example of a targeted intervention with great potential impact. There is broad consensus that education on AIDS and HIV should be combined with that on other STIs and integrated within general sex and/or health education curricula.

In the Netherlands, prostitute contact centers have been set up for street prostitutes to rest, have coffee, talk with colleagues, or consult with a health worker or doctor about STIs. Information materials and condoms are distributed. Homosexual groups have organized safe-sex parties as an alternative to homosexual saunas and backrooms, where anonymous, often unsafe sex took place. Group counseling has been offered to HIV-seropositive people so they may learn how to cope with their situation and how to prevent infecting others.

Examples of interventions directed at defined groups. Condom use has been promoted among immigrants in Santo Domingo (30). Although not an industrialized country, the Dominican Republic developed a very sophisticated Santo Domingo-based intervention for Haitian-Creole immigrant agricultural workers. It utilized local radio station broadcasts of AIDS prevention messages in conjunction with mobile education units and training of community health committees to form a comprehensive HIV prevention strategy. Subsidized condoms were made available at grocery stores, and an annual collective baptism of the condom was conducted during Easter Gaga rites. The baptism is done to advance condom use as a culturally acceptable behavior. Pre- and posttest knowledge, attitudes, and practices were measured to evaluate the program in each community. AIDS awareness and condom use reportedly have increased significantly in each community.

Discussion groups have been established for homosexual and bisexual men in California (22). The California-based AIDS prevention program, "Stop AIDS," offered one-time, 3.5-h discussion groups to homosexual and bisexual men, focusing on information, attitudes, and behaviors associated with HIV infection. These were assessed in a presession survey, while commitment to behavior change was measured in the postsession survey ($n = 148$). Very small but significant improvements in information, attitudes, and behavior were observed; however, there was no correlation among information, attitudes, and commitment to behavior change. Only pretest behavior correlated with the crucial outcome of posttest intended behavior. It was unclear which elements of the intervention, if any, were effective. A follow-up survey is regarded by the authors as essential to determine how much commitment to change is actualized.

Seven in-depth group sessions for homosexual men have been run (20). A similar but more in-depth study enrolled 15 homosexual men with a history of high-risk sexual activities. They attended seven group sessions that provided education and skills training and completed measures of knowledge and sexual practices for the preceding 4 months. Role playing was used to assess behavioral assertiveness skills for resisting pressure to engage in high-risk practices.

Comparing mean occurrences for the 4-month periods before and 4 to 8 months after the program, unprotected anal intercourse decreased from 0.93 to 0.21, oral-anal contact decreased from 0.80 to 0.07, and oral-genital contact involving sexual fluid exchange decreased from 0.67 to 0.50. The proportion of all intercourse occasions when condoms were used increased from 72 to 90%, while the number of partners with whom high-risk activities took place declined from 1.3 to 0.6. The participants themselves evaluated the program as extremely successful. The authors noted that the sample was small and that an experimental control group was not employed. Also, as usual, self-reported sexual practices could not be validated.

School education in the Netherlands has targeted STIs (9). Dutch Educational Television developed an AIDS education package for use in secondary schools that was evaluated by the State University of Limburg. The package consisted of three television broadcasts, a classroom session, a magazine, and a teacher's manual. The evaluation was conducted among 168 students divided into experimental and control groups and used a questionnaire.

Overall, the program was evaluated positively by teachers as well as by students, but the effect of the package was very limited. Although there was a significant increase in knowledge, the program did not have an impact on the respondent's attitudes, intentions, and behaviors related to prevention of HIV infection. The authors suggested that this could be explained by their limited understanding of the behavioral determinants.

An educational campaign was run for Greek registered prostitutes (27). After 3.4% of 350 registered Greek prostitutes were found to be HIV seropositive in 1984 and 1985, an intensive educational campaign was conducted. Registered prostitutes were counseled and advised to use condoms and to refuse clients from central Africa. They were regularly checked for STIs, and screened for anti-HIV antibody every 3 months. From November 1985 to October 1986, two new seroconversions occurred in 270 prostitutes. Further infections were not detected among 282 prostitutes monitored until 1988. Condom use with clients increased from 66% in 1984 to 98% by the end of 1987. Syphilis incidence decreased from 17.1% in 1985 to 3.2% in 1987, and since 1986, there have been no new cases of gonorrhea.

This study has been criticized because there were indications that women who practiced high-risk behavior were dropped from the study and because there was no control group. Furthermore, most prostitutes in Greece are illegal, nonregistered sex workers and therefore were not eligible for the study. Infections in them are thought to be much more common.

Many of the information, education, and communication activities for defined groups are unidirectional (brochures, advertisements, etc.). More bidirectional personal communication is needed to make people aware of their own personal risk, to persuade them of the necessity to change their behavior, and to teach them necessary practical and communication skills. This often requires behavioral interventions directed at the individual.

Interventions directed at the individual

Most behavioral intervention activities for disease prevention are not part of a professional service. Parents tell their children to be careful, friends talk together, partners ask questions. To maintain or improve the impact of this informal but individual education, it is important to regularly update the general public about STIs, including HIV infection.

Our focus, however, is on behavioral interventions by professional health workers, such as physicians, nurses, and counselors. Most individual behavioral interventions take place at sites for STI diagnosis and treatment and/or HIV testing and counseling, in many cases a private doctor's office or a specialized clinic. Patients are particularly open to counseling and behavioral change at the moment of personal confrontation with the diagnosis of an STI. This is also the rationale behind the huge efforts in the United States and other industrialized countries to provide voluntary, free, high-quality HIV testing and counseling and for integrating them into STD clinical services.

Not much is known about behavioral interventions by private physicians.

Horsburgh et al. (13) developed recommendations for STI prevention interventions to be performed by primary care physicians. The need is clear because, according to Milne and Keen (23), general practioners in Britain lacked the knowledge and willingness to advise their patients on AIDS prevention, and in a study of 3,427 U.S. general practioners, Rhodes et al. (28) identified as barriers to appropriate HIV education difficulties in discussing sexual behavior, particularly homosexual behavior; negative attitudes toward intravenous drug users; inadequate knowledge about AIDS and HIV; and the absence of guidelines for confidentiality and informed consent. Among 3,460 workers in the United States, the few people who received information on AIDS from a physician did not value it positively (34).

In STD clinics, there usually are trained health workers who inform patients about their disease, how to prevent transmission, the importance of warning partners, and how to avoid infection in the future. They often support their individual counseling with printed information. Importantly, many STD clinic patients are members of so-called high-prevalence STI and/or high-risk behavior core groups, and mathematical modeling suggests that treatment or prevention of an STI in a core group member has far greater impact on disease incidence than prevention of an STI in a non-core group member (see chapters by Anderson and by Brunham and Ronald, this volume).

An individual behavioral intervention approach provides the opportunity to personalize information and education to fit individual needs, beliefs, levels of knowledge, sexual preference, and perceived and true risk of infection. An HIV-seropositive man presenting with gonorrhea clearly needs a different approach than a 19-year-old girl who contracted herpes during her first sexual encounter.

Given the high cost of individual behavioral interventions, top priority should go to those with high-risk sexual behaviors who come from high-prevalence environments. In most industrialized countries, they belong to the following groups: patients with STIs, homosexual men, injecting drug users, prostitutes, poor inner city ethnic minorities, and migrant workers.

Individual counseling also can take place within a group, usually through voluntary workers who receive special training. Several types of community-based individual interventions have emerged during the HIV epidemic.

The most experience with interventions to alter individual sexual behavior through professional counseling has been with members of groups with high-risk behaviors for HIV infections. Increasingly, these interventions begin with HIV testing and counseling, which in the United States has quickly evolved into a federally funded program costing hundreds of millions of dollars a year. The underlying premise is that personal counseling could convince HIV-positive individuals to avoid infecting others and HIV-negative individuals to avoid becoming infected. Although it is widely believed that these services are effective, studies to date can only suggest that counseling plus testing leads to slightly greater behavioral changes than counseling alone (4).

A number of studies and programs have offered repetitive and intensive long-term individual counseling to members of groups with high-risk behaviors;

initially most were homosexual men. These studies have shown desired changes in many measures of risk behavior, but critical questions remain unanswered about the magnitude of the changes in behavior attributable to the interventions, sustainability, generalizability beyond predominantly educated, middle-class and upper-middle-class white homosexual men, and cost. The most important examples of this approach have been through the Centers for Disease Control-funded AIDS Community-Based Demonstration Projects, which consist of seven research centers (Denver, Dallas, Seattle, Albany, Long Beach, Chicago, New York) established in 1986 and 1987 to develop, implement, and evaluate interventions to prevent transmission of HIV.

During phase I (1985 to 1989), most interventions were directed to self-identified homosexual men. At the broadest level, the interventions convey factual information about HIV infection and AIDS and create the impression that prevailing social norms support changes to lower-risk behaviors. At the individual level, interventions are more intensive and based on the provision of HIV counseling and testing services. In the typical case, counseling employs a single pretest session to gain voluntary informed consent and a single posttest session to discuss the implications of the individual's HIV status. Appropriate referral and follow-up to measure behavioral impact are also standard. At the most intensive level, interventions include a variety of messages and skills training targeted to individuals resistant to behavioral change, those requiring additional skills to make changes, and those having trouble maintaining the lower-risk behavioral patterns they had adopted.

Important summary findings of phase I include the following. (i) Emphasis on community-peer influence. The data support the theory that interventions directed at influencing prevailing social norms are crucial for HIV prevention. Community-based programs have formed the foundation for delivering effective HIV prevention messages in a culturally sensitive manner acceptable to target populations.

(ii) Effect of learning HIV status. Even the relatively superficial interventions of HIV testing followed by a one-time counseling session were effective in their primary goal of helping individuals to realize the implications of their HIV infection status. Of homosexual men who chose to enroll in ongoing cohort studies, safer sexual behavior changes were initiated to a slightly greater extent among those who were HIV positive than among those who were HIV negative. There is a need to continue making HIV counseling and testing programs available as an important first step in helping to initiate safer sexual behavior changes, even in settings in which a high proportion of individuals in a community already know their antibody status.

(iii) Risky sex relapse. Within any 6-month interval, approximately 20% of homosexual male cohort study participants who had initially reported making safer sexual practices reverted to sporadic unsafe practices. As a result, HIV prevention programs have developed more intensive individual and group counseling sessions that reinforce safer behavior on a regular basis.

Phase II began in 1989 and has been oriented to specific hard-to-reach populations including men who have sex with men but do not identify themselves as homosexuals, intravenous drug users not in treatment, female sex partners of intravenous drug users and homosexual men, male and female prostitutes, and street youths. Interventions are based on social persuasion models, and members of communities with a high prevalence of risk-taking behavior help to identify barriers to risk reduction and to develop and deliver intervention activities.

Consistent condom use and/or needle hygiene are the behavioral goals. Initial data indicate that most members of target groups are not using condoms regularly and that intravenous drug users are not cleaning their needles and syringes regularly.

Efficacy is being evaluated through a three-step process: formative evaluation (developing the most appropriate interventions and assessment tools), process evaluation (documentation of the quantity and quality of the intervention), and outcome evaluation (matched intervention and control communities with baseline and postintervention data).

Interventions to Reduce Infectiousness and Secondary Transmission

Although there is much potential in interventions to enhance early recognition of risk of infection and/or symptoms, temporary cessation of sexual activities, and seeking early diagnosis and/or treatment, there has been little formal study. Recently, a program was developed in the United States to instruct women in performing periodic partial genital self-examinations for signs and symptoms of STIs. Wide-scale implementation and evaluation have not occurred. In addition, women with multiple partners, prostitutes, homosexual men with high-risk behavior, persons with a prior history of STIs, and persons from high-prevalence groups have long been encouraged to seek periodic examinations for STIs irrespective of symptoms. In some societies, the taboo character of a promiscuous life-style may act as a powerful deterrent to seeking timely advice (21).

From a compliance standpoint, by far the largest numbers of publications in the pre-AIDS era were on methods to obtain higher test of cure visit return rates, usually following gonorrhea treatment. Test-of-cure visits were felt to be important to ascertain cures and detect resistant organisms (5). This is perhaps ironic in that recent recommendations for treatment of gonorrhea with highly effective single-dose regimens, such as ceftriaxone, 125 or 250 mg, have abandoned routine test-of-cure visits as unnecessary and cost ineffective. Most studies demonstrated small to moderate improvements in compliance, often at considerable cost in counseling time (19). Rarely did such interventions become operational, and a common outcome was that the intervention would completely disappear some months before publication of the successful findings. In general, the data supported the commonly held belief about medication-compliance behavior: approximately one-third of patients will conscientiously adhere to instructions and need no counseling; one-third can be influenced to do better with variable amounts of counseling; and one-third will be resistant to all counseling efforts.

Partner notification of exposure to an STI coupled with the offer of testing, treatment, and/or counseling has been practiced extensively for syphilis control and to a lesser extent for gonorrhea, chancroid outbreaks, pelvic inflammatory disease, chlamydial infections, and, most recently, HIV infections. It is an inherently voluntary intervention that depends on patient compliance. By personalizing infection risk and delivering highly individualized prevention messages, it may initiate changes to safer sexual behavior. Partner notification has long been one of the most important services managed by the Division of STD/HIV Prevention of the U.S. Centers for Disease Control. During the AIDS era, the United Kingdom, Holland, and Canada have emphasized patient-initiated notification (referral) of partners exposed to HIV, while Belgium, Norway, and Sweden have used provider referral. The approach in the United States has varied from state to state.

The Oslo, Norway, experience of J. E. Kristoffersen summarized by Toomey and Cates (31) is representative of provider referral outcome. Of 639 index patients with HIV infection, 190 were interviewed for partner information. These patients reported a total of 225 identifiable contacts, of whom 172 (76%) were tested. Sixty-five individuals (38%) previously not known to be infected with HIV were identified through the partner notification process; of these, 30 (46%) would not otherwise have volunteered for HIV testing.

Similar results were obtained by the Colorado Department of Health (17). The first 504 HIV-positive persons interviewed named 768 at-risk partners, of whom 641 (83%) were located and counseled. Of the 452 (71%) not previously tested, 68 (15%) were HIV positive. The investigators conducted a cost-benefit analysis, and by even the most conservative assumptions about numbers of HIV infections prevented, the provider-initiated partner notification system was judged to be cost saving.

Nonetheless, provider referral remains incompletely evaluated and, especially for HIV infections, somewhat controversial. The most frequently voiced concerns are about cost-effectiveness relative to other behavioral interventions and the potential to invade privacy.

Interventions to Improve Behavior of Care Providers

A full review of behavioral interventions to improve STI health care provider behavior is beyond the mandate for this chapter. Related material appears in the chapter by Amaro and Gornemann, this volume. It is important to note, however, that in recent years the Division of STD/HIV Prevention of the Centers for Disease Control has been placing increasing emphasis on developing improved STI curricula for medical and nursing students and on regional STD and HIV training and prevention centers to provide various levels of training to physicians, nurses, physician extenders, and laboratory technologists involved in STI diagnosis and treatment. Also, a pharmaceutical company in the United States is developing a simple STI awareness and patient risk assessment instrument for use by private physicians who only occasionally see patients with STIs.

In the United Kingdom, a network of genitourinary clinics is viewed as the backbone of STI control efforts and is staffed by genitourinary medicine specialists. Similar roles are filled by dermatovenereologists in many other industrialized countries. The strengths of genitourinary specialists seem to derive from formal training, a sense of professional worth, and the resultant positive attitudes towards patients and their infections. Unfortunately, there has been less attention to standardization and quality control. Hart and colleagues (11) report that wide discrepancies exist in criteria used to diagnose and report various diseases and that treatment is often inappropriate.

To address similar problems in the United States, the Centers for Disease Control have developed "Quality Assurance Guidelines for Clinical Services" and on-site STI program review procedures, but evaluation of the effect of training on individual provider behavior, much less STI prevention, thus far has proved to be problematic.

Public Laws to Reduce Transmission of STIs

Although many public health professionals believe that imposition of legal standards for sexual behavior is counterproductive and likely to discourage cooperation with other programs designed to prevent STIs, most industrialized countries have not legalized prostitution (29). The most common laws to control prostitution are directed at the act of solicitation rather than at the sexual act. This is both because solicitation is easier to identify and because the community goal is to keep prostitution off the streets and out of sight. Enforcement is generally weak but depends on the priority that local governments give to suppression of prostitution.

Some laws provide only for fines and/or restrictive measures, while others have legalized or partially legalized sex work through a registration system that usually is linked with periodic health examinations for STIs. A compromise policy practiced in Denver and other communities utilizes a "health hold order" system. Sex workers who are arrested for solicitation are given a choice between defending themselves against the charges or reporting to a designated STD clinic for examination and, if indicated, treatment. Other than certifying in writing that the sex worker has complied with the health hold order (valid for 30 days), a sex worker receives the same care as other patients (15). The fact that most sex workers subsequently return to the clinic on a voluntary basis implies their acceptance of the high-quality services and supportive attitude of the clinic staff.

There have been no wholly adequate evaluations of any of these laws as to their impact on sex worker behavior or control of STIs. One example is a report from Poland that systematic screening and treatment of prostitutes in several big cities "decreased the prevalence of gonorrhea from approximately 50% in 1970 to 18% in 1983 and the prevalence of syphilis from 18% to a fraction of a percent in the same time-period" (11). These conclusions are based mainly on temporal associations.

In general, prevalence and incidence of STIs in sex workers of industrialized countries correlate best with rates in their noncommercial sexual partners and the communities in which they practice. Thus, predominantly white, middle-class, legally sanctioned Las Vegas (Nevada) female prostitutes who have sex mainly with white middle-class tourists and significant others will predictably experience comparatively low rates of STIs regardless of the legal and public health determinants of behavior.

The term "massage parlor" covers a variety of establishments that range from purveyors of legitimate physiotherapy to flagrant prostitution. Some governments have attempted to regulate massage parlors to exclude sex work, while others have simply banned them altogether.

Bathhouses for homosexual men flourished in many cities of industrialized countries during the 1970s and early 1980s. Although occasionally raided by law enforcement officers on dubious legal grounds, they were largely ignored until the AIDS epidemic. A conflict soon emerged between certain homosexual rights activists, who argued that government had no authority to regulate sexual activities of consenting adults anywhere, and public health and safety officials who argued that government had both legal and moral obligations to prevent new cases of AIDS, particularly within licensed (usually for food, swimming pool, and rooming functions) establishments open to the public. Some cities did nothing, some closed the bathhouses, and others, such as Denver, attempted to regulate out "unsafe sexual activities" and mandate provision of prevention information and condoms (18).

A direct evaluation of the effectiveness of the regulations was never undertaken; however, monthly unannounced inspections of Denver's three bathhouses indicated that they were conscientiously adhering to most requirements, and gonorrhea or syphilis cases diagnosed in the Denver Metro STD Clinic and traceable to sexual contact in the bathhouses became a very rare occurrence. As the AIDS epidemic worsened, many bathhouses simply closed for lack of customers and liability insurance.

BEHAVIORAL INTERVENTIONS RESEARCH: FUTURE DIRECTIONS AND PRIORITIES

Based on our experiences and a selective review of a disparate literature, it is clear that even in industrialized countries behavioral interventions have not been effectively applied to STI control. Rarely have interventions been designed around an established behavioral model, taken into account the complex interplay of behavioral and biological determinants, or stated which specific behavior(s) was to be modified. All too often, evaluative criteria either have been nonexistent or could not prove that the desired outcome was caused by the intervention.

Table 2 provides a framework for analyzing prior behavioral interventions and understanding why they may or may not have succeeded. It also points the way to developing more scientifically sound and sophisticated behavioral intervention research in the future. Although a thorough discussion of behavioral theory is left to other chapters, there are several relevant aspects of sexual, health care-seeking and compliance, and health care provider behaviors that deserve additional emphasis.

Sexual Behavior

Interventions directed at sexual behavior will always be challenging because this behavior has instinctive, pleasurable, and habituating components. Sexual behavior is much too important to the survival of a species to be left only to learning. Natural selection, in turn, ensures that there will be intraspecies variations in inherited sexual behavior (2). Recently, sociobiologists have offered detailed teleological explanations as to how these as well as gender differences in behavior are selected for. With the advancement of scientific knowledge, it appears that more and more of the fundamental determinants of human behavior are under some element of genetic control (drive or trait model). While a genetic influence on behavior is not a reason to be fatalistic about behavioral interventions, it does need to be considered.

Sexual orgasm has a habituating nature and, even when expressed as frequent masturbation or large numbers of same-sex anonymous male partners, represents nature's way of positively reinforcing reproductive behavior. This is better explained by behaviorist and drive or trait models than by cognitive models. As with physical addictions, it can be highly resistant to change.

Among the many cognitive determinants of sexual behavior in industrialized countries, fear of AIDS has been by far the most important behavioral intervention in recent history, beginning in 1982 for homosexual men and in 1985 for heterosexual men and women. The fear effect on sexual behavior has been greatest for those who have personally known someone with AIDS, but it also has been heavily influenced by mass media coverage of the epidemic. In the United States, this may have contributed to a 95% or greater reduction in the incidence of gonorrhea in homosexual men and up to 50% reductions in middle- and upper-middle-class heterosexual whites (16). Of importance to behavioral research, interpretation of interventions such as safe-sex campaigns and focused counseling can be hopelessly confounded by changes unrelated to the intervention.

The behavior of sexual partners is a determinant because most sexual behavior results from the interacting behaviors of two individuals. Thus, behavioral interventions that are directed at only one half of the sexual dyad may be less effective than expected in influencing, for example, acceptance of condoms or refusal of receptive anal intercourse. Research on improving communications between partners about safer sex is needed.

Use of addictive substances that alter mood and judgment has had variable adverse effects on STI control efforts in industrialized countries. Most important are the disinhibiting action of alcohol and the short-lived, hypersexual euphoria of cocaine followed by an equally intense depression and the need to relieve it with more drug. Poor inner city men may acquire drugs through theft or pimping and women through prostitution. From a behavioral intervention standpoint, expensive counseling to develop refusal skills and safe-sex practices will fail until the underlying drug problem is addressed.

There are many public laws that have the potential to influence sexual behavior. Whether or not a given law produces the outcome intended by society and whether or not that outcome is seen as good or bad are beyond the scope of this chapter. Clearly, however, laws that prohibit homosexual contact, anal intercourse, prostitution, solicitation for prostitution, public indecency, and condom distribution or advertising or that require disease reporting, partner notification, or restrictive measures can act both as direct behavioral interventions and as effect modifiers of other interventions and may have unintended, negative effects. Obviously, the impact of a law will depend on the extent to which it is enforced and understood by the population subject to the behavioral intervention. It is important to evaluate through research both beneficial and adverse consequences of such laws.

Health Care-Seeking and Compliance Behavior

In industrialized countries that are able to offer well-developed services for STIs including diagnosis, treatment, counseling, partner notification, and provision of condoms, patient behavior in seeking these services and complying with treatment and prevention recommendations can have a profound effect on overall efforts to control STIs.

HIV testing and counseling have been a cornerstone of many AIDS prevention programs; however, demand for this service always depended far more on perception of personal risk (i.e., fear) of AIDS than on knowledge about AIDS. It also depended on community norms, and in industrialized countries, at least for a while, HIV testing and counseling were viewed by some homosexual men as more of a threat to privacy than an aid to treatment and prevention (18).

Social norms for health care vary considerably among different sociocultural groups. In some, it can be the norm not to seek care until symptoms have failed to resolve on their own. In others, care will be avidly sought even when there are no symptoms and the risk of infection is small.

Individuals with serious substance abuse problems may not place a high priority on present or future health and tend to comply poorly with treatment and counseling recommendations. Finally, laws that require voluntary notification of partners exposed to STIs or periodic examination and/or treatment of prostitutes may serve to augment health care-seeking and compliance behavior.

Health Care Provider Behavior

An essential component of any STI control program is the provision of barrier-free high-quality clinical services. If individuals at risk of STIs believe that available services are effective, supportive, free (or at least affordable), and associated with a reasonable waiting time, their health care-seeking and compliance behaviors will be enhanced and the prevalence and incidence of STIs will be reduced (11, 15).

Health care provider behavior is a function of training, attitudes, skills, and resources that quite often reflect a community's health care priorities and attitudes toward STIs. It also can be shaped by the public laws noted previously. The extent to which providers comply with these laws depends not only on enforcement efforts but also on the feasibility and acceptability of compliance and the perceived benefits to provider, patient, and society.

CONCLUSIONS

Taking a very broad overview of research related to behavioral interventions to prevent STIs in industrialized countries, there are two large areas that stand out as potentially producing the greatest research payoff. One lies in evaluating the costs and benefits of placing high-quality, comprehensive, and affordable clinical and preventive STI services within easy reach of persons who most need them. The intent is to evaluate the effect of removing structural barriers to health care-seeking and compliance behavior on the numbers of patients receiving early diagnosis, treatment, and behavior modification messages. This approach has been most extensively developed in the United Kingdom, but there is not yet scientific proof that it has produced lower rates of STIs than other approaches have for comparable populations. In most industrialized countries, implementation of such an intervention is limited mainly by the low priority assigned to STIs within overall health care-funding schemes rather than by inadequate resources.

To avoid the many pitfalls of observational studies, there should be appropriate controls at a community service catchment level. Once well-defined full-scale clinical services interventions have been operating at equilibrium for a period, it should be possible to better evaluate more specific behavioral interventions such as negotiating skills counseling, partner notification, and condom provision. In measuring outcome, it is important to observe a hierarchy in which changes in incidence rates of specific infections in the intervention population are given the highest scientific value, followed by changes in prevalence rates, especially among young individuals just entering high-risk years. Much lower outcome value would be accorded to indirect measures such as self-reported changes in sexual behavior, condom sales, etc.

Because in our view high-risk sexual behavior falls more under normative than cognitive control, research to better define, understand, and modify social norms is the other priority study area. Much related work has been done with teenage pregnancies and substance addiction, including tobacco. Results to date reaffirm both the challenges and the promises of this research.

Specific Research Priorities

(i) Evaluate the costs and benefits of placing high-quality, comprehensive, affordable clinical and preventive STI services within easy reach of people who most need them to remove structural barriers to health care-seeking and compliance behavior. This should include comparisons of models that do and do not integrate STI services into other reproductive health services such as family planning, antenatal care, and school clinics.

(ii) Study sexual behavior in different groups and cultures to better understand the diversity of meanings and values attached to these behaviors. The goal is to develop more culturally specific and effective behavioral intervention strategies.

(iii) Better define the knowledge, attitudes, beliefs, and other behavioral determinants that underlie perceptions of personal risk and choices of risk-taking and risk-reduction behaviors, including those related to seeking early diagnosis and treatment.

(iv) Evaluate the relative efficacy of alternative strategies to reduce risk-taking behavior through controlled studies that are based on established behavioral models and use STI incidence and/or prevalence rates as outcome measures.

(v) Compare the effectiveness of different health promotion strategies in different countries, with particular emphasis on school-based approaches to reduce the incidence of adolescent STIs and pregnancies.

(vi) Evaluate the comparative costs and benefits of partner notification programs in controlling specific STIs.

(vii) Study the role of travellers and prostitutes in the national and global spread of STIs along with the possibilities for appropriate behavioral interventions.

(viii) Design and evaluate strategies to improve communication between sexual partners about safer sex.

LITERATURE CITED

1. **Anonymous.** 1989. *Assessment of AIDS Preventive Strategies*. Report on a workshop sponsored by the European Community Working Party on AIDS, Luzern (Switzerland), 28–29 November 1988. Institut Universitaire de Médecine Social et Préventive, Lausanne.
2. **Caldwell, J. C., and P. Caldwell.** 1990. High fertility in sub-Saharan Africa. *Sci. Am.* **May:**118–225.
3. **Campbell, M. J., and W. E. Waters.** 1987. Public knowledge about AIDS increasing. *Br. Med. J.* **294:**892–893.
4. **Cates, W., Jr., and H. H. Handsfield.** 1988. HIV counseling and testing: does it work? *Am. J. Public Health* **78:**1533–1534. (Editorial.)
5. **Center for Disease Control.** 1974. *Gonorrhea. CDC Recommended Treatment Schedules*. Center for Disease Control, Atlanta, Ga.
6. **Coates, T. J., and R. M. Greenblatt.** 1984. Behavioral change using interventions at the community level, p. 1075–1080. *In* K. K. Holmes, P.-A. Mardh, P. F. Sparling, and P. J. Wiesner (ed.), *Sexually Transmitted Diseases*. McGraw-Hill Book Co., New York.
7. **Cutler, J. C., and R. C. Arnold.** 1988. Venereal disease control by health departments in the past: lessons for the present. *Am. J. Public Health* **78:**372–376.
8. **de Vroome, E. M. M., M. E. M. Paalman, T. G. M. Sandfort, M. Sleutjes, K. J. M. de Vries, and R. A. P. Tielman.** 1990. AIDS in the Netherlands: the effects of several years of campaigning. *Int. J. AIDS* **1:**268–275.
9. **de Wit, J., G. J. Kok, C. Timmermans, and P. Wijnsma.** 1989. *De Effecten van het Voorlichtingsprogramma "AIDS, het komt je niet aanwaaien."* Rijksuniversiteit Limburg, Fac. Gezondheidswetenschappen, Vakgroep GVO, Maastricht, The Netherlands.
10. **Dubois-Arber, F., P. Lehmann, and D. Hauser.** 1988. Towards improved action against AIDS: continuous evaluation of Switzerland's control programmes provides guidance on how to make it more effective. *World Health Forum* **9:**376–381.
11. **Hart, G., M. W. Adler, A. Stapinski, T. F. Mroczkowski, and P. J. Wiesner.** 1984. Evaluation of sexually transmitted diseases control programs in industrialized countries,

p. 1031–1040. *In* K. K. Holmes, P.-A. Mardh, P. F. Sparling, and P. J. Wiesner (ed.), *Sexually Transmitted Diseases*. McGraw-Hill Book Co., New York.

12. **Hauser, D., P. Lehmann, F. Dubois-Arber, and F. Gutzwiller.** 1988. Effectiveness of the AIDS prevention campaigns in Switzerland, p. 219–228. *In* A. F. Fleming, M. Carballo, D. W. Fitz Simons, M. R. Bailey, and J. Mann (ed.), *The Global Impact of AIDS: Proceedings of the First International Conference on the Global Impact of AIDS*. Cosponsored by the WHO and the London School of Hygiene and Tropical Medicine, London, March 8–10, 1988. Alan R. Liss, New York.
13. **Horsburgh, C. R., J. M. Douglas, and F. M. LaForce.** 1987. Preventive strategies in sexually transmitted diseases for the primary care physician. *J. Am. Med. Assoc.* **258:**815–821.
14. **Judson, F. N.** 1989. Effectiveness of condoms for prevention of HIV infections. *AIDS Updates* **2:**1–8.
15. **Judson, F. N.** 1984. Clinical facilities for sexually transmitted diseases control, p. 1047–1055. *In* K. K. Holmes, P.-A. Mardh, P. F. Sparling, and P. J. Wiesner (ed.), *Sexually Transmitted Diseases*. McGraw-Hill Book Co., New York.
16. **Judson, F. N.** 1990. Gonorrhea. *Med. Clin. North Am.* **74:**1353–1366.
17. **Judson, F. N.** 1990. Partner notification for HIV control. *Hosp. Pract.* **December 15:**63–73.
18. **Judson, F. N., and T. M. Vernon, Jr.** 1988. The impact of AIDS on state and local health departments: issues and a few answers. *Am. J. Public Health* **78:**387–393.
19. **Judson, F. N., and F. C. Wolf.** 1979. Rescreening for gonorrhoea: an evaluation of compliance methods and results. *Am. J. Public Health* **69:**1178–1180.
20. **Kelly, J. A., J. S. St. Lawrence, R. Betts, T. L. Brasfield, and A. V. Hood.** 1990. Skills-training group intervention model to assist persons in reducing risk behavior for HIV infection. *AIDS Educ. Prev.* **2:**24–35.
21. **Leenaars, P. E. M., and A. J. P. Schrijvers.** 1990. Een soa-hulpvraag uitstellen, maar toch gaan (patient delay and STDs). Vakgroep Algemene Gezondheidszorg en Epidemiologie, Utrecht, The Netherlands.
22. **Miller, T. E., C. Booraem, J. V. Flowers, and A. E. Iversen.** 1990. Changes in knowledge, attitudes, and behavior as a result of a community-based AIDS prevention program. *AIDS Educ. Prev.* **2:**12–23.
23. **Milne, R. I. G., and M. Keen.** 1988. Are general practitioners ready to prevent the spread of HIV? *Br. Med. J.* **296:**533–535.
24. **National Commission on AIDS Control.** 1989. *Main Conclusions of First European AIDS-Hotline Conference*, 7–9 April 1989, Amsterdam. National Commission on AIDS Control, Amsterdam.
25. **Office of Technology Assessment.** 1988. *How Effective Is AIDS Education?* Office of Technology Assessment, Washington, D.C.
26. **Paalman, M., and T. Sandfort.** 1990. Promoting safer sex among the public at large, p. 199–216. *In* M. Paalman (ed.), *Promoting Safer Sex: Prevention of Sexual Transmission of AIDS and Other STD*. Proceedings of an International Workshop, May 1989. Dutch Foundation for STD Control, The Netherlands. Swets & Zeitlinger, Amsterdam.
27. **Papaevangelou, G., A. Roumeliotou, G. Kallinikos, G. Papoutsakis, E. Trichopoulou, and T. Stefanou.** 1988. Education in preventing HIV infection in Greek registered prostitutes. *J. Acquired Immune Defic. Syndr.* **1:**386–389.
28. **Rhodes, T., M. Gallagher, C. Foy, P. Philips, and J. Bond.** 1989. Prevention in practice: obstacles and opportunities. *AIDS Care* **1:**257–267.
29. **Richards, E. P., and D. C. Brass.** 1990. Legal aspects of STD control: public duties and private rights, p. 1101–1108. *In* K. K. Holmes, P.-A. Mardh, P. F. Sparling, P. J. Wiesner, W. Cates, Jr., S. M. Lemon, and W. E. Stamm (ed.), *Sexually Transmitted Diseases*, 2nd ed. McGraw-Hill Book Co., New York.
30. **Stoller, E. J., and G. W. Rutherford.** 1989. Evaluation of AIDS prevention and control programs. *AIDS* **3**(Suppl.)**:**S289–S296.
31. **Toomey, K. E., and W. Cates, Jr.** 1989. Partner notification for the prevention of HIV infection. *AIDS* **3**(Suppl.)**:**S57–S62.

32. **Turner, C. F., H. G. Miller, and L. E. Moses (ed.).** 1989. *AIDS: Sexual Behavior and Intravenous Drug Use*. National Academy Press, Washington, D.C.
33. **Vincent, M., A. F. Clearie, and M. D. Schluchter.** 1987. Reducing adolescent pregnancy through school and community based education. *J. Am. Med. Assoc.* **257:**3382–3386.
34. **Warshaw, L. J., and J. K. Barr.** 1990. The role of physicians in educating patients about AIDS. *N. Engl. J. Med.* **322:**1822.
35. **Wober, J. M.** 1988. Informing the British public about AIDS. *Health Educ. Res.* **3:**19–24.

Behavioral Interventions in Developing Countries

King K. Holmes and Sevgi O. Aral

Do prevention and control of sexually transmitted infections (STIs) work? If so, what are the relative contributions of behavioral versus other clinical and public health interventions? How may the relative roles of behavioral and nonbehavioral interventions differ in developing and industrialized countries? In the least-developed and developing countries, study of sexual behaviors has only recently begun in earnest, surveillance of STIs is virtually nonexistent, and STI prevention and control programs are undeveloped. Therefore, we turn first to the experience of the industrialized countries for an assessment of the potential impact of STI prevention and control.

LESSONS FROM INDUSTRIALIZED COUNTRIES

Two broad conclusions appear warranted. First, all industrialized countries experienced epidemic increases of STIs during the 1960s, and in some countries the increase continued through the 1970s and early 1980s. Second, all but one of the industrialized countries have brought the curable STIs under steadily improving control during the AIDS era. In many industrialized countries, certain STIs, such as chancroid, donovanosis, and lymphogranuloma venereum, had all but disappeared, except as imported infections, during the 1940s and 1950s. Trichomoniasis declined rapidly after the 1950s, and rates of gonorrhea and syphilis actually began to decline rapidly during the 1970s, well before the AIDS epidemic. During the AIDS era, gonorrhea and syphilis have become increasingly uncommon diseases in most industrialized countries, and a growing proportion of cases of gonorrhea and syphilis that do occur can be directly traced to an infection imported from a developing country.

The single exception to the success of prevention and control of curable STIs among the industrialized countries during the AIDS era has been the United States, where chancroid and syphilis have been increasing at epidemic rates in black and Hispanic populations in areas of concentrated poverty, and the incidence of gonorrhea remains at high levels. Within these minority populations, the resurgence of curable STIs has been closely linked not only to poverty but also to exchange of sex for money or drugs such as crack cocaine; to sustained high birth rates, leading to relatively large proportions in these populations of the adolescent

---

King K. Holmes – Center for AIDS and STD, Seattle, Washington 98122. ***Sevgi O. Aral*** – Behavioral and Prevention Research Branch, Division of STD/HIV Prevention, Centers for Disease Control, Atlanta, Georgia 30333.

and young adult ages; and to a breakdown in clinical and public health services for STIs in several metropolitan areas (3).

The epidemic of STIs in the industrialized countries during the 1960s was temporally related to the introduction of oral contraceptives; many surveys, especially in the United States, showed increases in premarital sex and number of sex partners, especially among women, during the 1960s and 1970s (2). However, at least in the United States, these increases appear to have been part of a long-term trend toward earlier premarital sexual activity throughout the 20th century. The sexual revolution involving homosexual men has been less well studied over time but clearly contributed to the epidemics of syphilis, hepatitis B, and human immunodeficiency virus (HIV) infection during the 1960s, 1970s, and early 1980s in the industrialized countries.

The impressive control of STIs that began in the mid-1970s in heterosexual populations in nearly all industrialized countries provides objective evidence of the effectiveness of intensified public health measures. In the West, these measures included strengthening of diagnosis and treatment efforts, expanded general public health education concerning STIs, and behavioral interventions focused on individuals and groups at high risk for STIs. It is difficult to define the relative contribution of these three approaches and the additional contribution of underlying social and demographic trends, such as the aging of the baby boom generation. However, the accelerated decline of gonorrhea and syphilis during the AIDS era in most industrialized countries attests to the contributions of general public education as well as of focused behavioral interventions involving homosexual men. The unique resurgence of STIs in poverty-stricken groups of blacks and Hispanics from 1985 to 1991 in the United States provides the exception that proves the rule—an exception that highlights the important impact both of behavioral factors and of clinical and public health services on STI incidence. It was the concurrence of two phenomena, both the changing behavioral risk factors (e.g., increasing exchange of sex for drugs or money) and the decline in public health services for STI control, that appears to be correlated with this new epidemic of STIs in the United States.

In summary, it is clear that strengthened clinical and behavioral interventions for STI prevention and control over the past 25 years have been associated with an impressive reduction in STI morbidity in the industrialized countries and that a resurgence of STIs has been seen where behavioral risks increase while clinical services deteriorate. Although data are lacking concerning the relative contribution of behavioral and nonbehavioral interventions versus that of underlying sociodemographic trends, the experience of industrialized countries strongly supports the strengthening of balanced programs for STI control, based on behavioral interventions, together with development of conventional clinical and public health services for STI control.

THE DEVELOPING COUNTRIES: HETEROGENEOUS PATTERNS OF SEXUAL BEHAVIOR

In 1985, the world population was nearly 5 billion people, and over three-fourths lived in developing countries. Of the total, 58% lived in Asia, 11% in Africa,

10% in Europe, 8% in Latin America, 6% in the USSR, 5% in North America, and 0.5% in Oceània (30). The developing countries comprise all those of Africa, Latin America, Asia (excepting Japan), and Oceania (excepting Australia and New Zealand). The United Nations further subdivides the developing countries into those that are "least developed" (largely concentrated in Africa) and those that are "developing" (concentrated in Asia and Latin America). In this chapter, the term "developing countries" includes both categories of development.

In this volume, Carballo and colleagues address cross-cultural comparisons of sexual behaviors. Major differences in sexual behaviors and patterns of occurrence of STIs have been seen among various groups within countries, between countries within continental and regional areas, and between continental regions. It is likely that patterns of sexual behavior are more heterogeneous in the developing countries than in the industrialized Western world, where common historical roots, together with today's economic interdependence and extensive networks of communication, produce more homogeneous social systems, culture, and shared values and beliefs.

Thus, generalizations are difficult. However, examples are useful to illustrate patterns that have been discerned. For example, in sub-Saharan Africa, homosexual partnerships among men have been difficult to find and appear to be relatively uncommon. Larson (14) has described two prototypes of heterosexual networking. In pattern 1, marital stability is strong, women tend to be very dependent on their husbands, social structure often tends to be patrilineal, and men frequently have premarital and extramarital sex with a relatively small number of women who themselves have many sex partners. In pattern 2, marital stability is weaker, and women are more independent, may be better educated, and may return more easily with their children to their original families; both men and women have relatively fluid networks of sexual partnerships, and the role of prostitution in these partnerships is less apparent.

Recognition of these patterns could guide the design of interventions. Pattern 1 is represented by Kigali, Rwanda, where the prevalence of HIV infection in young adults has risen to 20% or higher, while pattern 2 is represented by Kinshasa, Zaire, where the prevalence of HIV infection has leveled off at 7 to 8% in young adults.

In Asia, Latin America, and some countries of North Africa and the Middle East, there are long-standing double standards of sexual activity (25). Fewer women than men have extramarital sex (although this is changing in many Latin American countries, in particular). Prototypes for such patterns in Asia would include Thailand, the Philippines, Taiwan, and Hong Kong, with large and well-established international sex industries, and India and Indonesia, with established national sex industries. In such settings, the gender difference in sexual behavior is great. There is anecdotal evidence that in some of these same regions, where a double standard of sexual behavior is very apparent, bisexuality among men is rather common; among women, the mean rate of partner change is low, but the variance in rate of change is very large. From these perspectives, pattern 1, which presents a higher variance in the mean rate of partner change within the female population, may have a higher reproductive rate for STIs (see below), and behavioral interventions that target prostitutes and their clients may be relatively more important than in settings where pattern 2 predominates.

Because patterns of sexual behavior help determine the rate and extent of spread of STIs and can suggest different targets for intervention, quantitative as well as qualitative research on these patterns is needed to guide interventions. It is important to better understand not only what determines qualitative differences in patterns of sexual behavior but also what determines quantitative differences in the mean and variance in rates of partner change within societies conforming more or less to the same pattern. To what extent, for example, do differences in per capita income and economic development, rates of social evolution and devolution, birth rates, and status of women set the mean and variance in rates of partner change at different levels in different countries and populations? Since similar factors also influence the health care infrastructure that is essential for removal of STIs from the population, these factors may have complex influences on country-to-country differences in rates of STIs.

WHAT CHANGES IN BEHAVIORS ARE SOUGHT THROUGH BEHAVIORAL INTERVENTIONS?

For the prevention and control of the curable STIs (e.g., gonorrhea, syphilis, chancroid, chlamydial infection, donovanosis, and vaginal trichomoniasis), both sexual behaviors (including choice and number of partners, sexual practices, and use of condoms) and health care-seeking behaviors are important. For the viral STIs (e.g., infections with HIV, herpes simplex virus, hepatitis B virus, or human papillomavirus), health care-seeking behaviors currently are less important, since these infections are incurable, and treatment (seldom available in developing countries, in any case) cannot interrupt the chain of transmission of infection. However, even for viral STIs, health care seeking provides the opportunity for sexual behavioral interventions.

The specific behaviors that are sought have been listed in Table 3 of the chapter by Judson and Paalman in this volume. This table lists three categories of objectives of behavioral interventions: (i) reduce risk of exposure to and acquisition of STIs through changes in sexual behavior; (ii) reduce risk of transmission and complications of STIs through improvements in health care-seeking and compliance behavior; and (iii) improve health care provider behavior to increase the accessibility and effectiveness of STI services. The latter issues have also been discussed in detail by Amaro and Gornemann (this volume). This list of behaviors from Table 3 of Judson and Paalman seems equally applicable as objectives for behavioral interventions in developing countries. However, because of the frequency of polygamous marriages in developing countries, we would add the objective of closed relationships within polygamous or monogamous relationships as a further objective of sexual behavior change.

The behavioral interventions listed by Judson and Paalman (this volume) can be viewed as those that will reduce the reproductive rate, R_0, of an STI. As discussed by Anderson and by Brunham and Ronald, elsewhere in this volume,

$R_0 = \beta \times [m + (\sigma^2/m)] \times D$. R_0 represents the average number of secondary cases of an STI generated by one primary case in a susceptible population, and if R_0 is >1, the infection will spread until R_0 reaches equilibrium at 1 in the population. β is the efficiency of transmission, m is the mean rate of partner change, σ^2 is the variance in rate of sex partner change, and D is the duration of infectiousness. The three factors that directly determine R_0 represent the three points of attack in prevention of an STI. It is important to recognize that behavioral interventions can influence all three factors. For example, the mean efficiency of transmission per contact or per sexual partner relationship, β, for most STIs can be reduced by condom use, and for HIV (10, 18) and probably for hepatitis B virus (22), the efficiency of transmission of infection can be reduced by avoiding receptive anorectal intercourse. Epidemiological research also suggests that for HIV infection, β might be reduced by male circumcision, by avoiding vaginal intercourse during menses, and by reducing the prevalence of several other STIs (in part through behavioral interventions). Delay in onset of intercourse for women may be an important way to decrease β for certain STIs because the susceptibility of the cervix (e.g., to chlamydial or HIV infection) may be greater in teenage women than in older women (11, 16).

As discussed by Anderson (this volume), the mean rate of partner change (m) and the variance in rate of partner change (σ^2) in the population, as well as the patterns of partner mixing within the population, are all directly related to R_0. It can be shown that for any given mean rate of partner change in a community, values of R_0, and the ultimate equilibrium prevalence of STIs, can be greatly increased by the existence of a high variance in rate of partner change, owing to core groups with large numbers of partners, who frequently acquire and transmit STIs. Thus, targeted behavioral change among core group members would have much greater impact than behavioral change in non-core group members.

Finally, for the curable STIs, the duration of infectiousness, D, is strongly influenced by health care-seeking behavior. For example, in a 1985 study conducted in a slum area of Nairobi, 40% of prostitutes undergoing screening examinations were found to have genital ulceration, usually resulting from chancroid (13). The women had continued to engage in commercial sex despite the presence of genital ulcers. This indicated extraordinarily poor health care-seeking behavior and/or lack of access to health care for this condition at that time. Earlier consultation would have resulted in curative treatment, shorter duration of infection, and smaller R_0 for chancroid in the population. Behavioral interventions that reduce D by encouraging early diagnosis and treatment interrupt the chain of transmission of the curable STIs such as chancroid and thus result in primary prevention of the curable STIs (just as would behavioral intervention directed at β [e.g., condom use], or at m, the mean number of partners), as well as secondary prevention of the disease complications of these STIs.

A few additional specific comments are warranted on the behaviors listed in Table 3 of Judson and Paalman (this volume). First, the avoidance of high-risk partners may be relatively easier for men than for women. For example, a man can choose not to have sex with a prostitute, whereas in societies in which most women do not have extramarital sex but men may have sex with prostitutes, a woman's risk is less related to her own number of partners than to her partner's number and choice of partners (1, 5).

Second, we are unaware of concerted health promotion efforts having been initiated as a result of epidemiological data linking the lack of circumcision to increased risk of acquiring STIs, including chancroid, HIV, and perhaps other infections. What further data are needed before health promotion efforts include the promotion of circumcision? Is it time for intervention trials comparing risks of STIs in men randomized to groups of circumcision or no circumcision? Are such trials feasible? Should we proceed to advocate circumcision without further epidemiological data or intervention trials? While these questions are being asked, there is anecdotal evidence that in industrialized countries some parents and pediatricians are already electing circumcision to reduce subsequent risk of HIV infection, while in developing countries with high rates of HIV infection, some adult men now express interest in circumcisions to prevent HIV (E. M. Ankrah, S. Wangalwa, and A. Abura, Vth Int. Conf. AIDS Afr., abstr. WPA 3, p. 90, 1990).

Third, concerning condom use, the recent condom promotion campaigns in developing countries have generally suffered from lack of clear focus on objectives (prevention of HIV infection versus prevention of all STIs versus contraception) and from ambiguity regarding target groups (high-risk versus general population). Piot and Laga (this volume) cite the extraordinarily good cost-effectiveness of a condom promotion program conducted with Nairobi prostitutes for prevention of STIs at a time when 80% or more of the prostitutes had HIV infection (17). On the other hand, in most of the world (e.g., North Africa and the Middle East, Nigeria, most of Asia, Oceania, Europe, and the Americas), where the prevalence of HIV infection in the general population of young adults is $<1\%$, the promotion of condom use with every sexual encounter to prevent transmission of HIV infection is unrealistic. It may have been politically expedient, if inaccurate, to argue that everyone is at equal risk of HIV infection, in order to avoid stigmatizing particular high-risk groups and to encourage the broadest support for AIDS services, research, and prevention programs, but it does not follow that condom use should be widely promoted to prevent HIV infection, regardless of actual risk.

An alternative definition of objectives of condom promotion in settings in which prevention of STIs is at least as important as preventing pregnancy (e.g., where safe abortion is available) might be the prevention of all STIs, together with contraception, for individuals engaging in casual sex. Where contraception was the paramount concern, condoms could be promoted for sex with high-risk partners together with a more effective means of contraception. Promotion strategies would then differ for different target groups and in different settings. Public health education for schools and for the general public would lead to awareness of condoms and of the effectiveness of condoms in preventing STIs, including HIV, the effectiveness of condoms as contraceptives, and the appropriateness of condoms as prophylaxis and as contraception for individuals with casual or known high-risk partners. This approach could change social norms and make condom use acceptable in appropriate circumstances without advocating unrealistic condom use when the risk of STIs is low. Focused promotion of condom use—specifically during sex with prostitutes or for men who have sex with men—could be combined with skills training in condom use and offered to men likely to have sex with prostitutes (e.g., military personnel, truck drivers), to men in brothels or bars or other settings frequented by prostitutes and their clients or by homosexual men, or to men seeking treatment for STIs. This would further enable prostitutes to negotiate condom use with clients, yet would have much less potential for stigmatizing prostitutes than would a population-wide campaign to avoid prostitutes, for example. These would be rational objectives even in countries of Latin America, Asia, Oceania, and parts of Africa where HIV infection remains uncommon in the general population but where other STIs are widely prevalent.

Strategies for Achieving Improved Health Care Behaviors to Reduce Transmission and Complications of STIs

Strategies for health promotion to improve health care behavior and reduce transmission of STIs can include promotion of knowledge of the common manifestations of STIs; the belief that STIs are curable but can cause serious complications, including sterility and infant death, if not treated by qualified health care providers; the development of appropriate, adequate, and acceptable clinical services for STIs; and informing people about how to access these services. A sense of the individual's responsibility for the sexual and reproductive health of his or her sexual partner and the related health of his or her children should be promoted at the earliest possible stage of psychosocial development. Amaro and Gornemann provide a comprehensive discussion of these issues elsewhere in this volume.

UNIQUE PROBLEMS FOR PREVENTION AND CONTROL OF STIs IN DEVELOPING COUNTRIES

Developing countries present particular challenges to public health in general, and to prevention and control of STIs in particular, as a result of their specific demographic, economic, and educational profiles. In this section, we review the relevant aspects of these profiles in developing countries, and in the subsequent section, we review the issues raised by these profiles and the implications for prevention and control of STIs.

The Demographic Transition and the Population Age Pyramid

One major development relevant to the current epidemiology of STIs was the explosive growth in world population following World War II. Advances in medical science, childhood immunizations, and sanitation contributed to widespread improvement in health conditions. As a result, mortality rates declined sharply. Fertility rates also declined, but at a slower rate, especially in developing countries. The result has been a doubling of the world's population over the span of a generation. Most of this population increase was concentrated in developing countries, and the increase has been most striking in sub-Saharan Africa, the only region of the world where fertility rates have not declined during the past 20 years (7).

This pattern of demographic transition—falling child mortality with sustained birth rates in many developing countries—could be the single most important factor fueling the epidemic spread of STIs, including HIV infection, in the developing countries. The combination of relatively high birth rates and low death rates results in youthful populations in which the number of infants, children, and young adults exceeds the proportion of older adults (20). The youthful age structure has many implications, including a large and increasingly sexually active population.

The absolute increase in number of younger people leads to an absolute increase in numbers of STI cases in the population and to an increase in overall incidence of STIs (since a higher proportion of the total population belongs to the age groups at highest risk). In addition, age-specific rates of STIs may also increase for several reasons. For example, populations in which younger age groups outnumber older age groups are marked by a shift in the balance of power and values from older, more stable and conservative members of the population to the younger groups. The burden of socializing the upcoming generation poses a greater challenge for the older generation (4). We postulate a critical mass phenomenon, in which the increasing proportion of the population belonging to younger ages together with the removal of the restraining influence of older members of the population leads to more frequent interactions among youths that lead to sexual intercourse. Further, given the widespread practice of sexual unions between younger women and older men, the relative scarcity of older men contributes to increased promiscuity among older men. The absolute and relative increase in youthful populations leads to overburdening of public health facilities for STIs as well as other youth-oriented facilities. Finally, the formation of rural-to-urban migration streams of young, single adults in response to population pressure clearly has an additional effect on increasing rates of STIs (19).

The fundamental failure of the demographic transition in developing countries to balance the reduction in child mortality with a reduction in birth rates has had important implications (28). Prevention and control of STIs must now be coupled with new and innovative programs of reproductive health and family survival which link child survival with family planning, prenatal care, and prevention and control of reproductive tract infections, leading to preservation of fertility and improved health of women.

Economic Underdevelopment

The period following World War II was also marked by major economic and technological growth. Between 1955 and 1980, the world economic output tripled and per capita income doubled. However, economic growth was not distributed uniformly. In less developed countries, pressures from population growth were strong, and expansion of the industrial sector was not adequate to absorb the increases in the labor force. Consequently, unemployment and underemployment grew in these countries. Owing to pressures resulting from the unprecedented growth of the population in developing countries, the per capita income disparity between industrialized and developing countries has continued to widen during recent decades, despite overall economic growth (28).

Economic growth rates varied widely among developing countries as well. Oil-producing countries and several countries in the Far East and Latin America had rapid growth rates, while the poorest countries continued to drop further behind. During the 1970s, Africa's gains in per capita income were less than half the average for all developing countries, and by the early 1980s, the growth rate had become negative (31). The variation in economic growth rates across countries resulted in large-scale migrations of people seeking work from countries with slow economic growth to countries with rapid economic growth. According to the estimates of the International Labor Organization, by 1980, there were 20 to 22 million international migrants working in foreign countries (12).

The economic transformation that followed World War II was also marked by a decline in the relative importance of agriculture. In 1950, the agricultural sector of the world economy had employed almost two-thirds of the world's paid labor force; by 1980, this proportion was less than one-half of the total. Employment in industry and services grew twice as fast as in agriculture.

The situation of the poorest countries and their most vulnerable subpopulations was further worsened through the world recession of the early 1980s. The recession was marked by large-scale unemployment and a high rate of price inflation (23).

The implications of economic underdevelopment for prevention of STIs are twofold: (i) promotion of an integrated program of reproductive health, encompassing family planning and STIs, as discussed above, will help address the root causes of underdevelopment, while at the same time addressing the root causes of STIs, and (ii) structural constraints on both behavioral and nonbehavioral interventions must be considered in the design of behavioral interventions for preventing STIs in developing countries.

Education in Underdeveloped Countries

Low levels of literacy and education are an additional problem in the less developed countries. Despite unprecedented increases in literacy rates from the 1960s through the mid-1980s, only 78% of adult men and 68% of adult women in the world were able to read and write. In developing countries, the literacy average was 68% for men and 50% for women (26). Low literacy rates are strongly associated with poverty, with the lowest literacy rates being observed in the world's least-developed countries, especially in Africa and South Asia.

Basic elementary education is still unavailable to many children in the world. One-fourth of children of primary school age are not in school. In Africa, in 1980, 4 of 10 eligible children could not be enrolled in school (26). When first and second levels of education are considered together, the percentage not enrolled in schools increases further. In all developing countries, girls are less likely than boys to attend school; almost 60% of girls between 5 and 19 years of age are not in school. In rural areas, especially, the advantages to the family of girls' work at home can often override the benefits seen in female education (23).

Women's Social Status

Globally, women have become increasingly self-sufficient economically during the recent decades, but progress has been slow (6). By 1985, one in two women between the ages of 15 and 64 were in the paid labor force. In industrialized countries, women made up 40% of the total paid labor force, and in developing countries, they constituted 32% of the paid labor force, up slightly from 38 and 28%, respectively, in 1950. There is, however, marked divergence among the regions of the world in women's participation in the labor force. In Eastern Europe and the USSR in 1985, women's representation in paid employment was 90% of the men's. In contrast, in the Middle East, where women's activities outside the household are limited, this ratio was only 29% (23). In northern Africa and Latin America, women's economic activities are similarly limited.

In general, the rates of unemployment and underemployment among women are higher than those among men. In addition, the amount of hidden unemployment appears to be greater among women. In 1980, the International Labor Organization estimated the unemployment rates in developing countries to be 7.8% for women and 5.2% for men (12). Great proportions of women in developing countries are self-employed; therefore, estimating the extent to which they are being underutilized is difficult.

Women tend to be highly concentrated in a narrow range of fields and in jobs that are considered to require lower responsibility and skill. This is especially true in developing countries. Such concentration results in a substantial and persistent gap in earnings between men and women (6). Women's occupational concentration is also associated with lower status, longer hours, fewer or no fringe benefits, and less security.

In both industrialized and developing countries, the feminization of poverty has been observed. Women living in rural areas of less developed countries are in the worst socioeconomic situation. Migration of men to urban areas and to other countries in search of better-paying jobs leaves women in rural areas with the economic burden of families and a lack of resources. In many countries, laws and social institutions that do not give women any independent status further limit their ability to cope. They may have no rights to own, lease, buy, or sell property or to have access to credit. Modernization of agriculture has increased women's dependency because mechanization and related training have been primarily directed at men. Commercialization of agriculture has increased women's workload but reduced their opportunities for independent cash earnings, since men generally control the marketing of cash crops.

The legal system in many countries is not equally protective of men's and women's rights. Although by the end of the 1980s most countries had established constitutional or legislative provisions asserting the equality of the sexes, defining the scope and content of sexual equality and achieving equality are long-run processes. Matters such as divorce and family planning gradually became the subject of public regulation. For example, until the 1920s, English laws gave husbands the right to divorce their wives on grounds of adultery, while wives needed additional grounds, such as assault, to divorce their husbands. In France and Spain, female adultery was grounds for imprisonment, but male adultery was not (23).

In countries where traditional social and religious practices have strictly enforced women's subordinate status, the legal system has been slow to provide equal rights for women. For example, in countries with large Islamic populations, traditional holy law often takes precedence over secular law. Islamic law permits polygamy and divorce by the husband without court formalities. It also decrees that a woman must be under a male guardian and should not leave the house unless accompanied by a male relative and that a daughter inherits only half as much as a son. Adherence to Islamic law varies across countries. In Saudi Arabia, gender segregation is the law, while in Tunisia and Turkey, civil law follows principles of equality as enunciated in the United Nations Convention on Women's Rights (23, 27).

Customary law still takes precedence in many sub-Saharan African countries (23). For example, Kenya exempted inheritance of property from its constitutional provision on equality; Somalia conferred legal equality but continued to permit customs such as female circumcision; Burundi's family code allows the wife to work only if the husband consents to it; in India, wives are not recognized as joint owners of property acquired during marriage; in Peru, women cannot act in commercial matters without the authorization of their husbands. Regardless of existing religious or customary law, social tradition can limit effectiveness of equality legislation.

The subordinate status of women in several developing countries has many implications for the prevention of STIs. First, current health promotion efforts cannot focus only on changing the behavior of women, who may not be free to change behavior, but must also involve men and the community. Second, efforts to empower women to effect behavior change are essential in health promotion to prevent STIs. Third, long-term strategies to control STIs must address strategies to improve the status of women.

Health Services: Gender Differences in Need, Access, and Utilization

Health services for prevention and control of STIs in developing countries are discussed by Piot and Laga elsewhere in this volume. It is clear that the morbidity caused by STIs other than HIV infection is generally greater for women than for men. Early childbearing and short birth intervals also pose considerable risk to the health of women. According to the World Health Organization, deaths from pregnancy-related causes are among the five leading causes of death for women between the ages of 15 and 44; in one-third of the developing countries, pregnancy-related causes occupy the first or second position in overall causes of death (29, 30).

Gender differentials in the provision and use of health services are sizable (21). Despite women's childbearing function, men have a higher rate of hospital bed occupancy. Women's family responsibilities, lack of free time, and social and financial dependence limit their access to health care facilities, unless these are very easily accessible. In the past 20 years, major changes have been initiated in government health programs to place greater emphasis on primary health care and community-based health systems and to serve two target groups—children and reproductive-age women. These new programs may produce greater equality between men and women living in less developed countries with respect to access to and utilization of health services.

On the other hand, the emphasis on maternal and child health services at the primary health care level could be associated with underutilization of public primary health care services by men. In particular, men with STIs commonly seek treatment for STIs from pharmacies or the informal health sector, rather than from primary health services. Conversely, where categorical STI clinics do exist in developing countries, they commonly serve predominantly men, or sometimes predominantly commercial sex workers.

Limited access to and utilization of public sector health services by certain groups of individuals with STIs have further public health implications for behavioral interventions. They limit the health educators' access to priority groups for health education concerning STIs. Where accessible, health service facilities provide a convenient point at which public health workers can interface with populations at risk for purposes of health education and behavioral intervention.

STRATEGIC ISSUES CONCERNING BEHAVIORAL INTERVENTIONS IN DEVELOPING COUNTRIES

Differences between industrialized and developing countries have implications for the feasibility, acceptability, and potential effectiveness of interventions.

First, in developing countries, populations tend to be less educated, and greater proportions are illiterate. They also tend to be less responsive to written education materials and less experienced in responding to health education campaigns.

Second, culture in many developing countries dictates a greater dominance of the society, community, group, and family over the individual. In this respect, less developed countries constitute a marked contrast to the individualistic Western way of life.

Third, the existing infrastructure of STI services is very limited, as discussed further below. Technical and economic barriers in developing countries limit the implementation of the medical model of prevention and disease control. On the other hand, low levels of education, high levels of illiteracy, long traditions of fatalistic outlooks, and the communalistic (as opposed to individualistic) orientation limit the choice and implementation of behavioral models of prevention and control. Thus, modified versions of both behavioral and medical approaches to prevention are indicated in developing countries.

Interestingly, it is possible that such modified approaches, when implemented, may be uniquely effective in developing countries. The particular STIs that are highly prevalent and thus need to be controlled, such as chancroid and syphilis, are highly susceptible to the effects of health care-seeking behavioral intervention. In many developing countries, the patterns of sexual behavior involve core groups with clear boundaries; these target groups can be particularly responsive to focused interventions, and such interventions can be highly efficient in prevention of STIs. Finally, the nonindividualistic, nonwritten culture of the developing world may provide unusually effective avenues for communication. Verbally delivered messages coming from community leaders in communalistic societies may be very effective in bringing about preventive behavior change. For example, a review of Zimbabwean studies suggested that beliefs most predictive of HIV-preventive behaviors are "those least amenable to modification by the mass media or formal health education; instead, community-based, participative, small groups, face-to-face approaches," involving use of cultural approaches, such as drama and music, were thought to be needed (D. Wilson, R. Greenspan, and S. Lavelle, Vth Int. Conf. AIDS Afr., abstr. FPA 12, p. 262, 1990). One technique that appears acceptable and of interest to subjects involves the use of storytelling with visual aid flashcards to tell stories that are culturally relevant to raise issues concerning prostitution, premarital sex, HIV transmission, and condom use and female empowerment (G. Foster and F. Robinson, Vth Int. Conf. AIDS Afr., abstr. FPA 23, p. 265, 1990). The power of storytelling among indigenous populations of Peru has been vividly described by Mario Vargas Llosa in his novel, *The Storyteller* (15). Paradoxically, it is possible that economic, technological, and cultural changes inherent in development, by causing fragmentation of social and community influences, in some ways provide barriers to certain channels of communication. These new barriers may be as important as, if not precisely mirroring, those inherent in underdevelopment.

Limited Feasibility of Expanding Diagnostic and Treatment Services for Control of STIs in Least-Developed Countries: Implications for Behavioral Interventions

Piot and Laga (this volume) describe the objectives and constraints on development of clinical and public health services for STI control in developing countries. In particular, the lack of availability of diagnostic tests for cervical gonococcal and chlamydial infections greatly limits the potential for control of these infections, which have also been implicated as risk factors for acquisition of HIV infection by women. Constraints on some of the conventional clinical and public health approaches to STI control, particularly in the least-developed countries of Africa, place a greater burden on alternative approaches, such as behavioral interventions for both sexual and health care-seeking behaviors.

At first glance, it might appear that in settings in which public clinic services for diagnosis and treatment of certain STIs in women are negligible, there is no point in attempting to promote health care-seeking behavior. It has even been argued that it may be unwise to promote important health care-seeking behaviors for STIs in the absence of a well-established system for provision of clinical services. In fact, we believe that the opposite is the case. For example, because symptoms of STIs are less obvious in women than in men, in settings in which diagnostic services for women are not available, the development and recognition of typical symptoms in the man may offer the best opportunity for identifying female partners who are at risk. Thus, health promotion that encourages men to seek the highest possible level of health care (e.g., clinics or pharmacies rather than drug vendors or traditional healers) can lead to a more qualified diagnosis and more appropriate therapy; promotion of attitudes of responsibility for the sexual and reproductive health of the man's partner can facilitate notification of the partner; and innovative social marketing techniques (which would encourage clinics and pharmacists to treat exposed partners) could close the loop of partner notification.

Further, where clinical facilities for diagnosis and treatment of STIs are severely limited, focused interventions to change the sexual behavior of members of high-risk groups may be less feasible. This is because focused public health interventions for high-risk groups have often relied on STI clinical services to obtain access to high-risk groups and have relied on both condom promotion and STI diagnosis and treatment to motivate risk group members to participate in intervention programs. Focused behavioral intervention programs have often been implemented around existing or newly established clinical STI services for prostitutes or for men who are their clients. It is a common experience that where STI services are organized and available, participating prostitutes express interest in the STI services as a primary motivation for continued participation in ongoing behavioral intervention. However, behavioral interventions involving condom promotion for prostitutes are also being organized as community-based programs. Where STI services have been nonexistent (i.e., are unknown) for prostitutes, they may express less interest in obtaining STI clinical services as a motivation for continued participation in the community-based programs.

In summary, where well-organized systems for STI clinical services are lacking, alternative settings for interventions that aim to change sexual behavior could include those that do in fact offer treatment for STIs (e.g., primary care clinics, pharmacies, drug vendors). Such settings have been used effectively for condom distribution and sales in social marketing programs, for example, in Zaire (C. Ferreros, N. Mivumbi, K. Kakera, and J. Price, VIth Int. Conf. AIDS, abstr. SC 697, p. 263, 1990). The potential for greater use of these alternative settings and providers for health education, partner notification, and condom distribution should be further explored. Strengthening of clinical services in these and other settings, including community-based programs serving prostitutes, would not only complement but also strengthen these behavioral interventions.

Specific Strategies for Behavioral Interventions in Developing Countries: Considerations of Specific STIs, Focused Interventions (Targeting), and Type or Intensity of Intervention

The many strategies for prevention and control of STIs, including sexually transmitted HIV infection, follow three major approaches: (i) prevention of exposure to STIs by encouraging postponement of sexual debut, fewer sex partners, discrimination in choice of safer partners, and use of safer sex practices; (ii) use of condoms; and (iii) provision and appropriate utilization of services for diagnosis and treatment of STIs (this third approach potentially applies not only to prevention of the curable STIs, such as gonorrhea, syphilis, chlamydial infection, chancroid, and trichomoniasis, but also to HIV infection, because this infection appears to be transmitted more efficiently in the presence of these other curable STIs). Behavioral interventions that are directed towards any of these three approaches can be designed for the general population, special groups, or the individual and can utilize various channels and varying levels of intensity of communication. We believe that these three approaches, although overlapping, can be viewed as the three legs upon which rests the platform supporting all national and local programs for prevention and control of STIs, including sexually transmitted HIV infection. Use of only one or two of these approaches is insufficient to support such a program. However, the different STIs may respond differently to various behavioral interventions. The emphasis given to each of the three approaches, the choice of target population, and the intensity of interventions depends on the differing epidemiologies of various STIs, the availability of resources, and the prevalent patterns of sexual activity.

Relative Susceptibility of Various STIs to Health Care-Seeking Behavioral Interventions, and Relative Importance of Core Groups in Transmission

Relative susceptibility

The relative susceptibility of various STIs to specific behavioral interventions has not, to our knowledge, been formally compared and probably depends on the setting. For example, the power of specific sexual behavioral interventions for reducing the incidence of a specific STI (e.g., HIV infection) in an individual or in the population at large will depend on the availability and effectiveness of services or products that are to be promoted. For example, promotion of testing and counseling or treatment for the clinical carrier state (e.g., HIV infection or chlamydial infection) depends on the availability of these services. The success of condom promotion depends on the availability of condoms. Similarly, the impact of promotion of health care-seeking behaviors for symptoms suggestive of STIs may be much greater where diagnosis and treatments for the causes of these symptoms are available.

Nonetheless, based on the known clinical epidemiology of the various STIs, we can propose a relative rank ordering of susceptibility of STIs to those health care-seeking behavioral interventions that encompass recognition of symptoms and signs, avoiding sex when these are present, seeking health care, and notifying

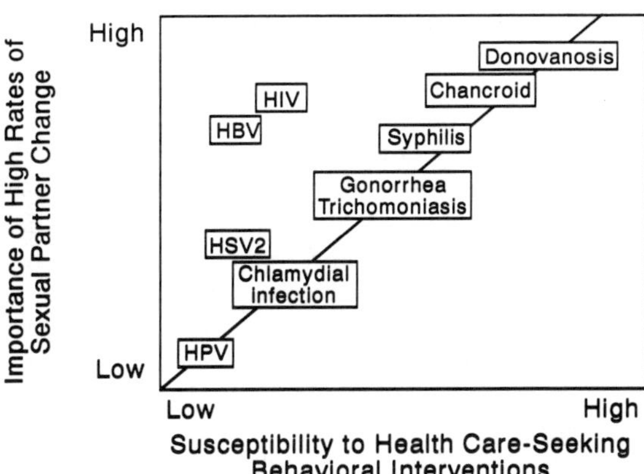

Figure 1. Estimates of relative ranking of STIs in terms of susceptibility to behavioral interventions and the relative importance of health care-seeking core groups that have high rates of sexual partner change. The curable STIs are susceptible to both sexual and health care behavioral intervention, while the viral STIs are, in general, only susceptible to sexual behavioral intervention. HBV, hepatitis B virus; HSV2, herpes simplex virus type 2; HPV, human papillomavirus.

partners. As shown in Fig. 1, those infections that produce easily recognized symptoms and signs in most infected persons and that are most easily diagnosed and potentially curable (e.g., donovanosis, chancroid, and syphilis) should be most susceptible to such interventions. In contrast, those STIs that usually do not produce characteristic symptoms and signs, are hard to diagnose, or are incurable would be least susceptible (e.g., human papillomavirus infection).

Importance of Core Groups

Furthermore, the importance of focusing interventions on core groups of individuals with many partners can also be inferred both from empirical observations on the role of core groups in outbreaks or in sustained transmission of STIs and from what is known about the efficiency of transmission and duration of infectivity for each STI (see Brunham and Ronald, this volume). According to the relationship $R_0 = \beta \times [m + (\sigma^2/m)] \times D$, it follows that for the STIs that have very low values for β and/or for D, the value for $m + (\sigma^2/m)$ must be relatively high if R_0 is to have a value greater than unity: core groups of highly sexually active individuals would be important for sustained spread of these diseases. For STIs that have intrinsically high values for β and D, the value for $m + (\sigma^2/m)$ required to sustain R_0 greater than unity could be much lower, and core groups would be relatively unimportant.

For the viral STIs, the mean duration of infectivity, D, is influenced very little or not at all by behavioral interventions because treatments are either unavailable or have little influence on duration of infectiousness. On the other hand, D could be strongly influenced by health care-seeking behaviors for the curable STIs, especially for those that usually produce obvious symptoms and are easily diagnosed and treated but that would have a long duration of infectiousness without treatment. Thus, for the easily recognized and curable STIs, the duration of infectivity should be low if knowledge and access to care are good; however, in developing countries, where core groups of individuals with high levels of sexual activity often have low knowledge concerning STIs and poor access to care (e.g., low socioeconomic status prostitutes), the influence of these factors would be multiplicative, leading to very high rates of spread of STIs but presenting great opportunities for intervention.

Interrelationships of the three determinants of R_0

We advance here the hypothesis that the three determinants of the reproductive rate for STIs, β, $m + (\sigma^2/m)$, and D, are actually highly interrelated rather than independent variables and that core groups of high-frequency transmitters of STIs tend to have higher than average values for all these determinants. There are several reasons for this. At the programmatic level, the duration of infection with curable STIs may tend to be longer than average in individuals and groups with very high rates of partner change (e.g., homosexual men during the 1970s, prostitutes, those who trade sex for drugs). This is partly because one of the key strategies for control of curable STIs, partner notification, is more difficult in these groups, and also because high rates of acquisition of STIs can overwhelm and clog up the public health clinical facilities for diagnosis and treatment, as is now the case in large inner cities of the United States. Further, the association of prostitution and homosexuality with stigma can inhibit development of health care systems serving these groups and at the individual level can reduce access to care. As discussed above, to the extent that poverty and social disintegration per se increase the mean and variance in rates of partner change, these same factors can preclude development of an infrastructure for diagnosis and treatment of STIs or, as in the case of Uganda, can lead to deterioration of an existing infrastructure. Finally, to the extent that drug addiction (e.g., cocaine or heroin use) contributes to high rates of partner change, a simultaneous effect on poor health care behavior can be postulated.

The efficiency of transmission of certain STIs also may be disproportionately higher in core group members with high rates of partner change. For example, among homosexual men, HIV spread rapidly not only because of high rates of partner change but also because of efficient transmission via receptive anorectal intercourse. High rates of coexistent anorectal herpes and syphilis (and perhaps other causes of proctitis) also may have made transmission more efficient (24). One can speculate that the epidemic of sexually transmitted hepatitis B virus infection among homosexual men during the 1970s may have had similar determinants. Among prostitutes and their clients, high rates of curable STIs again are associated with more efficient transmission and acquisition of HIV infection. Lack of access to effective health care for curable STIs and dependence on sex for income could lead to continued sex during the acute, highly infectious stages of STIs (as in the case of the Nairobi prostitutes with genital ulcers) and to lesser availability of condoms, resulting in efficient transmission.

We derive three conclusions from this discussion. First, for the curable STIs, the correlation of frequent transmission with delayed diagnosis and treatment helps to account for a postulated correlation between level of susceptibility to health care-seeking behavioral intervention and the important role of core groups with high rates of partner change in sustaining transmission (see below, and Fig. 1). Second, at least for the curable STIs, core groups tend to be characterized both by high rates of partner change and by relatively long duration of infectivity. Third, in settings in which the variance in sexual behavior is very high and core groups can be defined, both sexual and health care-seeking behavioral interventions could have great impact.

Figure 1 presents our estimates of the relative ranking of the various STIs, in terms of susceptibility to health care behavioral interventions on one axis and in terms of the potential importance of core groups in transmission on the other. Undeterred (and unfettered) by the absence of data, we postulate that the curable STIs are more susceptible than the viral STIs to health care behavioral interventions. We believe that the three bacterial genital ulcer diseases—donovanosis, chancroid, and syphilis—are likely to be highly susceptible to the promotion of good health care-seeking behavior, because they are the most easily recognized by the infected individual and among the most easily diagnosed and treated of all STIs. Further, because they also have the highest potential for focused interventions and persist only in core groups with high rates of partner change or with very poor use of or access to health care, and because health care behavior may be more susceptible to change than sexual behavior, as discussed below, we speculate that these three genital ulcer diseases should be viewed as hypersusceptible to behavioral intervention. Since genital ulcer diseases have repeatedly been implicated as risk factors for HIV transmission, and since syphilis causes considerable morbidity on its own, we would give very high priority to promoting health care-seeking behaviors for control of genital ulcer diseases, especially in populations having high rates of one or more of these STIs.

Lack of circumcision is also a factor in promoting efficient transmission of chancroid and, possibly, of donovanosis and syphilis as well. The clear link of outbreaks of sustained transmission of chancroid, or of individual cases of donovanosis, with sex with prostitutes in populations where male circumcision is not practiced is consistent with this scheme. So are the recent outbreaks of chancroid and syphilis in inner city U.S. minority populations during the AIDS era. While the precise role of circumcision as protection against sexual acquisition of HIV requires further study, the benefit of circumcision in reducing the risk of chancroid, itself a risk factor for HIV transmission, has become an important issue in health promotion. Circumcision is also protective against urinary tract infection in young boys.

The usual causes of vaginal discharge include trichomoniasis, gonorrhea, and chlamydial infection, STIs that are less readily recognized than genital ulcers by the infected person and therefore less readily diagnosed. These are therefore less susceptible to promotion of health care-seeking behaviors, especially in developing countries with limited diagnostic resources. Core groups have been somewhat less important in the transmission of these STIs than in the transmission of chancroid, donovanosis, and syphilis, especially in areas with limited diagnostic resources. This may be because the duration of infectiousness tends to be long for trichomoniasis, gonorrhea, and chlamydial infection, particularly in women in developing countries, and perhaps because the efficiency of transmission is somewhat higher for these infections than for the three bacterial genital ulcer diseases. Because trichomoniasis is easier to detect and to treat than gonorrhea, it is probably more susceptible to promotion of health care seeking and education of health care providers in most settings, whereas chlamydial infection is hardest to detect and therefore is less susceptible.

Among the viral STIs, all are less susceptible than the curable STIs to behavioral interventions, because promotion of health care seeking does not lead to interruption of the chain of transmission by curative treatment. However, for HIV, hepatitis B virus, and herpes simplex virus type 2 infections, health care seeking can lead to diagnostic testing and specific counseling on steps to be taken to avoid transmission. For HIV, although duration of infectiousness is long, the efficiency of sexual transmission is low (especially in heterosexuals without underlying risk factors for sexual transmission, such as other STIs), and therefore high rates of partner change and core groups are important in spread of infection. Susceptibility to behavioral intervention may be greater for HIV infection than for the other viral STIs, to the extent that sexual transmission of HIV is more efficient in the presence of curable STIs, and the curable STIs are susceptible to behavioral interventions that promote health care seeking.

Relative Responsiveness of Behaviors to Interventions

Behaviors vary in their responsiveness to interventions. For example, among adolescents in the United States, age at sexual debut has proved less responsive than condom use to AIDS prevention messages (8, 9). Similarly, among drug users, injecting behaviors appear to be more responsive to behavioral intervention than sexual behaviors (8). While systematic data are not available on relative responsiveness of specific sexual and health behaviors to preventive interventions, observations over a variety of studies coupled with deductive thinking lead us to hypothesize that type of behavior, type of sexual dyad, ages of sex partners, cost, whether the intervention can be implemented by one member of the dyad alone, and whether the intervention needs to be implemented by the man or the woman all influence the responsiveness of risk behaviors to behavioral interventions. Further, if health care-seeking behaviors are more responsive to behavioral intervention than certain sexual behaviors, the responsiveness of health care-seeking behaviors would depend on the availability of clinical services in general and on access to the specific services being marketed in particular. We would expect that the behaviors of long-term couples might be more responsive to interventions than are the behaviors of short-term sexual dyads; for example, use of condoms to prevent transmission of a chronic viral STI might be more easily effected in couples with shared values and commitment to the relationship than in the casual sexual encounters of an individual with a chronic STI. Similarly, certain behaviors of older individuals, such as avoiding high-risk practices or partners, might be more responsive to change efforts than those of younger individuals because of a greater sense of invulnerability and greater impulsiveness associated with sexual behavior among the latter. We would hypothesize that interventions that require only one member of the couple to change his or her behavior might be easier to implement than those that require both members to change and that women's behaviors might

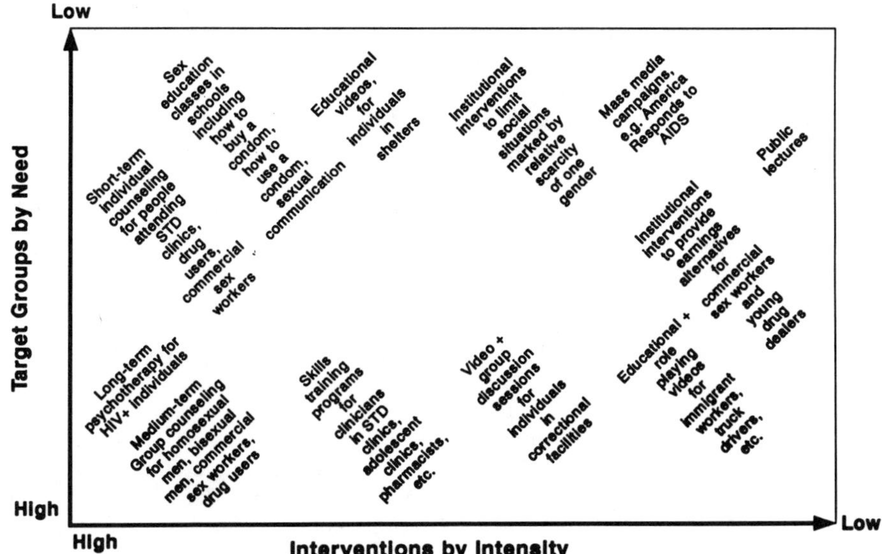

Figure 2. Behavioral interventions by need of target group and intensity of intervention.

be more responsive to intervention than men's behaviors, partly because of the greater risks of many STIs for women.

Balancing Targeting and Intensity of Intervention to Needs and Opportunities

Although Anderson (this volume) has observed a constant relationship between the mean and variance in rate of partner change in several reported studies, we suspect that sampling in a larger variety of countries and adequate representation of those with many partners (e.g., prostitutes and clients) would show important exceptions, especially among women. In general, in societies in which, for example, among women, the mean rate of partner change is very low but the variance in rate of partner change is very large, the needs and opportunities for behavioral interventions for the general female population are relatively low, and these should be of low intensity (e.g., posters, billboards, messages in mass media). On the other hand, the need for intervention in prostitutes and their clients is great, opportunities for intervention are provided at points of contact (e.g., bars and brothels) and where services for STIs are provided, and the intensity of intervention should be great (Fig. 2).

In contrast, in a country such as Uganda, where the countrywide prevalence of HIV infection has reached 10%, yet patterns of sexual networking may more closely resemble Larson's (14) pattern 2 than pattern 1, it may be that mean rates of partner change and efficiency of transmission of HIV are sufficiently high that intensive, population-wide behavioral interventions are necessary and most appropriate. Intensive interventions targeting all children, in and out of school, are important everywhere, but nowhere more so than in such countries.

Other important target groups with high rates of STIs in many developing countries include military personnel, who often are readily accessible and have relatively well organized systems for development of STI clinical services, and other mobile occupation groups, such as truck drivers, who can be reached with innovative programs for behavioral interventions, as reported in Kenya (M. A. Omari, J. J. Bwayo, A. N. Mutere, et al., *East. Afr. Med. J.*, in press).

RECOMMENDATIONS FOR BEHAVIORAL INTERVENTIONS IN DEVELOPING COUNTRIES

The major task involved in the prevention and control of STIs in developing countries is the definition and implementation of cost-effective control programs that would work in resource-poor settings, each with unique demographic, social, and cultural profiles. While these unique profiles may render the biomedical and behavioral intervention strategies developed in industrialized countries inappropriate, modified versions of these biomedical and behavioral strategies could prove even more effective in the developing world because of the high susceptibility of certain widely prevalent STIs to behavioral and focused interventions. The limited resources, the urgency of the need, and the variation in relevant parameters require that an algorithm be developed for the planning, implementation, and evaluation of a unique mix of integrated biomedical and behavioral intervention strategies for the prevention of STIs in each country.

For reasons outlined in this chapter, we believe that the definition of a control program best tailored to the needs and opportunities existing in each developing country depends on careful consideration of the following local factors: (i) epidemiology of STIs, (ii) epidemiology of sexual behaviors, (iii) epidemiology of health behaviors, (iv) patterns of existing and planned health care services for STIs, and (v) sociocultural factors that exert the most powerful influences on behavior and determine effective modes and channels of communication. An assessment of these factors, in conjunction with a clear understanding of the relative responsiveness of behaviors to interventions and the relative susceptibility of different STIs to interventions, can help determine the priorities for particular target groups, interventions, and intervention intensity that would maximize impact. On the other hand, to assess the essential needs and opportunities for integrated behavioral and biomedical interventions, it is not necessary to spend years developing a survey instrument, to send a team of ethnographers to define the sexual behavior of every individual member of society, or to identify every case of every STI in every remote sector of the country.

The assessment of the local epidemiology of STIs, sexual behaviors, and health behaviors should be an ongoing process because epidemiological patterns change and because one set of findings inevitably suggests other or better ways of looking at the problem. Thus, the absence of definitive, comprehensive, or even broadly representative data must not inhibit or paralyze the process of initiating, refining, and extending behavioral and clinical interventions. To get started, in fact, we believe that prevention priorities and the broad outlines for behavioral and biomedical interventions can be set on the basis of very simple and obvious data that can be obtained during a short time. The evaluation should be conducted by individuals with clinical, epidemiological, and health education skills. A simple needs assessment instrument is required to quickly assess the disease spectrum; services available in the public, private, and informal sectors; STI control program or organizational structure (if any); relevant policies; what is already known about sexual behavioral patterns; availability of management guidelines, diagnostic testing, and antimicrobial agents; existing health education initiatives for STIs; availability of condoms, etc. For example, concerning the epidemiology of STIs, if a specialized clinical service exists for STIs, it will be known whether genital ulcer disease is common or uncommon relative to other STIs in men or women, although the relative frequency of different causes of genital ulcers still has not been established in some areas. If common, priority should clearly go to promoting health care-seeking behaviors and services that will lead to early diagnosis and treatment of such diseases. If no specialized service exists, even in major urban areas, clinicians in related specialities (e.g., obstetrics and gynecology, urology, dermatology) can provide similar information. The availability of treatment for STIs from pharmacies without prescription can be easily and quickly assessed.

Similarly, concerning the epidemiology of sexual behaviors, the location and points of contact between prostitutes and their clients are already sufficiently well known in most cities of the world to begin to focus behavioral interventions for these groups. Experience with community-based targeted interventions involving prostitutes is growing on all continents, although experience with client-oriented health education is more limited.

Increasing amounts of data from surveys of knowledge, attitudes, beliefs, and practices and from ethnographic studies are becoming available in many regions; although analyses are still often incomplete, available information can be sought to help guide behavioral interventions. Health education materials have been developed in many settings but have been primarily aimed at preventing HIV infection. For such materials, there is by now considerable experience with the use of various media and with channels of communication for general public health education in developing countries; there remains a need for networking within and among countries and sharing of materials and experience and for evaluation of the process and outcome of the behavioral interventions.

However, important aspects of behavioral interventions have so far been neglected in developing countries. Explicit interventions for targeted audiences have even now still not been widely implemented in most developing countries, nearly 10 years after the recognition of AIDS. Furthermore, available materials generally do not concern STIs other than HIV infection and do not address what we believe may be the most modifiable behavior, namely, health care seeking for curable STIs. In most developing countries, there has been no promotion of health

Table 1. Examples of 10 health education messages for prevention of STIs in developing countries

1. Sexually transmitted infections have become very common and are often silent (you may not know you have one). Casual sexual partners are more likely than not to have at least one.
2. Condoms can prevent all dangerous sexually transmitted infections and should be used, for example, when you have sex with other partners or someone you don't know well.
3. Discharges (from penis or vagina) are sexually transmitted infections.
4. Genital ulcers are sexually transmitted infections.
5. If you develop a genital discharge or genital ulcer, see a doctor promptly, because early treatment prevents complications, and stop having sex until you go to the doctor.
6. When you get a sexually transmitted infection, you are responsible to get treatment for both yourself and your partner(s).
7. The most serious complications of sexually transmitted infections occur in women: infertility and cervical cancer.
8. Sexually transmitted infections in pregnant women will damage the fetus or newborn: abortion or stillbirth, infant death, blindness or deafness, or brain damage.
9. Only the AIDS virus (HIV) causes AIDS; however, other sexually transmitted infections can make you more susceptible to catching the AIDS virus if you are sexually exposed to someone infected with the AIDS virus.
10. In this city, you can get tested and treated for sexually transmitted infections at the following locations: ________, ________ . . .

care-seeking behaviors for STIs (or related promotion of improved health care services for STIs); no targeted health education (especially for male clients of prostitutes, such as men seeking treatment for STIs); and few well-conceptualized condom promotion programs. It seems extraordinary that in 1991, such programs are not in place and that in many developmental programs, there has been no meaningful planning, funding, or training for STI health education programs other than information concerning AIDS directed at the general public.

As discussed earlier, the three main approaches to prevention and control of STIs include promotion of safer sex, promotion of condoms, and provision and utilization of services for diagnosis and treatment of STIs. The target of behavioral interventions can be the general population, specific core groups, or high-risk individuals. Because general public health education has generally not contained information on STIs other than HIV infection and has generally not attempted to change health care-seeking behavior, and because focused core group interventions have been implemented only as isolated research or demonstration projects, we believe that health education for prevention of STIs, including HIV infection, remains in its early infancy in developing countries. There remains an urgent need for further development and evaluation of materials and strategies for behavioral interventions for prevention of all STIs. Examples of basic health education messages that are currently not included in the campaigns of many national AIDS or STI programs are listed in Table 1. The priority given to each message will vary from country to country. For example, the message "Condoms can prevent STI" is especially important today for the majority of the world's heterosexual population

Table 2. Priorities for behavioral interventions in developing countries

1. Develop health education messages for prevention and control of STIs appropriate to the local epidemiological situation, health care infrastructure, and sociocultural context.
2. Provide general public with health education, with community involvement, including (a) health education on STIs and (b) promoting early diagnosis and treatment of curable STIs, especially genital ulcer diseases, if common.
3. Identify target groups and develop community-based programs that include:
   (a) Health education on STIs.
   (b) Promotion of health care-seeking behavior for genital ulcer disease and abnormal genital discharges.
   (c) Providing access to health care for STIs.
   (d) Promotion of condoms.
   (e) Identification and special counseling of those with HIV infection.
4. Provide clinical services and national treatment guidelines for STIs, together with health education, condom promotion, and partner notification in settings that include but are not limited to:
   (a) At least one special clinic in a major urban center, affiliated with a medical school or teaching hospital, if possible, for training purposes.
   (b) Selected private physicians, who are trained and assisted in following national guidelines for STI management, health education, partner notification, and condom promotion.
   (c) Primary care clinics, especially those serving women, such as family planning and prenatal clinics.
   (d) Pharmacies in countries where pharmacies treat a large proportion of men with STIs. Primary care clinics and pharmacies must be encouraged and enabled to follow national guidelines.

(e.g., in most of Asia, Europe, and North America), where other STIs may be much more common and cause much more morbidity than HIV infection. Messages concerning genital ulcers would be important in sub-Saharan Africa, where chancroid is widely prevalent, or southern India, where donovanosis also occurs, but much less important in most of Europe, where curable forms of genital ulcers are rare.

Table 2 provides a generic list of priorities for behavioral interventions for prevention and control of STIs in developing countries. The program manager should be responsible for developing simple national STI management guidelines (in general, follow the available World Health Organization guidelines) and (with the AIDS program managers and health educators) for developing simple general and focused (including clinic-based) health education and condom promotion programs. The manager should set specific goals (e.g., involve a specific, achievable, and increasing percentage of school children in the program with each successive year and provide individual health education messages and condoms to a specific, achievable, and increasing percentage of patients attending public clinics for STIs within a set time, etc.).

We would regard the four priorities listed in Table 2 as such basic needs that the "research" component of developing these behavioral interventions would initially address evaluation and operational research methodologies. The evaluation should begin with the program manager setting specific, measurable, and attainable process goals and should proceed to evaluation of the process (e.g., numbers educated, quality and acceptability of the education) and of easily measured outcomes (e.g., knowledge gained from information provided).

A second level of behavioral research with immediate operational relevance to coordinated biomedical and behavioral interventions could address perceptions and acceptability and utilization of various models for delivery of clinical services for STIs. This area of behavioral research has been largely neglected. For example, what do men feel about obtaining treatment for STIs in primary care clinics oriented toward maternal and child health care? What do women feel about obtaining treatment for STIs in categorical STI clinics? What do men, women, and providers feel about provision of STI services in family planning clinics? What do registered and unregistered prostitutes feel about provision of STI services, condoms, and education through various systems now in existence? A third level could concern surveys and qualitative research on knowledge, attitudes, and beliefs about STIs other than HIV infection—a largely neglected subject until now, and one that is important in refining future health education efforts. More basic behavioral research questions and methodologies, as outlined elsewhere in this book, would proceed further from, and build on, this basic starting point. Small-scale and local studies that are derivative may be more persuasive to local policymakers than the original, more definitive research done elsewhere.

CONCLUSIONS

In most industrialized countries, the curable STIs have come under increasing control during the past 10 to 20 years, even as the incurable viral STIs have been increasing in incidence. The decline in curable STIs was coincidental with intensified public health measures, including integrated behavioral and biomedical interventions. Although it cannot be proved that these measures caused the decline in curable STIs, the experience of industrialized countries offers strong encouragement for development of similar measures in developing countries. The patterns of sexual behaviors of developing countries appear to be quite heterogeneous, offering differing needs and opportunities for targeted behavioral interventions. The three determinants of rate and extent of spread of STIs are the efficiency of transmission, the mean rates and variance in rates of partner change and patterns of partner networking, and the duration of infectivity. These three determinants are the three points of attack for prevention and control of STIs. These three determinants are closely interrelated, and all are susceptible to behavioral interventions.

Unique problems for prevention and control of STIs in developing countries include the demographic transition and rapid growth in the adolescent young adult population, economic and educational underdevelopment, the subordinate status of women, and the weak health infrastructure, particularly neglected services for STIs. Most of these problems parallel the problems among impoverished minority populations in the United States.

There is a growing consensus that strategies for behavioral interventions for prevention and control of STIs in developing countries should employ multiple channels of communications which are reinforcing. These channels include mass media, community organizations, peer group counseling, individual counseling, and entertainment. Nonindividualistic, nonwritten approaches and communalistic avenues of communication seem especially appropriate in developing countries. Innovative strategies should include promotion of health care seeking with existing health care services, together with strengthening of STI services for more balanced intervention programs. A typology has been developed for defining the relative susceptibility of various STIs to prevention and control, and the relative susceptibility of relevant behaviors has been considered. All STIs, including HIV infection, can be addressed by interventions directed at sexual behaviors and condom use. Interventions that target core groups of high-frequency transmitters can be highly cost-effective. In addition, promotion of health care-seeking behaviors, especially those targeting core groups, could be even more effective in prevention and control of certain curable STIs, particularly the bacterial genital ulcer diseases. Such behavioral interventions should receive very high priority in developing countries, especially where genital ulcer diseases contribute to the sexual transmission of HIV infection.

The local STI and behavioral parameters should dictate the specifics of the control program. However, the synergistic interactions between the biomedical and behavioral interventions and their effects are universal. Therefore, in all countries, the control programs should include both clinical and behavioral components (rather than one or the other) and should carefully plan the interactions between the two components to maximize their combined impact on the disease problem.

Finally, it is clear that no type of intervention—neither behavioral nor nonbehavioral—has been formally shown to be effective in prevention of STIs in developing countries. It will ultimately probably be much easier to demonstrate effective prevention of other STIs than to demonstrate effective prevention of HIV infection in most settings, simply because in many settings HIV is less common and more difficult to assess for sociopolitical reasons. It is essential to develop formal research to show efficacy of behavioral and nonbehavioral interventions but even more important to first establish the most basic and obviously needed services for clinical and behavioral interventions and begin with evaluation of delivery of these services.

LITERATURE CITED

1. **Aral, S. O.** 1990. The changing epidemiology of sexually transmitted diseases. *Curr. Opin. Infect. Dis.* **3:**20–23.
2. **Aral, S. O., and K. K. Holmes.** 1984. Epidemiology of sexually transmitted diseases, p. 127–144. *In* K. K. Holmes, P.-A. Mardh, P. F. Sparling, and P. J. Wiesner (ed.), *Sexually Transmitted Diseases.* McGraw-Hill Book Co., New York.
3. **Aral, S. O., and K. K. Holmes.** 1991. Epidemiology of sexually transmitted diseases, p. 126–141. *In* K. K. Holmes, P.-A. Mardh, P. F. Sparling, P. J. Wiesner, W. Cates, Jr., S. M. Lemon, and W. E. Stamm (ed.), *Sexually Transmitted Diseases,* 2nd ed. McGraw-Hill Book Co., New York.
4. **Aral, S. O., R. E. Johnson, A. Zaidi, R. Fichtner, and G. Reynolds.** 1983. Demographic effects on sexually transmitted diseases in the 70's: the problem could be worse. *Sex. Transm. Dis.* **10:**100–101.
5. **Aral, S. O., V. Soskolne, R. M. Joesoef, and K. R. O'Reilly.** 1991. Sex partner selection as risk factor for STD: clustering of risky modes. *Sex. Transm. Dis.* **18:**10–17.

6. **Boulding, E.** 1976. *Handbook of International Data on Women.* Sage Publications, Newbury Park, Calif.
7. **Caldwell, J., and P. Caldwell.** 1990. High fertility sub-Saharan Africa. *Sci. Am.* **264:**118–125.
8. **Centers for Disease Control, Division of STD/HIV Prevention.** 1990. *Annual Report, 1990.* Centers for Disease Control, Atlanta.
9. **Centers for Disease Control.** 1991. Premarital sexual experience among adolescent United States women, 1970–1988. *Morbid. Mortal. Weekly Rep.* **39:**929–932.
10. **European Study Group.** 1989. Risk factors for male-to-female transmission of HIV. *Br. Med. J.* **298:**411–415.
11. **Harrison, H. R., M. Costen, J. B. Meder, L. M. Bownds, D. A. Sim, M. Lewis, and E. R. Alexander.** 1985. Cervical *Chlamydia trachomatis* infection in university women. Relationship to history, contraception, ectopy, and cervicitis. *Am. J. Obstet. Gynecol.* **153:**244–251.
12. **International Labor Office.** 1984. *World Labour Report.* International Labor Office, Geneva.
13. **Kreiss, J. K., D. Koech, F. A. Plummer, K. K. Holmes, M. Lightfoote, P. Piot, A. R. Ronald, J. O. Ndinya-Achola, L. J. D'Costa, P. Roberts, E. N. Ngugi, and T. C. Quinn.** 1986. AIDS virus infection in Nairobi prostitutes: spread of the epidemic to East Africa. *N. Engl. J. Med.* **314:**414–417.
14. **Larson, A.** 1989. Social context of human immunodeficiency virus transmission in Africa: historical and cultural bases of East and Central African sexual relations. *Rev. Infect. Dis.* **11:**716–731.
15. **Llosa, M. V.** 1989. *The Storyteller.* (Translated by Helen Lane.) Penguin Books, New York.
16. **Louv, W. C., H. Austin, J. Perlman, and W. J. Alexander.** 1989. Oral contraceptive use and the risk of chlamydial and gonococcal infection. *Am. J. Obstet. Gynecol.* **160:**396–402.
17. **Moses, S., F. A. Plummer, P. Waiyaki, E. N. Ngugi, N. J. D. Nagelkerke, A. O. Anzala, and J. O. Ndinya-Achola.** 1991. Controlling HIV in Africa: effectiveness and cost of an intervention in a frequency STD transmitter core group. *AIDS* **5:**407–412.
18. **Padian, N., L. Marquis, D. P. Francis, R. E. Anderson, G. W. Rutherford, P. M. O'Malley, and W. Winkelstein, Jr.** 1987. Male-to-female transmission of human immunodeficiency virus. *J. Am. Med. Assoc.* **258:**788–790.
19. **Pan American Health Organization–United Nations.** 1966. *Demographic Yearbook, Issue 36.* Pan American Health Organization, Washington, D.C.
20. **Population Division of the Department of International Economic and Social Affairs.** 1987. World demographic trends. *World Health Stat. Q.* **40:**6–21.
21. **Royston, E.** 1982. The prevalence of nutritional anemia in women in developing countries: a critical review of available information. *World Health Stat. Q.* **35:**52–91.
22. **Schreeder, M. T., S. E. Thompson, S. C. Hadler, K. R. Berquist, A. Zaidi, J. E. Maynard, D. Ostrow, F. N. Judson, E. H. Braff, T. Nylund, J. N. Moore, Jr., P. Gardner, I. L. Doto, and G. Reynolds.** 1982. Hepatitis B in homosexual men. Prevalence of infection and factors related to transmission. *J. Infect. Dis.* **146:**7–15.
23. **Sivard, R. L.** 1987. *Women . . . a World Survey.* World Priorities, Inc., Washington, D.C.
24. **Stamm, W. E., H. H. Handsfield, A. M. Rompalo, R. L. Ashley, P. L. Roberts, and L. Corey.** 1988. The association between genital ulcer disease and acquisition of HIV infection in homosexual men. *J. Am. Med. Assoc.* **260:**1429–1433.
25. **Standing, H., and M. N. Kisekka.** 1989. *Sexual Behavior in Subsaharan Africa—a Review and Annotated Bibliography.* Overseas Development Administration, London.
26. **UNESCO.** 1982. *Trends and projections of enrollment by level of education and by age, 1960–2000.* UNESCO, Paris.
27. **UNESCO.** 1981. *Yearbook on Peace and Conflict Series, 1981.* UNESCO, Paris.
28. **United Nations.** 1982. *Demographic Indicators of Countries.* United Nations, New York.
29. **United Nations.** 1983. Infant mortality: world estimates and projects. *Popul. Bull.* **13:**1950–2025.
30. **United Nations.** 1986. *Demographic Yearbook, Issue 38.* United Nations, New York.
31. **World Bank.** 1984. *World Development Report.* Oxford University Press, New York.

Evaluation of Behavioral Interventions for Prevention and Control of Sexually Transmitted Diseases

Sylvan B. Green and A. Eugene Washington

As with any field of medical science, behavioral interventions for prevention and control of sexually transmitted diseases (STDs) should be investigated and evaluated in ways that lead to scientifically valid results. Studying such interventions presents special problems not present, for example, in conventional therapeutic trials. However, the principles that underlie clinical trials and observational epidemiological studies are applicable to this field, and we can benefit from considering how to apply these principles to the STD problem.

A first key step is to specify the research question. Although this seems like an obvious platitude, all too often studies suffer from unfocused hypotheses, from attempting to answer too many questions, or even from answering the wrong question (i.e., because of inadequate design, failing to answer the intended question reliably). This is not to say that one should not do exploratory studies to generate hypotheses or that one cannot study more than a single intervention in the same trial. There are appropriate ways to do these, but we should design for such purposes and not stumble into them.

Because of the urgency of making progress against serious public health problems, we should focus on important questions. Characteristics of a good research question are that it is ethical to study, feasible to investigate and to implement, interesting, and relevant to the problem.

Having identified the purposes of the study, one must select appropriate methods. These methods must be valid, so that we are likely to arrive at the correct conclusion, and defensible, so that we can convince others of the usefulness of the results. Errors in evaluating interventions can arise because of chance fluctuations and/or systematic biases. Clearly, the populations of individuals who are potential subjects for intervention are quite heterogeneous; selecting a small number to receive an intervention can by chance lead to quite different results than will be seen on average if the intervention is applied subsequently to large numbers of people. Furthermore, comparing two interventions (or comparing an intervention with no intervention) can be biased if the two groups being compared are inherently different. Therefore, adequate sample sizes and proper controls are required to produce good evidence.

The purpose of this chapter is to review general principles of study design and

Sylvan B. Green – Clinical and Diagnostic Trials Section, National Cancer Institute, Bethesda, Maryland 20892. *A. Eugene Washington* – Center for Reproductive Health Policy Research, School of Medicine, University of California, San Francisco, California 94143-0936.

on this basis to outline approaches for investigating behavioral interventions for STDs.

CATEGORIES OF STUDY DESIGN

Observational Studies

Observational studies can be recommended in the context of STD prevention and control primarily for identifying risk factors, with particular interest in risk behaviors. Such studies are valuable in developing interventions for future study, because they may provide relevant information about the acquisition and spread of disease and because they may identify behaviors to target. They may also be used to identify the appropriate subpopulations who would be candidates for intervention. In addition, observational data may provide suggestive evidence of benefit resulting from a change in behavior.

Possible approaches include cross-sectional studies, case-control studies, and cohort studies. The relative uses and merits of each method are described in epidemiological texts (4, 5).

Intervention Trials

In contrast to observational studies, intervention trials represent the experimental method and will be the focus of this chapter, which emphasizes the evaluation of behavioral interventions. Such trials allow the determination of the results of a behavioral intervention, thus testing the hypotheses that we may generate from observational studies or laboratory results. Although other types of studies may provide important information, it is the randomized controlled trial, in particular, that can provide the greatest strength of evidence concerning the efficacy of an intervention strategy.

Intervention trials for STDs can be characterized by their purpose into three broad categories. The first category includes trials aimed at the earliest intervention point, namely, prevention of infection. Moving a step later in the disease process, controlled trials can also be used to compare programs for screening and early detection of disease in populations at risk. The third category consists of conventional clinical trials comparing different drugs (or different therapeutic strategies) for treatment of specific infections. Although a common goal of behavioral intervention trials may be primary prevention, behavioral interventions may address more than one of the above purposes, for example, getting people to detect disease early and then preventing spread to partners.

TYPES OF INTERVENTION TRIALS

Traditional clinical trials have often been described as being of one of several types or phases. This approach has been used, for example, in trials of treatments for cancer, and there has been much recent discussion about corresponding phases for AIDS trials (3). In our view, it is instructive to consider this conceptual framework, previously formulated for treatment trials, and apply it to trials for behavioral modification.

Phase I: Formulation

Trials whose purpose is to investigate dosage and schedule of drugs, as well as to identify possible toxicity and perhaps determine the maximally tolerated dose, have been called phase I. Often these represent the first use of a drug in humans. In the STD context, this concept could be applied to studies investigating the logistics and acceptability of behavioral interventions. Phase I trials usually involve a relatively small number of subjects studied rather intensively. Phase I trials have usually been uncontrolled studies, although an argument can be made that randomization is appropriate even in this early phase, if it is known that more than one variation of the intervention will be investigated. Just as in the drug treatment setting in which basic laboratory research has preceded a phase I trial and pharmacokinetic studies may be part of the trial, so in the behavior modification context will basic behavioral research both precede and be part of the trial. Focus groups represent one of the techniques that might be used here. Basic research and phase I trials provide the foundation upon which large intervention trials are developed.

Phase II: Activity

The purpose of phase II trials is to look for evidence of "activity" of the intervention. For cancer trials this might be shrinkage of a measurable tumor; for AIDS trials this might be a favorable change in a surrogate or intermediate marker. In the context of STD prevention and control, the ability of an intervention to produce some relevant change in behavior would be an appropriate end point. Most often phase II trials have investigated a single intervention and have not included a control group. However, there are advantages to designs that randomize among competing interventions being studied for activity; such an approach allows an unbiased evaluation of which of the interventions is most promising, since the groups of subjects are comparable. In some situations, elements of phase I and II trials can be combined.

Phase III: Efficacy

Phase III trials are comparative, controlled trials that seek to determine the efficacy of intervention. The comparison may be of active intervention versus no intervention, or it may be of one intervention versus another. Efficacy is measured against some important "definitive" end point, which one can argue in the STD context should usually be a decrease in some measure of STD itself, such as incidence. Phase III trials are best done as randomized trials. The advantages of randomization (discussed below) are compelling.

Phase IV: Effectiveness

The term phase IV has been used in various contexts. Here we think it useful to denote as phase IV large trials that test the effectiveness of proven interventions in wide-scale use. The distinction here is that phase III trials test the *efficacy* of an intervention in an experimental situation (which may involve specific volunteers carefully monitored), while phase IV trials study the practical *effectiveness* of the intervention in large populations in which issues of cost and extent of use may be different. Expressed another way (perhaps oversimplistically), phase III shows that when done right something *can* work, while phase IV shows that in practice it *does* work. Depending on the nature of the intervention, the distinction between these two may be blurred.

DESIGNING AN INTERVENTION TRIAL

Study Subjects and Eligibility

The choice of study population will depend on the nature of the intervention and phase of the trial. Study subjects may represent volunteers or individuals otherwise accessible for recruitment (e.g., a clinic population), or the trial may attempt to sample from a large target population. Similarly, subjects may be recruited as individuals, or entire groups or communities may be asked to participate. For some interventions, the behavior change may be aimed, not at potential patients, but at health care providers, counselors, or educators.

The inclusion and exclusion criteria for a trial should be specified clearly. Although phase I and II trials may have special requirements, it is generally preferable (especially for later phases) to avoid the tendency to be overly restrictive in specifying eligibility.

Trial Outcomes

For each trial beyond phase I, it is usual to choose one outcome as the primary end point around which the trial is designed. Often, other outcomes will be studied as secondary end points, and various additional measurements will be made. A good collection of explanatory variables at baseline can be important for investigating prognosis and perhaps for adjusting analyses of differences between interventions. The decision about the amount of information to collect during the trial must balance two considerations. Collecting data on certain variables may be worthwhile to assess compliance or to assist in interpreting the results for the principal outcome. Conversely, especially for phases III and IV, too much data collection can degrade the quality of the data, can increase the cost, may discourage cooperation of the subjects, and may not be all that useful for the success of the trial. For example, in a phase III trial, randomization provides us with comparable groups. Using an "intention to treat" analysis, we include all randomized participants in the data analysis, counted according to their randomized intervention assignment, measure the major outcomes (certainly the primary end point and perhaps some secondary end points), and thus determine whether one overall intervention strategy is better than another (when one strategy may be no intervention at all). Details about what happens along the way, while possibly helpful in interpretation, may not be required to make a decision about which intervention strategy to recommend.

STD incidence, morbidity (e.g., symptomatic disease or adverse reproductive events), or mortality (for potentially fatal infections) provide definitive end points for phase III trials. Researchers addressing behavior must remember that these intervention trials are needed because of urgent public health problems, in the presence of limited resources, so a goal must be to determine what is truly efficacious and effective in controlling major STDs; with our current state of knowledge, demonstrating behavior change by itself is usually not sufficient. The exception is when there can be little doubt that behavioral change will produce a favorable health outcome (such as the arguments made in the area of behavioral trials for antismoking interventions). Whatever the end point, in comparative trials it is important to ensure that surveillance and identification of events occur equally in all groups, to avoid a biased assessment.

Unlike the situation for phase III trials, behavioral change will often be a sensible end point for the earlier phase II trials. Showing that a proposed intervention strategy does produce a desired change in behavior can indicate that the intervention has activity and is promising for study in larger comparative phase III trials. Also, behavior change may be useful as a secondary end point for interpreting results in phase III trials, particularly if the trial turns out negative with regard to impact on the primary STD end point. With a behavioral end point, we need to ensure that the assessment of the behavioral change does not itself affect the success of the intervention. Also, behavioral change is often self-reported rather than objectively observed, so we must consider the effect of the intervention on what gets reported, which may differ from the effect of the intervention on the behavior itself. For this reason, there are likely to be situations in which a further end point, beyond reported change in behavior, is necessary for concluding that an intervention leads to an actual behavioral modification.

Specific Trial Designs

Sometimes in comparative trials only two interventions will be compared. As noted above, depending on the setting, one of the intervention strategies may be specified as no intervention; i.e., compare a new intervention with what is happening anyway without that intervention. Such a comparison may be essential when the current situation is in flux, to avoid an incorrect interpretation of the effect of the intervention being studied. If things are improving during the trial (perhaps because of other activities within the community), in the absence of concurrent controls, we may falsely attribute a benefit to a worthless intervention. Conversely, if the situation is worsening (perhaps because of increased prevalence or virulence of an infection), we may fail to detect a benefit from a successful intervention, in the absence of which the results would have been even worse.

Sometimes, several intervention strategies are proposed for evaluation, so we design a multiarm trial to test these simultaneously. When different interventions can be applied either separately or in combination, then there are advantages to using a factorial design, in which all possible combinations of two or more interventions are studied. The simplest such design is a 2 × 2 factorial design, in which each of two interventions is either present or absent, forming four intervention groups among which randomization occurs: one intervention alone, the other, both, or neither. Sometimes, the possibility of an interaction between interventions is raised; interaction means that the effect of one intervention depends on whether the second intervention is given. In the absence of interaction, a factorial design is a very efficient way to study different interventions in a single trial. If an interaction does exist, then a factorial design is a very sensible way to detect and measure it.

Another type of design applicable to behavioral modification has been termed reciprocal control (1). This refers to the situation in which different intervention groups can receive programs targeted at different end points, so that one group can serve as the control for the others. For example, suppose we plan to study a behavioral modification program for the control of STDs, and in the same population we would like to study an antismoking program. If each of our interventions is thought to affect either the STD end point or the smoking end point, but not both, then we randomize participants to receive either anti-STD or antismoking intervention, and we use each group as the control for the other. We thereby answer two important public health questions in a single study, saving cost and time.

Randomization

There are many benefits that result from randomization (2). Randomization is advocated to avoid bias in comparisons of interventions. If investigators select which experimental intervention is given to which subjects, then differences in success rate may be due to inherent differences in the groups of subjects and not to differences in benefit from the interventions, thus leading to an erroneous conclusion. With randomization, risk factors will tend to be balanced (on average) across groups. This is true not only for risk factors we can identify and therefore adjust for imbalance but also for unknown or unmeasured factors, no matter how subtle. Randomization guarantees the validity of statistical tests used to provide statistical significance. In other words, we can quantify the probability of observing an apparent difference in outcome by chance alone (if, in fact, the interventions are equivalent in effect); if this probability is low enough (less than 0.05, for example), we consider a chance effect unlikely, and therefore we are more willing to believe that a true difference exists. Concurrent controls (whether randomized or not) provide the additional advantage, not present for formal historical controls or for informal comparisons with past experience, that an apparent intervention benefit is not spuriously produced (nor a real benefit hidden) by time trends, a danger very real in the area of STDs. Depending on the specific situation, relevant time trends might include changes in infection prevalence, virulence of the organism, sexual practices, other risk behaviors, diagnostic methods, effectiveness of treatments of disease once diagnosed, etc.

Given that a trial will use randomized assignment to intervention, there is a choice of unit of randomization. Most trials randomize individuals; this is statistically most efficient. However, there are situations when randomization by groups may be chosen; this will require a greater total number of individuals, and the data must be analyzed appropriately (taking into account the grouped randomization). Behavioral interventions for prevention and control seem more likely than therapeutic trials to suggest group randomization, with antismoking and dietary modification trials providing good examples, although the majority of such trials still involve (appropriately) randomization of individuals.

Units of grouped randomization may be communities, villages, factories, schools, religious groupings (e.g., churches), chapters of social organizations, clinical practices, etc. There are a number of reasons for considering group randomization. It may be impossible for political or practical reasons to randomize individuals or to deliver the intervention at the level of individuals. There may be cost savings that make a trial with group randomization feasible when an individually randomized study would not be. There may be ready-made end points available at a defined group level (e.g., group-wide incidence rate of STDs). It may be impossible to avoid contamination between individuals (i.e., people randomized to one behavioral intervention influencing others around them who had been randomized to a different intervention). Perhaps most important for certain behavioral modification trials, the nature of the intervention may be at the group level; by definition, the intervention may be delivered group-wide (for example, to a public school class). In the latter situation, contamination between individuals is not to be avoided but in fact may be an important part of the intervention. Just because individual randomization may be more difficult is not a reason to adopt randomization by group, but the above situations indicate when group randomization may be worth considering.

The issue of individuals versus groups applies to the unit of randomization, the unit of intervention, and the unit of outcome assessment. Sometimes, the decision for one of these aspects drives the others, but they need not always be the same. For example, people separately randomized as individuals may be referred to group counseling sessions, in which case the randomization determines to which group a person goes (or whether one goes at all). Likewise, interventions assigned by group randomization and then delivered on a group-wide basis may be assessed by considering individuals. This allows us to account for risk factors that vary at the level of individuals, but we must still take the grouped randomization into account in the statistical analysis.

Sample Size and Statistical Power

Using randomization addresses the issue of bias. The issue of randomness and variability across individuals is addressed by having a large enough sample size for the trial. Because of variability, the intervention effect (or difference of outcomes between intervention groups) observed during the trial is just an estimate of the "true" effect (the effect to be seen if the interventions were applied to the entire population of subjects, from which the actual participants are just a sample). The larger the sample size, the more precise the estimate. Suppose we are planning to test whether any difference observed during a trial is statistically significant (i.e., unlikely to be due solely to chance). Then the probability of getting a significant result, if some specified difference does truly exist, is the power of the study. Power increases with increasing sample size. The smaller the difference that we wish to detect, the larger the sample size required to obtain the desired power. Studies are commonly designed to have power of at least 0.80 (often 0.90) to detect worthwhile differences. Note that if a trial has a power of less than 0.50 to detect what is in fact the true difference between interventions, then the trial is more likely than not to fail to detect it (i.e., end up with a result that is not statistically significant). It is particularly important that the value of an otherwise well-designed trial not be jeopardized because of an inadequate number of subjects.

CONCLUSION

Investigators unfamiliar with principles of clinical trials may believe that a favorable result obtained in a small number of selected individuals demonstrates the efficacy of the intervention they have proposed. Perhaps if the results are dramatic and so different from all past experience that the observed benefit can be attributed only to the intervention, then the argument is correct. Because of possible errors due to chance and bias, however, in most cases more evidence will be required before concluding that an intervention is recommended for general use. Our purpose here has been to outline a number of considerations in evaluating behavioral interventions. Progress results from a variety of types of studies. We encourage the use of large, well-designed, randomized trials as one important approach to research on the prevention and control of STDs.

LITERATURE CITED

1. **Byar, D. P.** 1990. Factorial and reciprocal control designs. *Stat. Med.* **9:**55–64.
2. **Byar, D. P., R. M. Simon, W. T. Friedewald, J. J. Schlesselman, D. L. DeMets, J. H. Ellenberg, M. H. Gail, and J. H. Ware.** 1976. Randomized clinical trials: perspectives on some recent ideas. *N. Engl. J. Med.* **295:**74–80.
3. **Green, S. B., S. S. Ellenberg, D. Finkelstein, A. B. Forsythe, L. S. Freedman, K. Freeman, M. Lefkopoulou, D. Schoenfeld, and R. P. Smith.** 1990. Issues in the design of drug trials for AIDS. *Controlled Clin. Trials* **11:**80–87.
4. **Hulley, S. B., and S. R. Cummings (ed.).** 1988. *Designing Clinical Research: an Epidemiologic Approach.* The Williams & Wilkins Co., Baltimore.
5. **Kelsey, J. L., W. D. Thompson, and A. S. Evans.** 1986. *Methods in Observational Epidemiology.* Oxford University Press, New York.

Appendix I

Report of the NIAID Study Group on Integrated Behavioral Research for Prevention and Control of Sexually Transmitted Diseases†‡

In recognition of the crucial interplay between behavioral and biomedical risk factors for sexually transmitted diseases (STDs), the National Institute of Allergy and Infectious Diseases (NIAID) believes that there is an urgent need for focused, intervention-oriented behavioral research on STDs that draws on the experience of scientists from multiple disciplines. Few collaborations between social scientists and biomedical scientists exist currently in this field. Furthermore, the interface between behavioral and biomedical research on STDs remains ill defined, and specific research priorities and approaches have yet to be examined systematically.

As a result, on November 6–8, 1989, and April 11–12, 1990, the STD branch of the NIAID convened two interdisciplinary conferences on Integrated Behavioral Research for Prevention and Control of Sexually Transmitted Diseases. The goals of the conferences included the development of an agenda for intervention-oriented behavioral research on STDs and the definition of the NIAID's unique role in addressing that agenda. The three articles that follow comprise the report of the study group. They address crucial research issues in 1) defining behavioral risk factors and their distribution; 2) designing behavioral interventions; and 3) evaluating those interventions with respect to the prevention and control of STDs.

---

† Reprinted with permission from *Sexually Transmitted Diseases*, October-December 1990, vol. 17, no. 4, p. 200–210.

‡ The participants in the study group on Integrated Behavioral Research for Prevention and Control of STDs included: Hortensia Amaro, Boston University; Roy Anderson, University of London; Sevgi Aral, Centers for Disease Control; Robert Brunham, University of Manitoba; Manuel Carballo, World Health Organization; Anke Ehrhardt, Columbia University; Martin Fishbein, University of Illinois; Robert Fullilove, Columbia University; Sylvan Green, National Cancer Institute; King Holmes, World Health Organization; Edward Hook III, The Johns Hopkins University; Robert Hornik, University of Pennsylvania; Robert Jones, Indiana University School of Medicine; Franklyn Judson, World Health Organization; Marie Laga, Centers for Disease Control; Lucile Newman, Brown University; Maria Paalman, World Health Organization; Nancy Padian, San Francisco General Hospital; William Smith, The Academy for Educational Development; Frederick Sparling, University of North Carolina at Chapel Hill; and Eugene Washington, University of California at San Francisco. The director and staff of the NIAID greatly appreciate the time, energy, and insightful comments of these individuals. John La Montagne, Judith Wasserheit, and Penelope Hitchcock participated on behalf of the Institute.

Part I: Issues in Defining Behavioral Risk Factors and Their Distribution

NANCY PADIAN, PhD, MPH; PENELOPE J. HITCHCOCK, DVM, MS; ROBERT E. FULLILOVE III, EdD; VICTORIA KOHLSTADT, MPH; ROBERT BRUNHAM, MD; and the NIAID STUDY GROUP ON INTEGRATED BEHAVIORAL RESEARCH FOR PREVENTION AND CONTROL OF SEXUALLY TRANSMITTED DISEASES

From the Department of Epidemiology and Biostatistics, University of California, San Francisco; the National Institute of Allergy and Infectious Diseases, National Institutes of Health; HIV Center for Clinical and Behavioral Studies, College of Physicians and Surgeons, Columbia University; and the Department of Medical Microbiology, University of Manitoba.

The first objective of research on the prevention and control of sexually transmitted diseases (STDs) is to define the spectrum and prevalence of risk factors associated with an elevated frequency of disease. Such factors may be assessed in relation to increased risk of transmission of the infectious agent, or risk of progression to severe or irreversible sequelae. Some of these factors directly affect the risk of transmission or progression, whereas others have a more indirect effect, and thus, may be markers or surrogates for risk factors. For example, the use of alcohol during sexual intercourse may decrease the likelihood that condoms will be used. Therefore, alcohol use is associated with transmission, even though its primary effect is not direct. Factors may also be viewed as either increasing risk (e.g., anal intercourse) or as protective (e.g., condom use).

Such data are an essential prerequisite both for developing intervention strategies and for identifying target populations for those interventions. The model of May and Anderson (1) may be used as a conceptual framework to identify risk factors for transmission of STDs. This model, $R = \beta cD$, is based on the premise that the incidence of an STD is dependent on the transmissibility of the infectious agent, opportunity for exposure to the infectious agent, and duration of infectiousness.

Behavioral and/or biomedical risk factors determine each parameter in the model. "R" represents the reproductive rate of infection of a particular pathogen, i.e., the number of new infections transmitted by one infected person in a susceptible population. In epidemiological terms, this is known as the secondary infection rate. "R" depends on the three variables in the model. "β" represents the infectivity rate, the probability that infection results after exposure. Factors that affect "β" (such as age, gender, contraceptive method, circumcision status, and use of antibiotics) can also affect disease transmission. In this model, "c" represents the average rate and variability of new sexual partner selection, and "D" represents the duration of infectiousness. Each of these variables may be viewed as a category that encompasses certain classes of risk factors.

In addition to the three parameters defined by the model, it is also important to consider the sociocultural framework in which the model occurs. The context does not change the parameters defined by the model, but it can affect the relative weight and types of risk factors in each category, especially those pertaining to β and D. Although these sociocultural factors may exert their influence indirectly through other factors in the model, they are important to consider. Thus, the contextual foundation of the model defines a fourth category of risk factors. Risk factors from all four of these parameters must be evaluated when considering STD transmission in individuals and STD prevalence in populations. We thus discuss risk factors implicit in each of these four categories.

In considering risk factors for the development of sequelae after infection, we have no established mathematic model to use as a point of departure. However, with minimal modifications, the model described above can also be used as an initial conceptual framework for these risk factors.

Determinants of the probability of sequelae in infected persons include the intrinsic complication rate for each organism infection, the duration or stage of untreated infection, the nature of the host response to the infection, and a variety of factors specific to the individual syndrome (e.g., for infertility, oral contraceptive use in the setting of chlamydial cervicitis; for HIV infection, circumcision in the setting of chancroid; or for cervical cancer, smoking in the setting of HPV infection).

Table 1 summarizes some of the risk factors and risk markers that may affect transmission of STDs or development of sequelae within the framework outlined earlier. It is not comprehensive, but it may provide a starting point for examining risk factors and defining their prevalence.

The infectivity rate, β

The infectivity rate or the risk of acquiring infection after contact with an infected partner may consist of two separate components: those factors that define individual infectiousness and those that determine susceptibility. As with each parameter of the model, both biological and behavioral factors must be considered. Each pathogen or disease-causing agent has unique biological characteristics that affect transmissibility. The number of organisms necessary to establish infection, or the infectious dose, is an example. Gender, genetic susceptibility, age at exposure, co-infection with other infectious organisms, and immunologic status are examples of biologic host factors that affect β.

A number of behavioral risk factors and risk markers such as douching, contraceptive practices, circumcision, specific sexual practices, and use of drugs (including antibiotics) and alcohol all affect the infectivity rate. In turn, individual factors such as motivations, cognitive abilities to perceive risk, and past experiences

Table 1. Potential risk factors and risk markers for STDs

	Transmission	Sequelae
β (Transmission or Complication Rate)		
Risk factor	Infectivity of organism Genetic susceptibility Sexual practices*	Virulence of organism Genetic susceptibility
Risk factor or marker	Age Age of coital debut* Gender Contraceptive method* Circumcision status* Alcohol use* Drug use (IV & other)* Smoking* Prior/co-existing STDs Intravaginal or intra-anal preparations (including douching)*	Age Age of coital debut* Gender Contraceptive method* Circumcision status* Alcohol use* Drug use (IV & other)* Smoking* Prior/co-existing STDs Douching*
c (Rate and Nature of Partner Exchange)		
Risk factor	Number of partners/time* Type of partner* (eg, membership in core)	
Risk factor or marker	Age Age of coital debut* Gender	
D (Duration of Infectiousness or Active Infection)		
Risk factor	Infecting organism Host response Health care behaviors* Routine STD screening Early diagnosis & therapy of symptoms Compliance with therapy Compliance with partner notification Vaccine use Douching & other intravaginal preparations	Infecting organism Host response Health care behaviors* Routine STD screening Early diagnosis & therapy of symptoms Compliance with therapy Compliance with partner notification Vaccine use
S (Sociocultural Context)		
Risk marker	Race Ethnicity Religion* Marital status* Residence* Educational status* Socioeconomic status* Sexual preference* Temporal context	Race Ethnicity Religion* Marital status* Residence* Educational status* Socioeconomic status* Sexual preference* Temporal context

* Behavioral risk factor or risk marker.

all drive behavior. A hypothetical example would be an infectious agent that binds to host cell receptors found primarily on epithelial cells of rectal mucosa. People who have anal intercourse with infected individuals are more likely to acquire infection than those who are exposed through vaginal intercourse. Other similar examples can be constructed that illustrate the interplay of biological and behavioral factors that affect the likelihood of disease transmission or disease progression among infected persons.

The rate of new partner selection, c

The rate of new partner selection, in its most simple form, refers to the number of new partners a person chooses over a specified period. Because only a limited number of persons within a population are infected, greater numbers of partners increase the likelihood that any one randomly chosen partner is infected. Furthermore, Anderson has emphasized that variability in number of partners is the single most important determinant of the magnitude of an STD epidemic (2). However, the effect of number of partners can be defined further by whether the partners were encountered one at a time over a particular time interval (serial monogamy), or whether the person had multiple simultaneous partners. With diseases such as gonorrhea that have a short period of infectiousness, multiple simultaneous partners carry a greater risk of dissemination of infection than serial monogamous partners. For diseases such as AIDS with a long period of infectiousness, this distinction is less important.

Surveys have shown that most people have only a few sexual partners over their lifetime (3) and that the propagation of STD epidemics is actually attributable to a small group of high-frequency transmitters with large numbers of sexual partners, referred to as the core. The activities of core group members sustain hyperendemic levels of STDs within the core and, because the core is not a closed population, are also responsible for epidemics outside of the core. Mixing of core and noncore group members mediates transmission of STDs to the wider pool of partners in the general population.

Studies have defined some of the common characteristics of STD core members (4, 5). They include urban residence, low socioeconomic status, age between 15 and 30 years, membership in an ethnic minority, and participation in illicit drug use and prostitution. However, it is not clear to what extent these factors vary according to time, place, group, and pathogen. In addition, the size of the core group necessary to maintain an epidemic differs depending on the infectivity of the pathogen (β) as well as the duration of infectiousness (D, discussed later). The sociodemographic composition of the core might also vary depending on the pathogen and the characteristics of the affected population. Number of partners, per se, must therefore be qualified by information about the population from which the partner is selected. If the partner is part of the core, the likelihood that he or she is infected with an STD is increased.

Variables that may identify core members include the place where the partners met, elicitation of risk-related information from the partner, and length of the relationship before sexual activity occurred. Assessment of mixing among ethnic, social, and risk groups is another way of evaluating the permeable boundaries of core groups and the potential for disease transmission beyond the core. One example of this phenomenon would be a study of the frequency with which intravenous drug users (IVDU) choose non-IVDUs as sexual partners.

Duration of infectiousness, D

The duration of infectiousness is dictated by those factors that determine how long an individual is capable of transmitting infection. This category includes biological characteristics of the host and the pathogen. For example, the immune response to infection influences the duration of infection. However, fully protective natural immunity is rarely established against STD pathogens. In partially immune patients, the number of infectious organisms may be so low that the person is asymptomatic, but still remains infectious. Antimicrobial sensitivity is also important. If the organism is resistant, treatment failure may occur and the duration of infectiousness will be increased.

Behavioral factors that affect duration of infectiousness include health-seeking behaviors and access to health care. Health care includes screening programs, treatment protocols, partner notification systems, vaccine distribution programs, and behavior change programs. If infected persons and their partners are screened and treated appropriately for STDs and comply with therapy, then their ability to transmit disease is curtailed. However, some pathogens, such as *Chlamydia trachomatis*, commonly cause asymptomatic infections; infected persons often do not know they are infected and do not seek treatment. Thus, they remain sexually active carriers, still able to transmit disease. Access to health care is affected by the location of the clinic, the speed with which care can be obtained, and the cost of the services. The likelihood that an individual will use a health care facility is further influenced by such factors as the stigma associated with using the facility, the perceived quality of care, and the person's own assessment of his or her risk.

Changing biotechnologic developments play a major role in curtailing STD spread. Technologic aspects of treatment, screening, behavior change, and vaccine programs are relevant to all STDs, but their relative importance differs depending on the pathogen and the sex of the person. Effective treatment (including factors related to compliance, such as the number of doses and duration of therapy) is the obvious first step in prevention both of transmission and of development of sequelae for bacterial pathogens that usually cause symptomatic disease (e.g., *Neisseria gonorrhoeae* or *Haemophilus ducreyi*). For bacterial pathogens that frequently result in an asymptomatic carrier state (e.g., *C. trachomatis* or *Treponema pallidum*) screening and partner notification programs are more important because asymptomatic infected persons are not likely to seek treatment. Such screening programs are dependent on accurate, easy-to-use, inexpensive diagnostic tests. Behavior change programs (including programs that distribute effective, inexpensive, easy-to-use prophylaxis) are more important to prevent spread of viral pathogens for which there is currently no cure (e.g., HIV, hepatitis B virus, and herpes simplex virus).

Sociocultural context

The sociocultural context in which individuals and societies function includes factors that must be considered in the model. Variables in this class of behavioral and biological factors are defined on a population rather than an individual basis (e.g., societal and demographic influences); thus, they describe aggregate risk. They tend to have an indirect but important effect on other variables defined by the model. For example, depending on norms of sexual behavior, factors that influence the per contact infectivity rate may differ; likewise, duration of infectiousness clearly differs depending on accessibility and acceptability of health care that is, in part, mediated by cultural and social factors. This category includes, but is not limited to: social class, education (including gender development and socialization), ethnicity, race, neighborhood, urbanization, geographic region, transportation systems, population density, and religion.

By definition, social context is time dependent and thus may be viewed as an historical construct driven by political, economic, and biotechnologic forces. These population characteristics are the basis for individual and social or cultural norms. Thus, the overall qualities of the population define what is considered normal or acceptable. Ultimately, all of these factors dictate individual and institutional beliefs, values, intentions, and behaviors.

Research Needs and Opportunities

Risk factors from each of the parameters in the model may be considered as targets for interventions. For example, the use of condoms or other forms of barrier prophylaxis with casual partners would decrease β, the likelihood of transmission subsequent to exposure. D, the duration of infectiousness, can be modified by successful treatment of STDs. Thus, physical examinations and testing should be promoted if a person has multiple sexual partners or if symptoms occur. Sociocultural factors may also provide targets for behavioral intervention, and because of the ubiquitousness of these factors, the effect of interventions at this level may, in fact, far outweigh the effect of interventions directed at the individual. However, deeply rooted sociocultural factors may prove more difficult to modify than risk factors that operate at the level of the individual.

Additional research needs to be done both to identify the type and distribution of specific risk factors and to determine the prevalence of disease. To this end, three basic types of descriptive epidemiologic studies should be conducted to provide data for subsequent analytic studies. For each type of study, it will be important to survey high-prevalence as well as general populations.

1. A national survey of sexual practices similar to the one proposed by the National Institute of Child Health and Human Development is needed to assess the importance of behavioral risk factors in specific subpopulations and to define target populations for behavioral interventions.
2. Research is necessary to determine the true population rates for various

STDs. To this end, probability seroprevalence surveys are recommended in a variety of populations.

3. Natural history studies of the progression of disease among infected persons must be conducted to identify and describe long-term sequelae of STDs. For treatable STDs, including most bacterial infections, such studies may have to be cross-sectional, whereas prospective studies would be possible for untreatable (mostly viral) STDs.

These surveys will provide critical national data on the prevalence and distribution of sexual practices and STDs and their clinical manifestations in the American population. Such data will provide baseline information for the final research priority:

4. Subsequent analytic studies are needed to determine the strength of associations and attributable risks of factors with outcomes defined by the surveys. Such studies should also serve to refine our understanding of the biological mechanisms of transmission. In conducting these studies, comparisons should be made both at the neighborhood and the individual level.

Rational, scientifically sound decisions concerning which populations and behaviors to target for interventions can only be based on data collected from such studies. The STD Cooperative Research Centers will provide opportunities for behavioral studies.

References

1. May R, Anderson R. Transmission dynamics of HIV infection. Nature 1987; 326:137–142.
2. Anderson RM. The epidemiology of HIV infection: Variable incubation plus infectious periods and heterogeneity in sexual activity. J R Stat Soc 1988; 151:66.
3. Centers for Disease Control. Number of sex partners and potential risk of sexual exposure to Human Immunodeficiency Virus. MMWR 1988; 37:565–568.
4. Hethcote HW, Yorke JA. Gonorrhea transmission dynamics and control. Lecture Notes in Biomathematics No. 56, Springer-Verlag, 1984.
5. Hansfield H, Rice R, Roberts M, Holmes K. Localized outbreak of penicillinase-producing *Neisseria gonorrhoea*: Paradigm for introduction and spread of gonorrhea in a community. JAMA 1989; 261:2357–2361.

Part II: Issues In Designing Behavioral Interventions

ANKE A. EHRHARDT, PhD; MARTIN FISHBEIN, PhD; EUGENE WASHINGTON, MD; WILLIAM SMITH, EdD; KING K. HOLMES, MD, PhD; and the NIAID STUDY GROUP ON INTEGRATED BEHAVIORAL RESEARCH FOR PREVENTION AND CONTROL OF SEXUALLY TRANSMITTED DISEASES

From the Department of Psychiatry, College of Physicians & Surgeons, Columbia University; Department of Psychology, University of Illinois; Center of Reproductive Health Policy Research, School of Medicine, University of California at San Francisco; the Academy of Educational Development; and the Global Programme on AIDS, World Health Organization.

Preventing the acquisition and spread of sexually transmitted diseases (STDs) must be considered from a variety of perspectives. We will address intervention here in three sections: in a background statement (section I), we will define categories of biomedical disease prevention and behavioral intervention. In addition, we will suggest a theoretical framework for the design and execution of interventions. In section II, we will propose a number of research needs that will be linked to research opportunities. We will close by listing, in section III, specific recommendations for achieving and implementing an integrated approach to biomedical and behavioral intervention in the field of STDs.

Background

Definition of prevention

In medical and public health practice, three levels of prevention activity are recognized: primary, secondary, and tertiary (1). "Primary prevention" refers to the prevention of the occurrence of a disease. With primary prevention, measures are taken to promote good health and to protect individuals from contracting a disease or injury. Examples of primary prevention include health education, condom use, and vaccination.

"Secondary prevention" refers to activities directed at early detection and intervention (treatment) to prevent sequelae, limit disability, and for most STDs, prevent further transmission of infection. Examples of secondary prevention include screening programs, presumptive diagnosis and treatment, and partner notification. For communicable diseases such as STDs, secondary prevention has a direct effect on primary prevention in that early diagnosis and treatment limits exposure of susceptible persons to infected individuals.

"Tertiary prevention" refers to rehabilitation or efforts to minimize the effects of disease sequelae. An example of tertiary prevention is prompt treatment of pelvic inflammatory disease (a complication of untreated chlamydial or gonococcal cervical infection) to preserve fertility. In this report, we principally address primary and secondary prevention.

Strategies for prevention and control of STDs

Approaches to control of STDs vary by type of disease (2). For the curable bacterial STDs (e.g., gonorrhea, syphilis, chlamydia, and chancroid), the emphasis should be both on primary prevention and on early diagnosis and treatment. In cases of the incurable viral STDs (e.g., genital herpes, genital papillomavirus infection, and HIV), the most important efforts focus on primary prevention through health education and behavioral interventions. When available, however, effective vaccines (e.g., hepatitis B virus) can greatly facilitate primary prevention efforts.

Traditionally, the main components of a STD control program have included health education, routine screening, early consultation for diagnosis and treatment, effective therapy, compliance with therapy, and partner notification. For STDs, primary prevention activity has been limited in most areas. Secondary prevention activities or medical interventions, however, take place regularly throughout health departments, particularly in STD, family planning, and prenatal clinics. Medical intervention for STDs also occurs in many private practitioners' offices. STD control is mandated by law in most industrialized countries and has led to the establishment of a STD health care infrastructure. The effectiveness of the system is measured in disease indices that indicate whether the rates of a particular type of STD increase or decrease over time and for particular groups in the population.

In association with decreasing rates of a STD, effectiveness of the existing primary and secondary disease control is assumed. Since components of STD medical interventions (beyond diagnosis and pharmacologic therapy) are rarely tested for their specific contribution to STD disease control, we lack systematic and prospective research studies on their effectiveness.

Behavioral intervention can also be divided into primary and secondary levels. The goal of primary prevention is behavior change to interfere with acquiring the infection. Primary prevention consists of defining the risk behaviors for STDs (i.e., specific sexual behavior patterns and other transmission behaviors such as blood exchange) and designing appropriate intervention strategies for the population engaging in the targeted risk behavior.

Secondary intervention is focused on interfering with behavior patterns that exacerbate the infection or disease and spread STDs to partners. Behavioral interventions can be designed and implemented in a variety of approaches that will be described later. Although a new wave of behavioral interventions is focused on HIV (3, 4), the assessment of program effectiveness often lags behind or is lacking altogether.

The fact that homosexual men in some epicenters of AIDS in the United States have changed their behavior is, however, encouraging and suggests that aspects of sexual behavior can be modified within population groups who are at high risk of acquiring a specific STD.

Theoretical framework

In developing an intervention, many factors are considered (5). The goal of the intervention may be primary or secondary prevention. The objective of the intervention may be to increase knowledge and understanding, change behavior, influence attitudes, or affect a health outcome (e.g., reduce the incidence of STDs). Similarly, one may wish to consider whether the intervention should be directed toward providing information or some form of skill training (e.g., assertiveness, stress management) or a "nonpsychological" regimen (e.g., aerobics, dieting, relaxation). The target may be the person, the health care provider, or the institution.

Because many factors must be considered, it is useful to classify interventions in three major dimensions: intervention agent, intervention target, and type of intervention.

1. *Intervention agent.* Will the intervention be community based or will it rely on outside experts? That is, will the "change agents" be representatives of the community? Will the intervention take advantage of existing community organizations and services?
2. *Intervention target.* Will the intervention be directed at changing an individual, a group, or an institution? That is, will the intervention attempt to increase the likelihood that individual persons will use condoms (individual), will it try to change a general norm (or the perception of a norm) such as "everybody is expected to use condoms" (group), or will it attempt to change laws or policies such as those governing the advertising or distribution of condoms (institution)?
3. *Intervention type.* Will the intervention rely on interpersonal, institutional, or mass media communications? That is, will the intervention be analogous to therapy (either individual or group), to a program within an institution (e.g., the schools, the work place, an STD clinic), or to a mass media program?

The central focus, with respect to intervention type, concerns the nature of the relationship between the influencing agent and the target. With interpersonal interventions, one relies on one-to-one or small-group interactions where the influencing agent can change the intervention to respond to the particular needs of one's clients. At the institutional level (where there is a one-to-many relationship), one can still respond to questions raised by individual members of a group, but the program is more systematized and it is difficult (if not impossible) to modify the program to address the needs of each participant. Finally, at the mass media level, there is no direct contact between the influencing agent and the clients or target audience.

Models that combine elements of the third dimension are particularly promising (6). For example, mass media used to inform high-risk persons of new

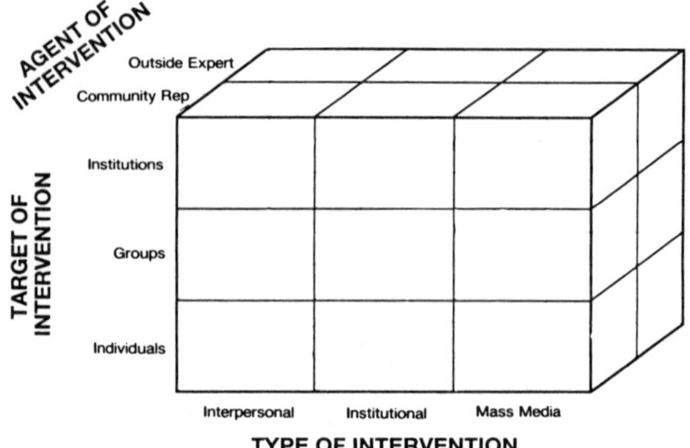

Figure 1. Three-dimensional taxonomy of interventions (from reference 5).

treatment services and to help create an atmosphere of trust and societal support are integrated with clinical services that include peer outreach, treatment, and psychosocial support to avoid re-infection.

Consideration of these three dimensions (i.e., agent, target, and type) suggests an intervention classification system such as that illustrated in Figure 1. It is interesting to note that, to date, almost all research concerned with evaluating the effectiveness of interventions designed to prevent the spread of AIDS and other STDs has taken place in the "outside expert-individual-interpersonal" cell of the figure. That is, most research in this area attempts to evaluate the effectiveness of therapeutic interventions carried out by professional experts and designed to change individual behavior. Although one can identify some ongoing programs using institutional and mass media interventions, these have typically not been researched, i.e., there has been no attempt to evaluate their effectiveness. Clearly, we need to develop and evaluate interventions in other cells of Figure 1.

Research Needs and Research Opportunities

When intervening with those who are at risk of acquiring or transmitting an STD or developing sequelae, the research needs in the areas of disease control and behavior change are numerous and multifaceted. In selecting priorities, the study group decided to take advantage of existing research opportunities to accelerate progress and to advance knowledge. It also seemed important to differentiate carefully between behavioral and disease control interventions, even though the ultimate goal may be the same. Furthermore, all interventions should reflect the cultural heterogeneity of the targeted populations. Suggested research strategies are discussed below.

STD clinic system

To describe, define, and evaluate the system and its components. To assess how the system works and whether its effectiveness can be documented.

Other health behavior intervention systems

1. To assess public health workers, counselors (disease intervention specialists)—what do they do, how good are they, are their techniques effective in getting people to change behaviors and in obtaining a lowered incidence of STDs?

2. To investigate legislative requirements for STDs and AIDS—what are they, what are they supposed to do, what do they do, and how effective are they (e.g., HIV curriculum from grades K–12 mandated at the state level; partner notification)?

3. To survey the procedures of existing maternal-child health programs (screening, counseling, testing, follow-up) and to develop a counseling package to be evaluated in one or several settings.

4. To survey existing STD prevention procedures in adolescent clinics (in schools or in adolescent medicine divisions in hospitals and family planning settings) and determine their effectiveness.

5. To assess contraceptive choices and their effect on STDs. It seems more important than ever to tailor contraceptive and disease barrier methods to individual choice. In addition, it must be acknowledged that the goals of pregnancy prevention and disease prevention may be antithetical. Specifically, disease protection cannot rely only on condom use but must also include the development of new barrier methods that women can control without being dependent on male cooperation (7).

6. To assess the use of hepatitis B vaccine. What are the barriers to its acceptance and how can a positive response to it be facilitated? This may be instructive for the planning and the use of future STD/HIV vaccines.

7. To assess potential, unexpected, adverse implications of education and intervention strategies for specific populations (e.g., encouragement of women to introduce condoms in sexual encounters may lead to physical abuse by their uncooperative male partners).

8. To assess the possibilities for the social marketing of STD prevention products and behaviors. For example, how can market segmentation and marketing strategies be used to improve specific prevention behavior?

All of the suggested research strategies should be addressed from the different perspectives defined by the dimensions discussed previously, (i.e., on interpersonal, institutional, and mass media levels). The outcome measures of all of these research strategies must include behavior change (e.g., from risk behaviors for acquiring STDs to safe behavior) and assessment of disease indices (e.g., measurement of the organism or antibodies to the organism).

Summary and Specific Research Recommendations

This section summarizes our recommendations and spells out possible mechanisms to foster interdisciplinary collaboration of medical specialists and behavioral scientists.

Behavioral research on STDs should be interdisciplinary

1. Creation of interdisciplinary STD research centers that include both biomedical and behavioral scientists collaborating on projects (8). These centers should

include both medical and basic science disciplines and the behavioral sciences. Behavioral sciences include a variety of strategies; in particular, social marketing and media experts should advise and collaborate on issues of health education and the development of educational programs. In addition, a mechanism must be established and documented to ensure a bidirectional exchange with the community of the targeted population (i.e., a system that facilitates input from the community to researchers and also provides a rapid feedback from the scientists to the targeted population in the community).

2. Establishment of an NIAID administrative structure to assure expert peer review of behavioral research.

3. Creation of a funding mechanism that facilitates maximum flexibility for interdisciplinary collaboration.

4. Establishment of a behavioral research branch to provide institutional expertise for expansion of integrated behavioral research activities.

Use the existing infrastructure (health services systems and research) to conduct behavioral research

5. Survey behavioral interventions in the existing infrastructure, especially STD clinics and schools, and assess their effectiveness. This could be achieved by grant or contract funding mechanisms in addition to the establishment of centers.

6. Interventions are needed in sexual behavior and health behavior, but emphasis should be placed on institutional and mass media approaches in study design and evaluation of both behavior change and public health impact.

Core group vs. non-core

7. Define core groups, and determine and compare the effectiveness and cost effectiveness of primary and secondary behavioral interventions in both core and non-core groups.

Practitioners: private vs. public sector

8. Define the current role of private practitioners in control efforts. Assess both private and public sector providers' attitudes and behavior related to the traditional components of STD prevention and control programs. Determine the effectiveness of behavioral interventions in both groups of providers.

References

1. Last JM. Scope and methods of prevention. In: Public Health and Preventive Medicine. 12th ed. Norwalk, Connecticut: Appleton-Century-Crofts, 1986:3–7.
2. Cates W Jr, Meheus A. Strategies for development of sexually transmitted diseases control programs. In: Holmes, Mardh, and Sparling, et al, eds. Sexually Transmitted Diseases. 2nd ed. New York: McGraw Hill, 1990: 1023–1029.
3. Smith WA. Lifestyle for Survival. Washington, DC: Academy for Educational Development, 1989.
4. Frederiksen LW, Solomon LJ, Brehony KA. Principles, techniques and applications. In: Marketing Health Behavior. New York: Plenum Press, 1984:120.

5. Fishbein M. Toward a taxonomy of intervention research. Working Paper, University of Illinois, 1989.
6. Rice RE, Atkin CK. Public Communication Campaigns. 2nd ed. Newbury Park, CA: Sage Publications, 1989.
7. Stein ZA. The need for methods women can use. Am J Public Health 1990; 80:460–462.
8. Ehrhardt AA. Preventing and treating AIDS: The expertise of the behavioral sciences. Bull NY Acad Med 1988; 64:513–519.

Part III: Issues In Evaluating Behavioral Interventions

SEVGI O. ARAL, PhD; JUDITH N. WASSERHEIT, MD, MPH; SYLVAN B. GREEN, MD; FRANKLYN N. JUDSON, MD; P. FREDERICK SPARLING, MD; and the NIAID STUDY GROUP ON INTEGRATED BEHAVIORAL RESEARCH FOR PREVENTION AND CONTROL OF SEXUALLY TRANSMITTED DISEASES

From the Behavioral Studies Section, Centers for Disease Control; Sexually Transmitted Diseases Branch, National Institutes of Health; Clinical and Diagnostic Trials Section, National Cancer Institute; Sexually Transmitted Diseases Programme, World Health Organization; and the Department of Medicine, University of North Carolina.

Behavioral research in sexually transmitted diseases (STDs) is marked by specific issues that must be considered in designing studies and in the interpretation of study findings. We discuss these issues in three categories: issues of measurement, issues relevant to epidemiologic studies, and issues relevant to intervention studies.

Issues of Measurement

Measurement of STD risk behaviors poses special problems in that most sexual, drug use, and health behaviors of interest do not lend themselves to objective measurement. Unobtrusive measures are rarely socially acceptable in the study of sexual and health behaviors. Investigations depend on self reports of these private behaviors.

In the absence of objective measures, validation of self-reported behavior is difficult. Past studies have relied on measures of reliability to reflect validity (1–3). Reliability is low for self reports of number of partners, frequency of particular sexual practices, and change in sexual behavior (3). Studies that assess the validity of self-reported sexual behavior data by comparing responses to the same questions made by both members of same-sex and mixed-sex couples find correlation coefficients on the order of 0.6 (4).

When all other conditions are constant, changes in the incidence of STDs in a closed population can be used to validate self-reported changes in sexual behavior. However, all other conditions are rarely constant; therefore, the use of incident STDs to validate sexual behavior data is rarely adequate.

The way data are collected influences the reliability and validity of self reports of risk behavior. For example, written responses to self-administered questionnaires may deviate from oral responses to interviews (5). Interviewer characteristics, as they influence measurement of sexual behavior, have not been systematically studied.

Experimental work in the measurement of other types of behavior indicates that status differences between interviewer and respondent are important (6, 7). Question wording is also important. The extreme variability in the wording is also important. The extreme variability in the wording of questions and in the periods covered in the questions have made it difficult to compare findings of epidemiologic studies. It is important to consider the study question and the particular STDs of interest in determining the period to be covered in the questions and their wording. For example, if currently incurable viral STDs such as genital herpes or human papillomavirus infection are the diseases of interest, longer time frames more appropriately capture the interval during which disease acquisition may have occurred. Unfortunately, longer time frames often result in greater recall bias.

Measurement of health outcome has been less problematic since sexually transmitted infections can be assessed objectively. Previous history of STDs can be measured based on medical records, but sometimes it is measured based on self reports. Self-reported history of previous STDs is subject to the same reliability and validity concerns as self-reported sexual or drug-use behavior. In epidemiologic and intervention studies it is important to note whether incidence or prevalence of infection is being measured. Some morbidity indicators, such as visits to a health care provider for a specific complaint, may capture a mixture of incident and prevalent STD cases.

Design Issues Relevant to Epidemiologic Studies

Behavioral risk factors for STDs and their complications are identified through cross-sectional, case–control, or cohort studies. These risk factors include behaviors that affect the risk of exposure to an infected partner and the risk of developing sequelae as a result of acquiring an STD as discussed elsewhere in this report (8). Most STDs are of low incidence in the general population. Therefore, cohort studies to investigate risk factors for STDs are expensive, time consuming, and rarely conducted. Case–control studies constitute the most frequent design choice. The choice of suitable control subjects may depend on the type of behavioral risk factor being studied. STD clinic control subjects may be appropriate in studies of behavioral risk factors. In studies focusing on risk factors for STD sequelae, infected STD clinic control subjects may help distinguish true risk factors for developing sequelae from risk factors for acquisition of uncomplicated infection. Control subjects recruited from the community may be more suitable in studies of behavioral risk factors for exposure to infected partners. For studying STD sequelae, cohort studies can play a role, as is being done with HIV infection.

In epidemiologic studies, it is important to account for possible confounders in attempting to identify true risk factors. However, STD risk behaviors overlap, and the resulting multicollinearity sometimes cannot be resolved. In such situations, controlled intervention trials may be the only viable alternative.

Design Issues Relevant to Intervention Studies

Interventions to control the transmission of STDs aim at preventing the risk behavior, lessening the risk associated with the behavior, or screening for early detection of curable infections leading to treatment.

Behavioral interventions may be evaluated in four phases, similar to the evaluation of drug therapies. Phase I studies focus on demonstrating the feasibility and safety of an intervention. In this phase, it is important to rule out any physical or socioemotional adverse outcomes that may result from the intervention. The main goal of phase I studies is to demonstrate that the intervention is acceptable to subjects. The outcome measure in these studies is behavioral. The behavior may be measured through self reports and, where possible, through observations. Feasibility studies usually involve small numbers of subjects and no controls.

Phase II studies are conducted to determine whether an intervention has any effect on behavior and to determine the optimal duration and frequency of the intervention. Those interventions that show evidence of "activity" in phase II studies are candidates for phase III studies. If more than one intervention is available for study in phase II, it makes sense to assign subjects randomly so that the interventions receive a comparable assessment. However, randomization is not absolutely required.

Phase III studies evaluate the efficacy of an intervention in comparison to no intervention or other interventions, under ideal study conditions. However, in contrast to phase II studies, control subjects and random assignment are important components of a phase III study design. The advantage of randomization is that bias is avoided, prognostic factors (whether known or unknown) tend to be balanced across intervention groups, and the validity of statistic tests of significance used to compare interventions is assured. In addition, the best outcome measure in a phase III study would be STD incidence. Behaviors should be measured to help interpret study findings. The efficacy of an intervention can only be evaluated based on the health outcome, but the interpretation of negative findings necessitates measurement of behavioral outcomes. Failure to change STD incidence cannot be assumed to result from failure to change behavior. Phase III studies are called randomized controlled trials or comparative efficacy studies. The unit of randomization may be the individual, the community, or some other group, depending on the nature of intervention and the feasibility of delivery. The unit of randomization may or may not be the same as the unit of the outcome measure.

Case–control studies can also provide information about the efficacy of an intervention. They may be particularly appropriate when randomization is not possible, programs are already in place, or evaluation of sustained efficacy is desired after completion of a randomized trial.

Three issues that are particularly important in behavioral intervention trials should be noted. First, behavioral measurement may influence the behavior itself, turning measurement into intervention. Second, contamination between intervention and control groups may be likely, and should be minimized. Third, generalizability of study findings across population subgroups cannot be assumed. Therefore, it is important to conduct behavioral intervention trials on those populations for which the intervention is being developed.

Phase IV studies are designed to test the real world effectiveness of interventions. These studies focus on external validity or generalizability. Randomization may not always be possible in phase IV studies, but it is desirable if possible.

Utility of Qualitative Data

Qualitative methods, for example, ethnographic assessment, focus groups, in-depth interviews, or immersion in a community, may be useful at several points in the research process. In the preliminary design phases, qualitative research may be important in framing research questions and preparing data collection instruments. During the investigation, qualitative approaches applied to subsamples may enrich our understanding of the meaning and social context of the behavior under study. Ongoing qualitative assessments may provide insight into unanticipated effects of interventions. This is particularly important for the study of poorly understood behaviors in heterogeneous cultural subgroups. However, these approaches do not contribute to establishing causality or efficacy.

Research Needs and Opportunities

Methodologic research on the measurement of risk behaviors and factors influencing the validity and reliability of such measurement is greatly needed. Mode of data collection, interviewer characteristics, question wording, and sequencing may influence the measurement of each risk behavior differently. Also, population subgroups may vary in their reactions to measurement strategies. As discussed elsewhere in this report, survey research to assess the magnitude and distribution of risk behaviors in the population and behavioral trials to define interventions that work are urgently needed. It will be important to use this unique opportunity to develop measurement instruments with known reliability and validity, and to conduct methodologic research on the measurement of sexual, drug use, and health behaviors.

References

1. Delameter J, MacCorquedale P. The effects of interview schedule variation on reported sexual behavior. Soc Meth Res 1975; 4:215–236.
2. Ehrmann WW. Premarital Dating Behavior. New York: Henry Holt, 1959.
3. Saltzmann SP, Stoddard AM, McCusker J, Moon MW, Mayer KH. Reliability of self reported sexual behavior risk factors for HIV infection in homosexual men. Public Health Reports. 1987; 102:692–697.
4. Coates RA, Calzavara LM, Soskolne CL, Reed SE, Fanning MM, Shepherd FA, Klein MH, Johnson KJ. Validity of sexual histories in a prospective study of male sexual contacts of men with AIDS or an AIDS related condition. Am J Epidemiol 1988; 128:719–728.
5. Aral SO, Magder LS, Bowen GS. HIV risk behavior screening: Concordance between assessments through interviews and questionnaires, V International Conference on AIDS, Montreal, Quebec, Canada, June 4–9, 1989:699.
6. National Center for Health Services Research. Advances in health survey research methods: Proceedings of a national invitational conference research proceedings series. Arlington, Virginia: U.S. Department of Health, Education and Welfare, 1975.
7. Potterat JJ, Phillips L, Muth JB. Lying to military physicians about risk factors for HIV infections. JAMA 1987; 257:1727.
8. Padian N. Issues in defining behavioral risk factors and their distribution. Sex Transm Dis 1990; 18.

Appendix II

Glossary

algorithm: any systematic process that consists of an ordered sequence of steps with each step depending on the outcome of the previous one. This approach makes use of branching logic and of all pertinent data, both about the patient and from epidemiological and other sources, to arrive at clinical management decisions that yield maximum benefit and minimum risk.

antibody: a molecule generated by the body, usually in response to a foreign agent or organism, as part of the host's defense.

antimicrobial sensitivity: the susceptibility of a specific organism to therapeutic agents.

attributable risk: the proportion of disease in a defined population resulting from a specific exposure or risk factor.

attitude: the interpretation or reaction of an individual to a particular situation that reflects the residue of previous experience developed from a complex system of social and environmental influences.

biovar: a term that describes a group of organisms that have in common the ability to cause a similar type of infection. Biovars are applied most commonly to *Chlamydia trachomatis*.

carrier: an individual who harbors in his or her body the specific organisms of a disease without manifest symptoms but who can still spread infection; the condition of such an individual is known as **carrier state**.

case finding: a form of disease detection in which individuals seeking health care for any reason are given additional tests to detect sexually transmitted disease (e.g., serological testing for syphilis of adult patients admitted to hospitals). This is in contrast to **screening**, in which testing is performed in apparently healthy individuals who are not seeking other health services.

cervicitis: inflammation of the cervix that may or may not be related to infectious causes.

chancroid: a painful ulcerative sexually transmitted disease that is often associated with enlarged and inflamed lymph nodes in the groin and is caused by *Haemophilus ducreyi*.

chemoprophylaxis: see **prophylaxis**.

chlamydia: a sexually transmitted disease caused by the organism *Chlamydia trachomatis* that results most commonly in abnormal vaginal and urethral discharge. *Chlamydia trachomatis* also causes eye disease and pneumonia in infants born to infected women.

chorioamnionitis: inflammation of fetal membranes most commonly caused by infectious agents. Chorioamnionitis is associated with premature delivery.

cirrhosis: liver disease characterized pathologically by loss of the normal microscopic architecture, scarring, and, ultimately, loss of normal liver function.

cognitive structure: organizations of conceptually related representations of objects, situations, and events derived from past experiences. They allow the perceiver to reduce an enormously complex environment to a manageable number of meaningful categories.

coital debut: first episode of sexual intercourse.

condyloma acuminatum (condylomata acuminata): genital warts caused by human papillomavirus (HPV).

confounding: the distortion of the apparent effect of an exposure on risk brought about by the association of both the risk factor and the outcome with yet another risk factor.

conjunctivitis: inflammation of the conjunctiva (the delicate membrane that lines the eyelids and covers the exposed surface of the white outer coat of the eyeball), generally consisting of redness and discharge. **Inclusion conjunctivitis** is caused by the organism *Chlamydia trachomatis* and is primarily found in newborns born to mothers with chlamydial genital infections.

control group: a subgroup of the study population that differs from the remaining study participants with respect to disease outcome or intervention received and that offers a basis for comparisons.

core group: a group of individuals who by virtue of their behavior contribute disproportionately to the transmission of sexually transmitted diseases in the population (e.g., young unmarried urban adults, prostitutes, and long-distance truck drivers).

Credé's prophylaxis: the placing of 1 drop of 2% solution of silver nitrate in each eye of a newborn child to prevent ophthalmia neonatorum (gonococcal eye infection).

dementia: a general designation for mental deterioration.

dependent variable: a manifestation or outcome whose variation we seek to explain or account for by the influence of other variables.

determinant: any factor, whether event, characteristic, or other definable entity, that brings about change in a health condition or other defined characteristic.

donovanosis: a progressively destructive bacterial sexually transmitted disease of the genital region. The most common synonyms are granuloma inguinale and granuloma venereum.

dimorphic: occurring in two distinct forms.

dysuria: painful urination.

ecological research design: a study in which the units of analysis are populations or groups of people, rather than individuals. An example is the study of association between median income and cancer mortality rates in administrative jurisdictions such as states and counties.

ectocervix or exocervix: the surface of the cervix that protrudes into the vaginal canal; in contrast to the **endocervix**, which is the passageway leading from the vaginal canal into the uterus.

ectopic pregnancy: development of the fetus outside the uterine cavity.

ectopy, zone of: the portion of columnar epithelium that lies in an exposed position on the ectocervix. It is usually maximal in extent in adolescence and gradually decreases through young adulthood. The zone of ectopy is important because it is believed to be a site of attachment for gonococci and chlamydiae.

endemic: the constant presence of a disease or infectious agent within a given geographic area or population group.

endocervix: the mucous membrane lining the canal that connects the vagina with the uterine cavity.

endogenous flora: the bacteria normally residing within a specific part of the body (e.g., the vagina).

endometritis: inflammation of the lining of the uterus, usually caused by infection.

enteric: pertaining to the intestines.

epididymitis: inflammation of the epididymis, the elongated cordlike structure along the posterior border of the testis, in the ducts of which the spermatozoa are stored. Epididymitis is most commonly due to infection.

epithelium: the covering of internal and external surfaces of the body, including the lining of vessels and other small cavities.
columnar: a type composed of tall prismatic cells.
cuboidal: a type composed of cells that are cuboidal.
stratified squamous: a type composed of flattened, platelike cells arranged in several layers.

ethnography: a descriptive form of investigation of a particular ethnic or social group that includes in-depth study of cultural context, ranges of interactive behavior within the group, values, attitudes, and perceptions in a particular community.

evaluation research: a process that attempts to determine as systematically and objectively as possible the relevance, effectiveness, and impact of activities in light of their objectives.

expectancy value model: a theory of rational choice predicting the anticipated satisfaction with an outcome.

focus group: a small discussion group designed to elicit views on a central point of attention or activity and to determine norms of behavior within the group.

genitourinary: pertaining to the genital and urinary organs.

glycogen: a polysaccharide, the chief carbohydrate storage material in animals. It is formed by and largely stored in the liver and to a lesser extent in the muscles, being converted to glucose and liberated as needed.

gonorrhea: a sexually transmitted disease that is caused by the organism *Neisseria gonorrhoeae* and that results most commonly in an abnormal vaginal or urethral discharge. Gonorrhea also causes eye disease in infants born to infected women.

Gram staining: a rapid, inexpensive staining procedure to detect bacteria.

high-frequency transmitters: see "**core group.**"

ideation: the process of forming ideas or concepts.

ideology: those modes of feeling, valuing, perceiving, and believing that have some relation to the maintenance of social power.

immunoglobulin: a protein of animal origin endowed with known antibody activity; plays a role in the body's defense mechanism.

incidence: the number of new cases of a disease in a defined population within a specified period.

incubation period: the time interval between exposure to an infectious agent and the appearance of symptomatic disease.

independent variable: the characteristic being observed or measured that is hypothesized to influence an event or manifestation (the dependent variable).

index case: the case in a family or other defined group that first comes to the attention of the investigator or health care provider.

infectiousness: a characteristic of the *disease* that concerns the relative ease with which it is transmitted to other hosts.

infectivity: the characteristic of the *disease agent* that embodies capability to enter, survive, and multiply in the host.

introitus: a general term for the entrance to a space or cavity.

in vitro: in a test tube; in an artificial environment.

in vivo: within the living body.

lactobacilli: organisms that are the major constituents of normal vaginal flora and that usually do not cause disease.

language elicitation: a form of investigation of a particular group directed to meanings of words or terms as understood by native speakers.

lymphadenopathy, generalized: enlargement of lymph nodes, often in response to infection. Generalized lymphadenopathy refers to involvement of lymph nodes throughout the body.

lymphocyte: a white blood cell that participates in both arms of the immune response (that due to antibodies and that due to cells).

lymphogranuloma venereum (LGV): a sexually transmitted disease caused by *Chlamydia trachomatis* that results in genital ulcers and lymph node enlargement.

mean: a measure of central tendency computed by summing all the individual values and dividing the resulting sum by the number of values.

median: a measure of central tendency obtained by identifying the middle value of an array of numbers (the value that divides the range of values in half).

menarche: the beginning of menstrual function.

meningitis: inflammation of the membranes that envelop the brain and spinal cord.

morbidity: the condition of being diseased or otherwise unhealthy.

mucous membrane: a thin, mucus-secreting layer of tissue that covers a surface, lines a cavity, or divides a space or organ.

mutation rate: the number of changes in form, quality, or some other characteristic over a given period.

natural history (of disease): the course of a disease from onset (inception) to resolution, including the development of complications.

neonatal: pertaining to the first 4 weeks after birth.

neoplasia: the formation of new and abnormal growth of a neoplasm or tumor that may be malignant or benign.

nerve, sensory: a peripheral nerve that conducts impulses from a sense organ to the spinal cord or brain.

nonkeratinized: lacking a specialized protein that is the principal constituent of skin, hair, and nails.

oncogenic: giving rise to tumors or causing tumor formation.

operational research: the systematic study, by observation and experiment, of the working of a system (e.g., health services), with a view to improvement.

ophthalmia neonatorum: infection of the conjunctiva (the delicate membrane that lines the eyelids and covers the exposed surface of the white outer coat of the eyeball) in the newborn, often acquired from the mother during birth. Major causes include gonococci and chlamydia.

opportunistic infection: the bodily invasion by and multiplication of microorganisms that usually do not produce disease in a normal immune-competent individual.

partner notification: the practice of informing sexual partners of individuals with sexually transmitted diseases that they may have been exposed to an infection. Partner notification may be performed by the patient or, for some sexually transmitted diseases, may be performed at the request of the patient, or, finally, may be conducted by trained staff who maintain the anonymity of the index patient. Partner notification is an important means of identifying individuals with untreated infection.

pathogen: any disease-producing organism.

patient management: patient care, including diagnosis, treatment, counseling, psychological support, and care of sex partners.

patrilineal: relating to, based on, or tracing descent through the male line.

pelvic inflammatory disease (PID): infection of the upper genital tract (uterus and fallopian tubes) in women; often leads to severe complications such as infertility and ectopic pregnancy.

perianal: located around the anus.

perinatal: pertaining to or occurring in the period shortly before and after birth.

pH: the symbol relating to the level of acidity of a substance.

polymerase chain reaction (PCR): an enzyme-based procedure for making many copies of a specific sequence of genetic material (nucleic acid).

prevalence: the number of persons with a disease or an attribute at a specified point in time.

prevention:

primary: prevention of infection in a population (e.g., condom use to prevent transmission of human immunodeficiency virus).

secondary: prevention of complications in infected individuals (e.g., early diagnosis and treatment of gonorrhea in women to prevent the development of salpingitis and infertility).

primary health care: a health system based on the following principles: (1) integration of health programs at the district level; (2) decentralization of health services management; (3) involvement of the community and of other sectors; (4) increased emphasis on health promotion and prevention; and (5) reduced inequity in access to health care.

process evaluation: examination of changes occurring during a program or study.

prodromal symptoms: premonitory symptoms indicating the onset of a disease.

programs/services:

categorical or vertical: a health system based on distinct services and programs for specific health problems starting at the primary care level (e.g., sexually transmitted disease clinics, mother and child services, etc.)

integrated or horizontal: health services that offer comprehensive care for patients with all types of diseases, as well as preventive activities at the primary health care level.

prophylaxis: use of an antibiotic or antiviral agent to prevent the development of a specific disease.

proctitis: inflammation of the rectum caused by infection.

prostitution: the practice of providing sexual stimulation for money, drugs, or other rewards.

protozoa: a group of unicellular organisms that range in size from submicroscopic to macroscopic, some of which are pathogenic (e.g., *Trichomonas vaginalis*).

puerperal: pertaining to the period or state of confinement after labor.

pustule: a visible collection of pus within or beneath the top layer of the skin, often in a hair follicle or sweat pore.

reactive syphilis serology: a positive syphilis test.

relative risk: the ratio of the risk of disease or death among the exposed to the risk among the unexposed; this usage is synonymous with risk ratio.

reservoir: an alternative host or passive carrier of a disease-producing organism that is significant as an ongoing source of infection.

risk factor/behavior: an aspect of personal behavior or life-style, an environmental exposure, or an inborn or inherited characteristic whose presence is associated with an increased probability of infection or disease development (this does not mean that all individuals with the risk factor become infected or that the absence of the risk factor ensures absence of infection).

risk group: a group of people whose behavioral features include risk factors for a specific disease (e.g., adolescents are a risk group for sexually transmitted diseases).

safer sex: any sexual practice that reduces the risk of passing sexually transmitted diseases from one person to another (e.g., a mutually faithful relationship between two uninfected partners; using a condom for all types of intercourse).

salience: a situation in which an individual is more focused on one portion of the environment than on others, resulting in a disproportionate weighting of that portion in subsequent decision-making.

screening: the testing of apparently healthy volunteers from the general population for the purpose of detecting disease. This is in contrast to **case finding**, in which tests are performed in individuals seeking health care for other reasons.

sensitivity: the proportion of individuals with a positive test among those who truly have the disease.

septic abortion: a serious postabortion infection of the uterus leading to generalized infection and often resulting in the death of the mother.

sequela: a complication of initial disease.

seroepidemiology: epidemiological study based on the detection of characteristic changes in the level of specific antibodies in the blood.

serology: examination of infection through testing of blood specimens for evidence of an immune (antibody) response.

social organization: the structure and function of groups and institutions around specific values, beliefs, and traditions.

socialization: the process by which the individual learns to adjust to the group by acquiring social behavior of which the group approves.

social marketing: the design, implementation, and control of programs seeking to increase the acceptability of a social idea or cause in a target group.

social network: a system of cooperating individuals.

social norm: a standard of behavior determined by members of a group (not necessarily all of them).

specificity: the proportion of truly nondiseased persons who are so identified by a test or other procedure.

squamocolumnar junction: the point of juncture between the simple columnar epithelial lining of the cervical canal and the stratified squamous epithelial covering of the part of the cervix that projects into the vagina.

subclinical: without signs or symptoms.

surface antigen: any substance that is capable, under appropriate conditions, of inducing the formation of an immune response.

surveillance: ongoing monitoring, generally using methods distinguished by their practicality, uniformity, and, frequently, their rapidity, rather than by complete accuracy. Its main purpose is to detect changes in trends in order to initiate investigative and/or control measures.

syndromic management: patient management based on a set of clinical manifestations (i.e., syndrome), as opposed to management based on an etiological, laboratory-based diagnosis.

syphilis: a sexually transmitted disease characterized initially by painless genital ulcers and caused by *Treponema pallidum*.

systemic: pertaining to or affecting the body as a whole.

traditional healers: health care providers who use diagnostic and therapeutic approaches that are not part of accepted modern medical management (e.g., herbal remedies, massage).

teleological: the use of an ultimate purpose or design as a means of explaining natural phenomena.

transparent phenotype: a growth characteristic of gonococci that is important because it is associated with invasive and/or systemic disease.

transmission, horizontal: the spread of an infectious agent from one individual to another, usually through contact with excreta (e.g., sputum).

temporal trends: variations or patterns in a parameter over time.

treponemes: spiral bacteria, some of which are pathogenic for humans (e.g., the causative agent of syphilis).

trichomoniasis: an infection associated with vaginal discharge, caused by a flagellated protozoon, *Trichomonas vaginalis*. This is most commonly a sexually transmitted disease.

urethra: the passage through which urine moves from the bladder to the exterior of the body.

vesicle: a small blister.

virus: one of a group of minute infectious agents, not resolved in the light microscope, and characterized by a lack of independent metabolism and by the ability to replicate only within living host cells.

Index